Rapidly Progressive Glomerulonephritis

Oxford Clinical Nephrology Series

Editorial board
Professor J. Stewart Cameron, Dr Tilman Drueke, Dr John Feehally,
Professor Leon G. Fine, Professor David Salant, and Dr Christopher
G. Winearls

*To subscribe to this series, see subscription information and order form at the back of this
book.*

Rapidly Progressive Glomerulonephritis

Edited by

CHARLES D. PUSEY and ANDREW J. REES

Department of Medicine
Royal Postgraduate Medical School
London
and
Department of Medicine and Therapeutics
University of Aberdeen

Oxford   New York   Tokyo
OXFORD UNIVERSITY PRESS
1998

Oxford University Press, Great Clarendon Street, Oxford OX2 6DP

Oxford   New York
Athens   Auckland   Bangkok   Bogota   Bombay   Buenos Aires
Calcutta   Cape Town   Dar es Salaam   Delhi   Florence   Hong Kong
Istanbul   Karachi   Kuala Lumpur   Madras   Madrid   Melbourne
Mexico City   Nairobi   Paris   Singapore   Taipei   Tokyo   Toronto   Warsaw

and associated companies in
Berlin   Ibadan

Oxford is a trade mark of Oxford University Press

Published in the United States
by Oxford University Press Inc., New York

A catalogue record for this book is available from the British Library

Library of Congress Cataloging in Publication Data
Rapidly progressive glomerulonephritis / edited by Charles D. Pusey
and Andres J. Rees.
(Oxford clinical nephrology series)
Includes bibliographical references and index.
ISBN 0 19 262636 1 (Hbk)
1. Glomerulonephritis.   I. Pusey, C. D.   II. Rees, A. J.
III. Series.
[DNLM: 1. Glomerulonephritis–pathology.   WJ 353 R218 1997]
RC918.G55R37   1997   616.6'12–dc21   97–16817

ISBN 0 19 262636 1

Typeset by EXPO Holdings, Malaysia

Printed in Great Britain by
Bookcraft (Bath) Ltd
Midsomer Norton, Avon

PREFACE

Rapidly progressive glomerulonephritis (RPGN) is one of the most exciting areas in renal medicine. The disease usually presents acutely, and leads to end-stage renal failure in weeks or months if untreated. However, appropriate immunosuppressive therapy can dramatically improve the prognosis in many cases, such that renal failure is avoided. It is now clear that various immunopathological processes are involved, and that an accurate diagnosis is of value in guiding management.

This volume aims to bring together current knowledge of both scientific and clinical aspects of RPGN. Recent advances in the immunology, inflammatory mechanisms, and pathology of RPGN are discussed. This is followed by consideration of the major causes of RPGN, which include Goodpasture's disease, primary systemic vasculitis, and systemic lupus erythematosus. RPGN secondary to other renal and systemic diseases, and RPGN in children are also described. Finally, new approaches to treatment are reviewed.

Although certain of these areas are covered in the larger textbooks of renal medicine, our aim is to provide a current overview of RPGN in a concise volume. This should be of particular interest to nephrologists and general physicians, including those in training, but may also be of value to pathologists, immunologists, and others studying the mechanisms of renal disease. We hope that this volume will help them in the management of patients with RPGN, or in planning their research into this condition.

London and Aberdeen   C.D.P.
October 1997   A.J.R.

CONTENTS

CONTRIBUTORS

Howard A. Austin III National Institute of Diabetes and Digestive and Kidney Diseases, Bethesda, Maryland, USA

James E. Balow National Institute of Diabetes and Digestive and Kidney Diseases, Bethesda, Maryland, USA

Dimitrious T. Boumpas National Institute of Diabetes and Digestive and Kidney Diseases, Bethesda, Maryland, USA

J. Stewart Cameron Clinical Science Laboratories, Guy's Hospital, London, UK

Michael J. Dillon Institute of Child Health, London, UK

Jonathan H. Ehrlich Department of Medicine, Monash University, Melbourne, Australia

Ronald J. Falk University of North Carolina School of Medicine, Chapel Hill, North Carolina, USA

Franco Ferrario Nephrology Division, S. Carlo Borromeo Hospital, Italy

Gillian Gaskin Department of Medicine, Royal Postgraduate Medical School, London, UK

Stephen R. Holdsworth Department of Medicine, Monash University, Melbourne, Australia

J. Charles Jennette University of North Carolina School of Medicine, Chapel Hill, North Carolina, USA

C. Martin Lockwood University of Cambridge, School of Clinical Medicine, Cambridge, UK

Peter W. Mathieson Academic Renal Unit, Southmead Hospital, Bristol, UK

Patrick Nachman University of North Carolina School of Medicine, Chapel Hill, North Carolina, USA

Charles D. Pusey Department of Medicine, Royal Postgraduate Medical School, London, UK

Maria Pia Rastaldi Nephrology Division, S. Carlo Borromeo Hospital, Italy

Andrew J. Rees Department of Medicine and Therapeutics, University of Aberdeen, Scotland, UK

Peter G. Tipping Department of Medicine, Monash University, Melbourne, Australia

A. Neil Turner Department of Medicine and Therapeutics, University of Aberdeen, Scotland, UK

Roger C. Wiggins University of Michigan, Ann Arbor, Michigan, USA

1

Historical background and concepts in rapidly progressive glomerulonephritis

Andrew J. Rees and Charles D. Pusey

Background

In 1914, Volhard and Fahr provided the classic description of what has come to be known as 'crescentic glomerulonephritis'. The glomeruli were severely damaged and the tuft was surrounded by a mass of cells filling Bowman's space. This was referred to as 'extracapillary' proliferation, but its appearance in cross-section on light microscopy led to the widespread use of the term 'crescentic' nephritis. It was appreciated that patients with crescentic nephritis usually died of renal failure within weeks of the apparent onset of the disease. Later, Ellis (1942) approached the same topic from a clinical standpoint and introduced the term 'rapidly progressive glomerulonephritis, type I' (subsequently condensed to 'rapidly progressive glomerulonephritis', 'RPGN') for patients with nephritis who developed renal failure within weeks or months. Most patients with RPGN were shown to have crescentic nephritis and were thought to have severe poststreptococcal disease.

In 1948, Davson, Ball, and Platt described a group of patients with systemic vasculitis involving small arteries, in whom 'epithelial crescent' formation was widespread and often associated with fibrinoid necrosis of the glomerular tuft. They called this condition the microscopic form of periarteritis nodosa, nowadays described as microscopic polyarteritis (or more accurately polyangiitis). Davson *et al.* distinguished microscopic polyarteritis from poststreptococcal disease and wondered whether some of Ellis' patients had this disorder rather than poststreptococcal nephritis; later, they and others made detailed comparisons of the two conditions (Davson and Platt 1949; Harrison *et al.* 1964). Harrison *et al.* also discussed the difficulty of diagnosing microscopic polyarteritis from renal biopsies, and described patients with crescentic nephritis on needle biopsy who were subsequently shown to have microscopic polyarteritis at autopsy. Nevertheless, the widespread use of renal biopsies enabled clinicopathological correlations to be made during life.

Throughout the 1960s, numerous studies of crescentic nephritis were published and have been summarized in several reviews (Pollak and Mendoza 1971; Couser 1982; Heaf *et al.* 1983; Glassock 1985). Bacani *et al.* (1968) clearly distinguished between poststreptococcal and other forms of the disease, and Scheer and Grossman (1964) showed that some patient with crescentic nephritis had antibodies to glomerular basement membrane (GBM). However, the observation with the greatest practical implication was that less than 10% of untreated patients survived and were independent of dialysis within months or a few years (see Couser 1982; Glassock 1985), the only apparent exception being those with poststreptococcal nephritis. It became clear that 'crescents' were a superadded feature found, more or less commonly, in many forms of nephritis and that 'crescentic' nephritis was a heterogeneous condition.

Types of crescentic nephritis

The lack of effective treatment meant that the principal purpose of reporting large series of patients treated during the 1960s and 1970s was to define prognostic features more accurately. However, they also revealed the variety of clinical contexts in which crescentic nephritis occurred (Whitworth *et al.* 1976; Beirne *et al.* 1977; McLeish *et al.* 1978; Morrin *et al.* 1978; Davis *et al.* 1979; Stilmant *et al.* 1979; Neild *et al.* 1983), and enabled crescentic nephritis to be categorized into three groups depending on the immunofluorescence findings: (1) patients with linear staining due to anti-glomerular basement membrane antibodies; (2) those in whom glomerular immunoglobulins were scanty or absent; (3) those with prominent granular deposits.

At the time these differences had little effect on prognosis, and so attention was concentrated on better ways to assess the outcome. The severity of renal failure at presentation was immediately recognized as indicating a bad prognosis, whether assessed by the presence of oliguria or the need for dialysis (Whitworth *et al.* 1976; Beirne *et al.* 1977; Morrin *et al.* 1978). Patients with preceding infection (Whitworth *et al.* 1976; Beaufils *et al.* 1976), or with systemic evidence of vasculitis, were said to fare better. Proliferation within the glomerular tuft was also said to be associated with a better prognosis, but the most important factor appeared to be the proportion of glomeruli surrounded by crescents (Elfenbein *et al.* 1975; Whitworth *et al.* 1976; Morrin *et al.* 1978). Patients with less than half the glomeruli affected by crescents fared much better than those with 50–79% affected, who in turn had a better prognosis than those with more than 80% crescents.

The importance of crescent scores for prognosis led to detailed discussions of how crescents should be defined, and how crescent scores should be calculated. This focused on three main issues: (1) whether the denominator used to calculate a crescent score should be the total number of glomeruli in the biopsy or only those that were not sclerosed; (2) the minimum number of glomeruli in a biopsy needed to calculate a crescent score; and (3) the extent of extracapillary proliferation that was needed before it was appropriate to use the term 'a crescent'. With hindsight, these discussions seem almost irrelevant, especially as needle biopsies take such small samples, and because the plane through which glomeruli are cut can have a tremendous influence on the apparent extent of extracapillary proliferation.

It was also at this stage that terminology became thoroughly confused, especially with regard to so-called 'idiopathic' crescentic glomerulonephritis. This term has been used to describe at least three subtly different sets of patients: (1) those with crescentic glomerulonephritis without extrarenal disease (Glassock 1985); (2) those with crescentic glomerulonephritis, irrespective of the pathogenesis, in whom another specific diagnosis such as vasculitis, mesangial IgA disease, or poststreptococcal nephritis cannot be made (Beirne *et al.* 1977); and (3) crescentic nephritis with either granular or scanty immune deposits (Couser 1982). Although confusing, this had no practical consequences until the development of treatments the effectiveness of which was influenced by the pathogenesis and associated diagnosis. Thus, severe anti-GBM disease has a worse prognosis than other types of crescentic nephritis of comparable severity (Beirne *et al.* 1977; McLeish *et al.* 1978; Hind *et al.* 1983), a fact not recognized in the protocols of some trials of treatment in crescentic nephritis (Glockner *et al.* 1988; Keller *et al.* 1989).

The confusion over terminology was easily resolved in patients with anti-GBM disease, who could be diagnosed unequivocally by serology or by immunofluorescence. Using this approach, Goodpasture's disease (nephritis and pulmonary haemorrhage) and isolated anti-GBM antibody-induced nephritis were shown to be different clinical expressions of the same disease. An analogous situation almost certainly exists in the case of crescentic glomerulonephritis with scanty immune deposits, also known as 'no immune deposits' (Couser 1982) or as 'pauci-immune' crescentic nephritis (Jennette *et al.* 1989). Comparisons of clinical (Serra *et al.* 1984; Couser 1988), histological (Velosa 1987), and serological data (Falk and Jennette 1988; Cohen Tervaert *et al.* 1990; Andrassy *et al.* 1986; Ferrario *et al.* 1985) suggest that microscopic polyarteritis and idiopathic 'pauci-immune' crescentic nephritis are the same or very similar diseases. The group of patients with obvious glomerular immune deposits is much more heterogeneous, but most have pre-existing nephritis or systemic immune complex disease complicated by the development of crescents. Thus, it is important to consider patients in pathogenetically defined groups when considering the response to trials of therapy, rather than relying on similarities of crescent scores. The immune mechanisms underlying the development of RPGN have been reviewed recently (Pusey and Peters 1993).

The other semantic issue that has caused considerable confusion is the definition of the term '*crescentic* nephritis'. This has often been applied only to patients with a greater than specified proportion of crescents on a renal biopsy. Crescents occur when breaks in glomerular capillaries allow leakage of cells and plasma proteins into Bowman's space, and so it is not surprising that occasional crescents have been described in many chronic renal diseases, including those that do not primarily affect the glomerulus. Widespread crescent formation, however, requires active and specific attack on glomerular capillaries. Clinical (Gill *et al.* 1997; Rees *et al.* 1977; Juncos *et al.* 1979; Fairley *et al.* 1987) and experimental (Wilson and Dixon 1986) studies have shown that glomerular inflammation can evolve very rapidly, and that an individual with no crescents one day can have 100% as little as five days later. Obviously, effective treatment should be introduced at the earliest possible stage, even though the crescent score might not justify a diagnosis of crescentic glomerulonephritis by traditional criteria. For this reason, some (Parfrey *et al.* 1985; Weiss and Crissman 1985; Furlong *et al.* 1987) have used the name 'focal necrotizing glomerulonephritis', whereas others rediscovered the term 'renal microscopic polyarteritis' (Serra *et al.* 1984; Savage *et al.* 1985; Coward *et al.* 1986; Croker *et al.* 1987).

Epidemiology

Crescentic glomerulonephritis affects patients of all races and of all ages, except perhaps infants. The diversity of conditions that cause crescentic nephritis means that descriptions of demography, epidemiology, and clinical presentation should be interpreted cautiously. Nevertheless, the proportion of patients with crescentic nephritis in unselected series of renal biopsies is remarkably consistent through-out the world. An incidence of 2–5% has been reported from France (Whitworth *et al.* 1976), the United Kingdom (Neild *et al.* 1983), the United States (Heilman *et al.* 1987), Africa (Dilma *et al.* 1981; Parag *et al.* 1988), India (Bhuyan *et al.* 1982; Date *et al.* 1987), and in the Chinese (Woo *et al.* 1986). There is an overall male predominance of approximately two to one. In adults, including the elderly (Potvliege *et al.* 1975; Montoliu *et al.* 1981; Kingswood *et al.* 1984; Stachura *et al.* 1984), anti-GBM disease accounts for 10–20% of patients with severe cres-centic nephritis, whereas the remainder is divided equally between those with scanty and those with granular deposits (Whitworth *et al.* 1976; Stilmant *et al.* 1979; Neild *et al.* 1983; Velosa 1987). Fewer children with crescentic nephritis have anti-GBM antibodies and a greater proportion have granular immune deposits (see Chapter 10).

There is relatively little information on the influence of race on susceptibility, but there is a strong clinical impression that the black races are less susceptible, at least to some types of crescentic nephritis. In a series of 110 patients with Wegener's granulomatosis and microscopic polyarteritis studied at Guy's Hospital (London), only one patient was black, compared with 6–11% of black patients in other categories of glomerular disease (J.S. Cameron, personal com-munication). Support for this idea comes from Parag *et al.* (1988) in a study of 24 patients in Natal. They provided population statistics for blacks, caucasoids, and Indians, which showed that poststreptococcal nephritis occurs in exactly the expected frequencies for the three populations, whereas anti-GBM disease and 'idiopathic' crescentic nephritis were more common than expected in caucasoids.

Management

A common approach to the management of crescentic nephritis was entirely rea-sonably in the 1960s, before the heterogeneity of the condition was appreciated and before any specific treatments were effective. This is illustrated by the fact that all the patients died in the series reported by Berlyne and Baker (1964), Bacani *et al.* (1968), and Lewis *et al.* (1971). Later, survival figures improved, probably because of increased availability of dialysis, and also because of the more widespread use of steroids. Even so, less than 25% of patients escaped the need for dialysis (Leonard *et al.* 1970; Striker *et al.* 1973; Beirne *et al.* 1977; Whitworth *et al.* 1976). Couser (1988) reviewed the early literature and calculated that 73% of 339 patients with idiopathic rapidly progressive glomerulonephritis reported at the time either died or went on to chronic dialysis. The only groups with a more encouraging prognosis were those with poststreptococcal nephritis (Leonard *et al.* 1970), and possibly those with crescentic nephritis associated with other types of infection (Beaufils *et al.* 1976; Whitworth *et al.* 1976). There are several possible explanations for this: first, treatment of infection could have eradicated the stimulus to crescent formation (i.e. the immunopathology); second, the patients tended to be younger; and third, the underlying inflammatory process was different in some way. Nevertheless, this observation encouraged the hope that renal function might recover in other types of crescentic nephritis, provided that treatment to abort the immunopathological process could be found.

Treatment in the acute stage has three objectives: (1) to control the immunopathology; (2) to suppress acute inflammation; and (3) to limit scarring. Such treatment needs to be introduced early to be successful, as even the most effective control of the immunopathology could not improve renal function of nephrons that had already been destroyed. These principles are illustrated by the effects of immunosuppression and plasma exchange on patients with anti-GBM disease. Concentrations of circulating anti-GBM antibodies can be reduced rapidly both in dialysis-dependent patients and in those who still have reasonable renal function, but renal function improves only in the latter group (Pusey and Lockwood 1984). Similar principles are likely to apply to other forms of crescentic nephritis, but are more difficult to demonstrate because of the uncertainties about pathogenesis, and because they seem to have a higher threshold above which treatment becomes ineffective (Hind *et al.* 1983). Thus, diagnosis needs to be made early, and this can be achieved by greater clinical awareness and the more widespread use of serological assays (Cassidy *et al.* 1990). Early diagnosis may explain in part the improved prognosis now being reported for both the kidney and the patient (Coward *et al.* 1986; Pusey and Lockwood 1984; Furlong *et al.* 1987; Bruns *et al.* 1989; Bolton and Sturgill 1989; Falk *et al.* 1990; Bindi *et al.* 1993; Ferrario *et al.* 1985).

Better immunosuppressive and anti-inflammatory regimens are almost certainly an important contributing factor to the better results currently reported, and it should now be an exception for renal function to continue to deteriorate once treatment has been started. Various treatments have been used in the past including anticoagulants and antiplatelet drugs (Cameron 1973; Brown *et al.* 1974; Suc *et al.* 1976); occasional patients with severe renal failure survived (Fischer and Blumberg 1978) but this was unusual. Most modern immunosuppressive regimens used for crescentic nephritis are 'cocktails' consisting of oral steroids and a cytotoxic drug, usually azathioprine or cyclophosphamide. These are often supplemented with pulses of methylprednisolone (Cole *et al.* 1976; Bolton and

Couser 1979; O'Neill *et al.* 1979; Oredugba *et al.* 1980; Adu *et al.* 1987; Bolton and Sturgill 1989), or with plasma exchange (Lockwood *et al.* 1976; Becker *et al.* 1977; Thysell *et al.* 1983; Pusey and Lockwood 1984; Walker *et al.* 1986; Burran *et al.* 1986). It is not easy to ascertain which components of these regimens are critical to success because most studies contain relatively small numbers of patients, with diseases of varying aetiologies treated with a variety of regimens. A few investigators have used a consistent approach, and have shown that the response to an individual therapy is influenced more by the immunopathogenesis than by crescent scores or other morphological markers of prognosis (Hind *et al.* 1983; Bolton and Sturgill 1989).

The studies already cited allude to the difficulties of assessing the prognosis of crescentic nephritis by morphology. The traditional approach has been to use the crescent score, which used to be a good guide (Whitworth *et al.* 1976; Neild *et al.* 1983) but is now relatively ineffective (Hind *et al.* 1983; Heilman *et al.* 1987), probably because current treatments have changed the outlook. Evans *et al.* (1986), in a detailed analysis of a large number of patients, found that outcome could still be predicted from the renal biopsy in anti-GBM disease, but not in other forms of crescentic nephritis, and these conclusions have recently found support from a prospective multi-centre European collaborative study (Bajema *et al.* 1996). Overall measurement of renal function is a better guide to immediate prognosis (i.e. to the response to treatment: Neild *et al.* 1983; Parfrey *et al.* 1985; Heilman *et al.* 1987; Hind *et al.* 1983), and has the additional advantage that it can be assessed more easily. Parfrey *et al.* (1985) and Heilman *et al.* (1987) reported that serum creatinine at presentation was a good prognostic indicator. Others have used the need for dialysis as the yardstick (Hind *et al.* 1983; Stevens *et al.* 1983; Serra *et al.* 1984; Bolton and Sturgill 1989). It now seems sensible to categorize patients by renal function as well as by disease when considering trials of therapy in crescentic nephritis (Pusey *et al.* 1991).

Conclusion

Over the past 20 years, developments in treatment have transformed the outlook for patients with crescentic nephritis in ways only equalled for those with systemic lupus erythematosus. In doing so, many of the guiding principles have changed. It is no longer possible to assert that glomeruli surrounded by crescents are inevitably destroyed; many will be, but the degree of recovery possible in poststreptococcal nephritis is proof against this. This suggests that effective control of the underlying immunopathology may allow resolution without scarring, and this perhaps underlies the effectiveness of current regimens for renal microscopic polyarteritis. Another cause for encouragement comes from studies in anti-GBM disease, which have shown the value of being able to relate injury directly to the presence of autoantibodies, so that treatment can be given and monitored in a rational way. The recent discovery that antineutrophil cytoplasmic antibody (ANCA) concentration is closely associated with injury in most patients with renal microscopic polyarteritis should lead to work into the pathogenesis of these diseases, which will enable them to be approached as rationally as anti-GBM disease (Rees 1996).

It is, however, disappointing that the immunosuppressive regimens in common use have changed little over the last 10–15 years. It is hoped that developments in understanding of the cellular and molecular mechanisms of autoimmunity, inflammation, and scarring should lead to the introduction of more specific and effective treatment strategies. The use of experimental models of nephritis has already allowed proof of concept for various approaches to treatment, for example, anti-T cell therapy for autoimmunity, modulation of the cytokine network for inflammation, and inhibition of growth factors for scarring. The assessment of these new approaches in human crescentic nephritis is one of our major challenges for the next few years.

References

Adu, D., Howie, A.J., Scott, D.G.I., Bacon, P.A., McGonigle, R.J.S., and Michael, J. (1987). Polyarteritis and the kidney. *Quarterly Journal of Medicine*, **239**, 221–37.

Andrassy, K., Koderisch, J., Rufer, M., Erb, A., Waldherr, R., and Ritz, E. (1986). Detection and clinical implication of anti-neutrophil cytoplasmic antibodies in Wegener's granulomatosis and rapidly progressive glomerulonephritis. *Clinical Nephrology*, **32**, 159–67.

Bacani, R.A., Velasquez, F., Kanter, A., Pirani, C.L., and Pollak, V.E. (1968). Rapidly progressive (non-streptococcal) glomerulonephritis. *Annals of Internal Medicine*, **69**, 463–85.

Bajema, I.M., Hagen, E.C., Hermans, J. *et al.* (1996). Predicting renal outcome in systemic vasculitis from the kidney biopsy: a clinico-pathological analysis of 157 patients. *Journal of the American Society of Nephrology*, **7**, 1770 (abstract).

Beaufils, M., Morel-Maroger, L., Sraer, J-D., Kanfer, A., Kourilsky, O., and Richet, G. (1976). Acute renal failure of glomerular origin during visceral abcesses. *New England Journal of Medicine*, **295**, 185–9.

Becker, G., Kincaid-Smith, P., D'Apice, A., and Walker, R.G. (1977). Plasmapheresis in the treatment of glomerulonephritis. *Medical Journal of Australia*, **2**, 693–6.

Beirne, G.J., Wagnild, J.P., Zimmerman, S.W., Mackem, P.D., and Burkholder, P.M. (1977). Idiopathic crescentic glomerulonephritis. *Medicine*, **56**, 349–81.

Berlyne, G. and Baker, J.S. (1964). Acute anuric glomerulonephritis. *Quarterly Journal of Medicine*, **33**, 105–15.

Bhuyan, U.N., Dash, S.C., Srivastava, R.N., Sharma, R.K., and Malhotra, K.K. (1982). Immunopathology, extent and course of glomerulonephritis with crescent formation. *Clinical Nephrology*, **18**, 280–5.

Bindi, P., Mougenot, B., Mentre, F., Noel, L.H., Peraldi, M.N., Vanhille, P. *et al.* (1993). Necrotizing crescentic glomerulonephritis without significant immune deposits: a clinical and serological study. *Quarterly Journal of Medicine*, **86**, 55–68.

Bolton, W.K. and Sturgill, B.C. (1989). Methylprednisolone therapy for acute crescentic rapidly progressive glomerulonephritis. *American Journal of Nephrology*, **9**, 368–75.

Bolton, W.K. and Couser, W.G. (1979). Intravenous pulse methylprednisolone therapy of acute crescentic rapidly progressive glomerulonephritis. *American Journal of Medicine*, **66**, 495–502.

Brown, C.B. *et al.* (1974). Combined immunosuppression and anticoagulation in rapidly progressive glomerulonephritis. *Lancet*, ii, 1166–72.

Bruns, F.J., Adler, S., Fraley, D.S., and Segel, D.P. (1989). Long-term follow-up of aggressively treated idiopathic rapidly progressive glomerulonephritis. *American Journal of Medicine*, 86, 400–6.

Burran, W.P., Avasthi, P., Smith, K.J., and Simon, T.L. (1986). Efficacy of plasma exchange in severe idiopathic rapidly progressive glomerulonephritis: A report of ten cases. *Transfusion*, 26, 382–7.

Cameron, J.S. (1973). Are anticoagulants beneficial in the treatment of rapidly progressive glomerulonephritis? *Proceedings of the European Dialysis and Transplant Association*, 10, 57–90.

Cassidy, M.J., Gaskin, G., Savill, J., Pusey, C.D., and Rees, A.J. (1990). Towards a more rapid diagnosis of rapidly progressive glomerulonephritis. *British Medical Journal*, 301, 329–31.

Cohen Tervaert, J.W. *et al.* (1990). Autoantibodies against myeloid lysosomal enzymes in crescentic glomerulonephritis. *Kidney International*, 37, 799–806.

Cole, B.R., Brocklebank, T.J., Keinstra, R.A., Kissane, J.M., and Robson, A.M. (1976). 'Pulse' methylprednisolone therapy in the treatment of severe glomerulonephritis. *Journal of Pediatrics*, 88, 302–14.

Couser, W.G. (1982). Idiopathic rapidly progressive glomerulonephritis. *American Journal of Nephrology*, 2, 57–69.

Couser, W.G. (1988). Rapidly progressive glomerulonephritis: Classification, pathogenetic mechanisms, and therapy. *American Journal of Kidney Diseases*, 11, 449–64.

Coward, R.A., Hamdy, N.A.T., Shortland, J.S., and Brown, C.B. (1986). Renal micropolyarteritis: A treatable condition. *Nephrology Dialysis Transplantation*, 1, 31–7.

Crocker, B.P., Lee, T., and Gunnells, J.C. (1987). Clinical and pathologic features of polyarteritis nodosa and its renal-limited variant: Primary crescentic and necrotizing glomerulonephritis. *Human Pathology*, 18, 38–44.

Date, A., Raghavan, R., John, J., Richard, J., Kirubakaran, M.G., and Shastry, J.G. (1987). Renal disease in adult Indians: A clinicopathological study of 2827 patients. *Quarterly Journal of Medicine*, 64, 729–37.

Davis, C.A., McAdams, A.J., Wyatt, R.J., Forristal, J., and McEnery, P.T. (1979). Idiopathic rapidly progressive glomerulonephritis with C3 nephritic factor and hypocomplementemia. *Journal of Pediatrics*, 94, 559–63.

Davson, J., Ball, J., and Platt, R. (1948). The kidney in periarteritis nodosa. *Quarterly Journal of Medicine*, 67, 175–202.

Davson, J. and Platt, R. (1949). A clinical and pathological study of renal disease: I. glomerulonephritis. *Quarterly Journal of Medicine*, 18, 149–71.

Dilma, M.G., Adhikari, M., and Coovadia, H.M. (1981). Rapidly progressive glomerulonephritis in black children: A report of 4 cases. *South African Medical Journal*, 60, 829–32.

Elfenbein, I.B., Baluarte, H.J., Cubillos-Rohas, M., Gruskin, A.B., Cote, M., and Cornfeld, D. (1975). Quantitative morphometry of glomerulonephritis with crescents: diagnostic and predictive value. *Laboratory Investigation*, 32, 56–64.

Ellis, A. (1942). Natural history of Bright's disease. Clinical, histological and experimental observations. *Lancet*, i, 34–6.

Evans, D.J., Savage, C.O.S., Winearls, C.G., Rees, A.J., Pusey, C.D., and Peters, D.K. (1986). Renal biopsy in prognosis of treated 'glomerulonephritis with crescents'. *Abstracts of the Xth International Congress of Nephrology*, p. 60.

Fairley, C., Mathewson, D.C., and Becker, G.J. (1987). Rapid development of diffuse crescents in post-streptococcal glomerulonephritis. *Clinical Nephrology*, **28**, 256–60.

Falk, R.J. and Jennette, J.C. (1988). Anti-neutrophil cytoplasmic autoantibodies with specificity for myeloperoxidase in patients with systemic vasculitis and idiopathic necrotizing and crescentic glomerulonephritis. *New England Journal of Medicine*, **318**, 1651–7.

Falk, R.J., Hogan, S., Carey, T.S., and Jennette, C. (1990). Clinical course of anti-neutrophil cytoplasmic autoantibody-associated glomerulonephritis and vasculitis. *Annals of Internal Medicine*, **113**, 656–63.

Ferrario, F. *et al.* (1985). The detection of monocytes in human glomerulonephritis. *Kidney International*, **28**, 513–19.

Fischer, E. and Blumberg, A. (1978). Prolonged anuria in Wegener's granulomatosis: Recovery of renal function. *Journal of the American Medical Association*, **240**, 1174–5.

Furlong, T.J., Ibels, L.S., and Eckstein, R.P. (1987). The clinical spectrum of necrotizing glomerulonephritis. *Medicine*, **66**, 192–201.

Glassock, R.J. (1985). Natural history and treatment of primary proliferative glomerulonephritis: A review. *Kidney International*, **17** (suppl.) 136–42.

Gill, D.G., Turner, D.R., Chantler, C., and Cameron, J.S. (1977). Progression of acute proliferative poststreptococcal glomerulonephritis to severe epithelial crescent formation. *Clinical Nephrology*, **8**, 449–52.

Glockner, W.M. *et al.* (1988). Plasma exchange and immunosuppression in rapidly progressive glomerulonephritis: A controlled, multi-center study. *Clinical Nephrology*, **29**, 1–8.

Harrison, C.V., Loughridge, L.W., and Milne, M.D. (1964). Acute oliguric renal failure in acute glomerulonephritis and polyarteritis. *Quarterly Journal of Medicine*, **129**, 39–55.

Heaf, J.G., Jorgensen, F., and Neilsen, L.P. (1983). Treatment and prognosis of extracapillary glomerulonephritis. *Nephron*, **35**, 217–24.

Heilman, R.L., Offord, K.P., Holley, K.E., and Velosa, J.A. (1987). Analysis of risk factors for patient and renal survival in crescentic glomerulonephritis. *American Journal of Kidney Diseases*, **9**, 98–107.

Hind, C.R., Paraskevakou, H., Lockwood, C.M., Evans, D.J., Peters, D.K., and Rees, A.J. (1983). Prognosis after immunosuppression of patients with crescentic nephritis requiring dialysis. *Lancet*, i, 263–5.

Jennette, J.C., Wilkman, A.S., and Falk, R.J. (1989). Anti-neutrophil cytoplasmic autoantibody-associated glomerulonephritis and vasculitis. *American Journal of Pathology*, **135**, 921–30.

Juncos, L.I., Alexander, R.W., and Marbury, T.C. (1979). Intravascular clotting preceding crescent formation in a patient with Wegener's granulomatosis and rapidly progressive glomerulonephritis. *Nephron*, **24**, 17–20.

Keller, F., Oehlenberg, B., Kunzendorf, U., Schwarz, A., and Offerman, G. (1989). Long-term treatment and prognosis of rapidly progressive glomerulonephritis. *Clinical Nephrology*, **31**, 190–7.

Kingswood, J.C., Banks, R.A., Tribe, C.R., Owen Jones, J., and MacKenzie, J.C. (1984). Renal biopsy in the elderly: clinicopathological correlations in 143 patients. *Clinical Nephrology*, **22**, 183–7.

Leonard, C.D., Nagle, R.B., Striker, G.E., Cutler, R.E., and Scribner, B.H. (1970). Acute glomerulonephritis with prolonged oliguria: An analysis of 29 cases. *Annals of Internal Medicine*, **73**, 703–11.

Lewis, E., Cavallo, T., Harrington, J.T., and Cotran, R.S. (1971). An immunopathological study of rapidly progressive glomerulonephritis in the adult. *Human Pathology*, **2**, 185–208.

Lockwood, C.M., Rees, A.J., Pearson, T., Evans, D.J., and Peters, D.K. (1976). Immunosuppression and plasma exchange in the treatment of Goodpasture's syndrome. *Lancet*, **i**, 711–15.

McLeish, K.R., Yum, M.N., and Luft, F.C. (1978). Rapidly progressive glomerulonephritis in adults: Clinical and histologic correlations. *Clinical Nephrology*, **10**, 43–50.

Montoliu, J., Darnell, A., Torras, A., and Revert, L. (1981). Acute and rapidly progressive forms of glomerulonephritis in the elderly. *Journal of the American Geriatric Society*, **29**, 108–16.

Morrin, P.A., Hinglais, N., Nabarra, B., and Kreis, H. (1978). Rapidly progressive glomerulonephritis. A clinical and pathologic study. *American Journal of Medicine*, **65**, 446–60.

Neild, G.H., Cameron, J.S., Ogg, C.S. *et al.* (1983). Rapidly progressive glomerulonephritis with extensive glomerular crescent formation. *Quarterly Journal of Medicine*, **52**, 395–416.

O'Neill, W.M., Jr., Etheridge, W.B., and Bloomer, H.A. (1979). High-dose corticosteroids: their use in treating idiopathic rapidly progressive glomerulonephritis. *Archives of Internal Medicine*, **139**, 514–18.

Oredugba, O., Mazumdar, D.C., Meyer, J.S., and Lubowitz, H. (1980). Pulse methylprednisolone therapy in idiopathic, rapidly progressive glomerulonephritis. *Annals of Internal Medicine*, **92**, 504–6.

Parag, K.B., Naran, A.D., Seedat, Y.K., Nathoo, B.C., Naicker, I.P., and Naicker, S. (1988). Profile of crescentic glomerulonephritis in Natal—a clinicopathological assessment. *Quarterly Journal of Medicine*, **68**, 629–36.

Parfrey, P.S., Hutchinson, T.A., Jothy, S., Cramer, B.C., Martin, J., and Seely, J.F. (1985). The spectrum of diseases associated with necrotizing glomerulonephritis and its prognosis. *American Journal of Kidney Diseases*, **6**, 387–96.

Pollak, V.E. and Mendoza, N. (1971). Rapidly progressive glomerulonephritis. *Medical Clinics of North America*, **55**, 1397–415.

Potvliege, P.R., De Roy, G., and Dupuis, F. (1975). Necropsy study on glomerulonephritis in the elderly. *Journal of Clinical Pathology*, **28**, 891–8.

Pusey, C.D. and Lockwood, C.M. (1984). Plasma exchange for glomerular disease. In *Nephrology* (ed. R.R. Robinson), pp. 1474–85. Springer, New York.

Pusey, C.D. and Peters, D.K. (1993). Immunopathology of glomular and interstitial disease. In *Diseases of the kidney* (5th edn), (ed. R.W. Schrier and C.W. Gottschalk), pp. 1647–80. Little Brown, Boston.

Pusey, C.D., Rees, A.J., Evans, D.J., Peters, D.K., and Lockwood, C.M. (1991). Plasma exchange in focal necrotizing glomerulonephritis without anti-GBM antibodies. *Kidney International*, **40**, 757–63.

Rees, A.J., Lockwood, C.M. and Peters, D.K. (1977). Enhanced allergic tissue damage in Goodpasture's syndrome by intercurrent bacterial infection. *British Medical Journal*, **2**, 723–6.

Rees, A.J. (1996). Renal vasculitis. *Current Opinion in Nephrology and Hypertension*, **5**, 273–81.

Savage, C.O.S., Winearls, C.G., Evans, D.J., Rees, A.J., and Lockwood, C.M. (1985). Microscopic polyarteritis: presentation, pathology and prognosis. *Quarterly Journal of Medicine*, **56**, 467–83.

Scheer, R.L. and Grossman, M.A. (1964). Immune aspects of glomerulonephritis associated with pulmonary haemorrhage. *Annals of Internal Medicine*, **60**, 1009–21.

Serra, A. *et al.* (1984). Vasculitis affecting the kidney: Presentation, histopathology and long-term outcome. *Quarterly Journal of Medicine*, **210**, 181–207.

Stachura, I., Si, L., and Whiteside, T.L. (1984). Mononuclear-cell subsets in human idiopathic crescentic glomerulonephritis (ICGN): analysis in tissue sections with monoclonal antibodies. *Journal of Clinical Immunology*, **4**, 202–8.

Stevens, M.E, McConnell, M., and Bone, J.M. (1983). Aggressive treatment with pulse methylprednisolone or plasma exchange is justified in rapidly progressive glomerulonephritis. *Proceedings of the European Dialysis and Transplantation Association*, **19**, 724–31.

Stilmant, M.M., Bolton, W.K., Sturgill, B.C., Schmitt, G.W., and Couser, W.G. (1979). Crescentic glomerulonephritis without immune deposits: clinicopathologic features. *Kidney International*, **15**, 184–95.

Striker, G., Cutler, R.E., Haung, T., and Benditt, E. (1973). Renal failure, epithelial cell hyperplasia. In *Glomerulonephritis*, (ed. P. Kincaid-Smith, R. Mathew, and E. Becker), pp. 657–75. Wiley, New York.

Suc, J.M., Durand, D., Conte, J. *et al.* (1976). The use of heparin in the treatment of idiopathic rapidly progressive glomerulonephritis. *Clinical Nephrology*, **5**, 9–13.

Thysell, H., Bygren, P., Bengtsson, U. *et al.* (1983). Improved outcome in rapidly progressive glomerulonephritis by plasma exchange treatment. *International Journal of Artificial Organs*, **6**, 11–14.

Velosa, J.A. (1987). Idiopathic crescentic glomerulonephritis or systemic vasculitis. *Mayo Clinic Proceedings*, **62**, 145–7.

Volhard, F. and Fahr, T. (1914). *Die Brightsche Nierenkrankheit*. Springer, Berlin.

Walker, R.G., Becker, G.J., D'Apice, A.J., and Kincaid-Smith, P. (1986). Plasma exchange in the treatment of glomerulonephritis and other renal diseases. *Australian and New Zealand Journal of Medicine*, **16**, 828–38.

Weiss, M.A. and Crissman, J.D. (1985). Segmental necrotizing glomerulonephritis: diagnostic, prognostic, and therapeutic significance. *American Journal of Kidney Diseases*, **6**, 199–211.

Whitworth, J.A., Morel-Maroger, L., Mignon, F., and Richet, G. (1976). The significance of extracapillary proliferation. Clinicopathological review of 60 patients. *Nephron*, **16**, 1–19.

Wilson, C.B. and Dixon, F.J. (1986). The renal response to immunological injury. In *The kidney* (ed. B.M. Brenner and F.C. Rector), pp. 800–900. Saunders, Philadelphia.

Woo, K.T., Chiang, G.S., Edmondson, R.P., Wu, A.Y., Lee E.J., and Pwee, H.S. (1986). Glomerulonephritis in Singapore: An overview. *Annals of Academy of Medicine, Singapore*, **15**, 20–31.

2

Immunopathogenesis of crescentic glomerulonephritis

Stephen R. Holdsworth, Jonathan H. Erlich, and Peter G. Tipping

The characteristic and unifying feature of crescentic glomerulonephritis is the extracapillary accumulation of cells within Bowman's space. The consequent shape of the accumulating cells within this space surrounding and compressing the residual capillary loop resembles that of a crescent when cut in section and viewed under the microscope.

Arbitrary definitions of 'crescents' allowing uniform diagnostic criteria have been proposed. These have included the requirement for a minimum number of cell layers overlying the parietal epithelium in Bowman's space. However, experimental evidence suggests that cellular crescents are but one phase in the evolution of crescent formation. At the onset of crescent formation, Bowman's space may be filled with fibrin forming an acellular or fibrinous crescent. The final outcome of crescent formation may be sclerosis with development of an acellular, collagenous scar. Thus, the presence of cells in Bowman's space is not an invariable feature of crescents.

Crescentic glomerulonephritis constitutes an important subgroup of glomerulonephritis which is often associated with a poor clinical outcome. Crescentic glomerulonephritis itself may be classified into distinct subgroups according to clinical, aetiological, and histological categories. The major subgroups are discussed in detail in the subsequent chapters of this book. A common feature of all these subgroups is the presence of crescents in a significant percentage of glomeruli. Although a precise definition is not agreed, traditionally the term 'crescentic glomerulonephritis' includes those forms of nephritis where the process of crescent formation involves the majority (>70%) of glomeruli (Bolton and Sturgill 1989; Glassock *et al.* 1991).

Crescent formation can be observed in a variety of clinical settings and is not a unique feature of any single clinical entity. However, our understanding of the immunopathogenesis of crescent formation suggests that a common sequence of inflammatory events is likely to underlie crescent formation. Crescents are an outcome of intense glomerular inflammation and typically reflect severe injury and poor outcome. Thus, the diagnosis of crescentic glomerulonephritis in general foreshadows a natural history of rapid deterioration in renal function and grave renal prognosis (Glassock *et al.* 1991). Paradoxically, these forms of glomerulonephritis often respond to treatment. However, the window of opportunity for sucessful therapeutic intervention is narrow, and early diagnosis remains a major clinical goal (Holzman and Wiggins 1991).

Immunological mechanisms in glomerulonephritis

In most situations, evidence from human observations and experimental models confirms that glomerulonephritis is the result of a local inflammatory process initiated by host immune responses to antigens in the glomeruli (Fig. 2.1). In the majority of cases, these are not intrinsic glomerular antigens, but are antigens carried to the kidney via the circulation and localized within glomeruli as a consequence of its high plasma flow and filtration function.

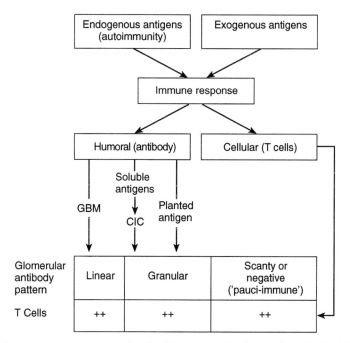

Fig. 2.1 Immune responses associated with crescentic glomerulonephritis (GN). Host immune responses to exogenous antigens or endogenous antigens (autoimmunity) generate antibody and T lymphocyte effector responses. Crescentic GN is often classified according to the pattern of glomerular antibody deposition. Anti-GBM antibodies give a *linear pattern*. ANCA-positive or vasculitis-associated GN has a *scanty pattern* of little (or absent) glomerular antibody. A *granular pattern* is associated with deposition of circulating immune complexes (CICs) but may theoretically be due to *in situ*-formed immune complexes. Evidence of the T cell effector arm of immunity can be seen in all types of crescentic GN.

Antigens involved in glomerulonephritis

Autoimmunity to constitutively expressed glomerular antigens is an uncommon mechanism for the initiation of glomerulonephritis. Anti-glomerular basement membrane (anti-GBM) glomerulonephritis represents the only clearly defined example in man (Lerner *et al.* 1967). This disease also rarely occurs spontaneously in animals (Banks 1967) but can be induced experimentally when immune tolerance is lost (Steblay 1962; Sapin *et al.* 1977). Autoimmunity to an epithelial cell antigen (Gp330 or megalin) can be induced in rats resulting in a form of glomerulonephritis (Heymann nephritis) with similar immunopathological features to human membranous glomerulonephritis (Heymann *et al.* 1959). However, evidence of an true autoimmune response in human membranous glomerulonephritis remains elusive.

In man, a large number of antigens have been implicated in the initiation of glomerulonephritis (Wilson 1991). The vast majority of the defined antigens initiating immune responses associated with glomerulonephritis are not intrinsic glomerular antigens but are exogenous antigens derived from bacteria or parasites. However, some endogenous human antigens have also been identified. The immune response in this situation thus represents failure of immunological tolerance, or a response to neoantigens or antigens previously in an immunologically privileged site.

Immune responses associated with glomerulonephritis

Although most attention has focused on the antigens involved in glomerulonephritis, the nature and intensity of the elicited immune response may be the most important determinant in the development of crescents. This point is well illustrated in chronic serum sickness nephritis (Dixon *et al.* 1961). Variations in immune responses are genetically determined and several studies have addressed the immunogenetics of glomerulonephritis.

In experimental glomerulonephritis, predisposition to anti-GBM autoantibody formation in response to mercuric chloride has a clear genetic component (Druet *et al.* 1977) as does the susceptibility to Heymann nephritis (Steinglen *et al.* 1978). Autoimmune immune complex disease with crescentic glomerulonephritis has been extensively studied in susceptible murine strains and strong genetic linkages have been found in NZB/NZW and MRL/lpr mice (Andrews *et al.* 1978).

In humans, genetic linkage with several forms of glomerulonephritis that exhibit crescent formation have been reported. The relative risk of developing anti-GBM glomerulonephritis for individuals with DR2 is 9.6 (Rees *et al.* 1978, 1984). Recent studies have shown a closer association with the DRw15 allele (Rees 1994). In Japan, IgA disease has been associated with DR4 although this has not been confirmed in Caucasians (Rees 1984). An association with DQB 0301 has been recently demonstrated in Caucasians (Li *et al.* 1991). Despite clear genetic associations in the murine model of systemic lupus erythematosus, genetic association with human lupus nephritis is controversial (Rees 1994; Drake and Kotzin 1992). Recent studies suggested an association between DR4 DQw7 and those forms of vasculitis associated with antineutrophil cytoplasmic antibody (ANCA) and crescentic glomerulonephritis (Spencer *et al.* 1992) but these results have not been confirmed by others (see chapter 7).

Mechanisms of glomerular immunoglobulin deposition

In most situations, immunoglobulins localize in glomeruli by one of two mechanisms: (1) deposition of circulating immune complexes; and (2) *in situ* immune complex formation. The understanding of these mechanisms is derived largely from experimental studies.

Glomerulonephritis induced by deposition of circulating immune complexes

Glomerulonephritis occurring in association with the therapeutic use of foreign serum was first observed in humans more than 100 years ago, but animal studies have provided a clear understanding of the immunopathogenic mechanisms involved. Injection of foreign serum protein leads to host antibody production over the subsequent 7–10 days. This immune response results in rapid clearance— 'immune elimination'—of persisting antigen by immune complex formation and vascular deposition, leading to widespread vasculitis and a transient glomerulonephritis.

Recurrent injection of foreign serum proteins may induce chronic serum sickness with a more persistent immune complex glomerulonephritis (Dixon *et al.* 1961). A variety of histological types of glomerulonephritis have been observed in this situation, but only a subgroup of animals develop crescents. Those animals which exhibit the greatest immune response with the greatest antigen load and the greatest levels of immune complex formation are the ones that develop glomerular crescents (Holdsworth *et al.* 1980*b*). In man, continuous intravascular persistence of foreign antigen is seen in bacterial endocarditis, infected shunts, and sequestered infections. All these conditions can be associated with the development of crescentic glomerulonephritis.

Glomerulonephritis associated with in situ *immune complex formation*

The injection of heterologous anti-GBM antibody can induce immediate but transient glomerular injury. A second phase of injury follows when the host mounts an immune response to this planted glomerular antigen (foreign anti-GBM antibody). This form of immune response regularly leads to glomerular crescent formation. While the development of crescents resulting from an immune response to heterologous anti-GBM antibodies is often referred to as a model of autoimmune human anti-GBM disease, in fact it represents a planted antigen model of glomerulonephritis. The propensity of this model to induce crescent formation is likely to reflect the intensity of the glomerular inflammation which results from the large quantities and the wide distribution of antigen deposited within the glomerular capillary loops.

In anti-GBM disease, the immunological specificity of the heterologous anti-GBM antibody ensures its localization to the glomerulus. However, other antigens with particular physico-chemical properties can also be specifically targeted to the glomerulus. Concanavalin A (con A) is a lectin that binds avidly to the endothelium. Selective renal infusion of con A into a sensitized host or passive transfer of anti-con A antibody to naive animals with this planted glomerular antigen can induce severe glomerular injury (Golbus and Wilson 1979). The net negative charge of the glomerular filter allows positively charged antigens such as cationic bovine serum albumin (BSA) to be planted selectively in the glomerulus, allowing a host immune response to result in *in situ* immune complex formation (Border *et al.* 1981). A range of modified (cationized) proteins have been employed in experimental models to confirm both the enhanced capacity of these molecules to localize in the glomerular filter (Wilson 1979) and the capacity of subsequent host immune responses to lead to severe glomerular injury (Couser 1986).

Microbial antigens with lectin properties or cationic charge, allowing them to localize in glomeruli, are associated with human glomerulonephritis. Several endogenous antigens also have the physico-chemical characteristics which potentially cause them to localize in glomeruli initiating *in situ* immune complex-induced injury. Such endogenous antigens may include DNA and other nuclear antigens (Lake *et al.* 1985) and components of neutrophil granules (Savage *et al.* 1993). Thus, the potential for *in situ* immune complex glomerulonephritis exists in systemic lupus erythematosus (SLE) and ANCA-associated vasculitis.

Initiation of immune injury within glomeruli

The effector arms of the immune response leading to glomerulonephritis may involve either humoral (B cell) or cellular (T cell) immunity. Typically, these act synergistically. However, most attention in the past has focused on the role of antibody in the initiation of disease. In crescentic glomerulonephritis, there is now good evidence of an important role for the cellular immune response. Thus, either deposition of immunoglobulin or glomerular localization of T cells may comprise the essential first step in the initiation of glomerular inflammation that leads to crescent formation.

Mediators of glomerular injury

Leucocytes, platelets, and intrinsic glomerular cells all have the potential to produce a variety of pro-inflammatory products which may contribute to glomerular injury. These include prostaglandins, leucotrienes, cytokines, growth factors, procoagulant molecules, fibrinolytic molecules and their inhibitors, degradative enzymes, reactive oxygen species, and nitric oxide. The relative abundance and timing of the production of these cell products may determine the severity of glomerular injury and its resolution or progression.

Initiation of an immune response in the glomerulus may activate a number of these inflammatory pathways. Deposition of autologous immunoglobulin itself does not usually cause injury but acts as a local initiator of inflammatory mediators. For example, conformational changes in immunoglobulin consequent on antigen binding reveal a variety of receptors on the Fc piece capable of binding and activating humoral and cellular mediator systems. In experimental models, anti-GBM antibodies administered in large amounts are capable of inducing injury in the absence of humoral or cellular mediators (Golbus and Wilson 1979; Boyce and Holdsworth 1985). It is not known if immunoglobulin deposition in these quantities occurs in human glomerulonephritis. Current evidence suggests that T cells do not directly induce glomerulonephritis, but also act by initation of secondary effector mechanisms, particularly macrophage recruitment.

The best defined humoral mediators of injury in glomerulonephritis include complement, leucocytes and coagulation proteins. Complement is the most prominent humoral mediator observed in human glomerulonephritis. Complement activation occurs primarily via the Fc piece of deposited antibody. However, autoantibodies to the C3 convertase (C3 nephritic factor) can induce chronic complement activation by rendering this convertase refractory to the action of regulatory control proteins. C3 nephritic factor is observed in certain forms of glomerulonephritis, including crescentic glomerulonephritis (West *et al.* 1973).

Many of the cleaved complement components have potent pro-inflammatory functions inducing effects on vessel permeability, chemotaxis, and activation of leucocytes. The relative involvement of classical, and alternative, pathways and the membrane attack complex (MAC) may vary between different types of glomerulonephritis. Neutrophil recruitment and degranulation appears to be a major effector pathway by which complement induces glomerular injury (Cochrane *et al.* 1965). However, leucocyte-independent complement-mediated glomerular injury can be induced by the assembly of the C5b-9 membranolytic terminal attack complex—the MAC (Groggel *et al.* 1983; 1985). A minor component of complement-mediated glomerular injury is both leucocyte- and MAC-independent (Tipping *et al.* 1989).

Neutrophil recruitment resulting from antibody-induced complement activation was the first demonstrated mechanism for leucocyte-mediated glomerular injury. Monocytes are now also recognized as potent mediators of glomerular injury and immunoglobulin deposition can induce monocyte recruitment via their Fc receptors (Holdsworth 1983). Endothelial cells may play an active role in leucocyte recruitment by expression of cell adhesion molecules (CAMs). A number of studies have shown that endothelial cell expression of adhesion molecules facilitates leucocyte-mediated injury, including experimental crescentic glomerulonephritis (Kawasaki *et al.* 1993; Nishikawa *et al.* 1993). CAMs are also a requisite component of antibody-initiated complement-independent, glomerular neutrophil recruitment (Tipping *et al.* 1994*b*). However, in situations where other signals, such as complement and Fc receptor-mediated adherence, determine neutrophil or macrophage influx their involvement may be redundant (Tipping *et al.* 1994*b*).

Intrinsic glomerular cells were once thought to be merely targets of immune inflammatory injury. It is now appreciated that they may be active contributors to the inflammatory process. Endothelial cells express many molecules normally maintaining an anticoagulant state in the circulation. However, in response to inflammatory signals, they may become procoagulant thereby facilitating glomerular fibrin deposition (Cotran 1987). Endothelial cells *in vitro* can act as antigen-presenting cells and may potentially play this role in glomerulonephritis (Savage 1994). These cells can also produce pro-inflammatory molecules, particularly those of the chemokine family, including interleukin 8 (IL-8), RANTES and monocyte chemotactic protein-1 (MCP-1) (Abbott *et al.* 1991; Kusner *et al.* 1991; Brown *et al.* 1991; Zoja *et al.* 1991; Sedor 1992) as well as participating in inflammatory cell recruitment via their capacity to express cell adhesion molecules.

Mesangial cells have been shown *in vitro* to be capable of responding to a number of pro-inflammatory signals, including immune complexes, complement components, and products of T cells and macrophages. These may alter mesangial cell phenotype and induce production of inflammatory mediators, including reactive oxygen species, cytokines, prostaglandins and leucotrienes (Sedor 1992), which may have a role in crescentic glomerulonephritis. Although intrinsic cells produce cytokines *in vitro*, in experimental anti-GBM glomerulonephritis, where macrophage infiltration is prominent, the relative contribution of intrinsic glomerular cells to glomerular production of interleukin-1 (IL-1) (Tipping *et al.* 1991*b*) and tumour necrosis factor-α (TNFα) (Tipping *et al.* 1991*a*) appears to be minor compared to that of macrophages. This is possibly because they are only two of many pro-inflammatory mediators produced by macrophages.

Immunopathological mechanisms in crescent formation

Crescent formation occurs exclusively in the context of inflammatory cell recruitment in glomeruli and is associated with proliferative forms of glomerulonephritis. Macrophages are the major inflammatory cells which accumulate in glomeruli and play a pivotal role in crescent formation. Recently, however, an important role for T lymphocytes has been suggested by both human and experimental studies. Neutrophils are also observed in crescents but their role in crescent formation has not been extensively studied. As well as bone marrow-derived leucocytes, intrinsic glomerular cells are also prominent participants in crescents. Epithelial cells, particularly from the parietal epithelium of Bowman's capsule, have been demonstrated to proliferate and contribute to the accumulation of cells in Bowman's space. Proliferation of mesangial cells or endothelial cells does not appear to contribute to glomerular crescent formation. However, although these cells do not directly contribute to the morphological structure of crescents, increasing evidence of their ability to participate in inflammatory events, including production of pro-inflammatory cytokines and expression of adhesion molecules, raises the possibility that they may play an important role in directing or modifying the inflammatory processes leading to crescent formation (Fig. 2.2).

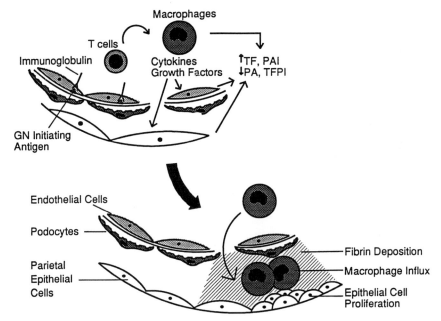

Fig. 2.2 Immunopathogenesis of crescent formation. The immune effector response to glomerular antigens includes both antibody and T cells that recruit and activate macrophages. These leucocytes produce cytokines and growth factors that act on intrinsic glomerular cells. These cell products produce a procoagulant state with enhanced glomerular expression of plasminogen activator inhibitor (PAI) and tissue factor (TF), and down-regulation of plasminogen activator (PA) and tissue factor pathway inhibitor (TFPI). The resulting fibrin deposition in Bowman's space induces macrophage migration, which, together with cytokine and growth factor-stimulated epithelial proliferation, forms crescents.

Cellular participants in crescent formation

A number of histological studies of human tissue have demonstrated the accumulation of macrophages and proliferation of epithelial cells in glomerular crescents. Macrophages have been demonstrated in crescents by electron microscopic studies (Magil and Wadsworth 1981, 1982), enzyme histochemistry (Holdsworth *et al.* al. 1980*a*), and immunocytochemistry (Hooke *et al.* 1984). Further evidence for an important role for these bone marrow-derived cells in glomerular crescent formation has come from studies in two male patients who developed crescentic glomerulonephritis in transplanted kidneys from female donors. The majority of the cells in their crescents were Y body-positive indicating that they were derived from the recipient not from the intrinsic glomerular cells (Schiffer and Michael 1978). Similar experimental transplantation studies using mice with a morphologically identifiable lysosomal abnormality (Chediak–Higashi mice) have demonstrated a prominent role for bone marrow-derived cells in glomerular crescent formation (Striker *et al.* 1979).

Experimental studies similarly indicate an important role for macrophages in glomerular crescent formation (Fig. 2.3). Glomerular macrophage accumulation is an early event in crescent formation in experimental models in rabbits (Kondo *et al.* 1972). Further studies which demonstrate that unilateral renal irradiation does not suppress crescent formation also suggest an important role for bone marrow-derived macrophages (Cattell and Jamieson 1978). In rats, which appear less susceptible to crescent formation, specific monoclonal anti-

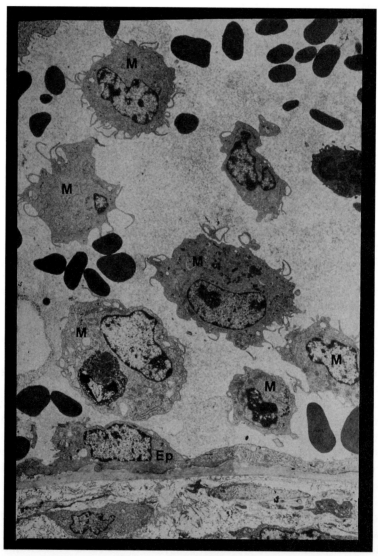

Fig. 2.3 An electron micrograph showing macrophages (M) accumulating in Bowman's space (above parietal epithelial cells, Ep) in a sheep developing crescentic glomerulonephritis.

macrophage antibodies have been used to demonstrate the participation of macrophages in crescents in anti-GBM antibody-initiated glomerulonephritis (Boyce *et al.* 1987).

Histological studies have demonstrated that proliferation of parietal epithelial cells also contributes to the cellular composition of crescents. In crescentic human glomerulonephritis, cytokeratin and vimentin, which are expressed in glomerular parietal epithelial cells, were demonstrated in a substantial number of cells within crescents (Hancock and Atkins 1984; Magil 1985). Although there has been debate over many years as to whether macrophages or epithelial cells are the major cellular contributor to glomerular crescent formation, this question cannot be easily answered. The participation of both cell types has been clearly established and their relative abundance may well vary according to the duration and severity of the glomerular injury and the stage of crescent formation. Macrophages may be more abundant in early crescents, whereas proliferation of epithelial cells may be more prominent in the later stages of crescent formation.

Fibrin as a mediator of crescent formation

Apart from accumulation of cells in Bowman's space, the other major feature of crescent formation is the local deposition of fibrin. Fibrin is a important mediator of glomerular injury in severe crescentic forms of glomerulonephritis. This has been best demonstrated in experimental models, in rabbits and mice, where anticoagulation (Thompson *et al.* 1975*a*; Humair *et al.* 1969*b*), defibrination (Briggs *et al.* 1969; Naish *et al.* 1975; Thomson *et al.* 1975*b*), or fibrinolytic therapy (Humair *et al.* 1969; Briggs *et al.* 1969; Tipping *et al.* 1986; Zoja *et al.* 1990) can protect renal function and prevent crescent formation after immune complex- or anti-GBM-mediated injury. In anti-GBM glomerulonephritis in rabbits, defibrination does not prevent the accumulation of macrophages in the glomerular tuft but prevents their accumulation in Bowman's space (Holdsworth *et al.* 1979), suggesting that fibrinogen/fibrin, or its split products, provide important chemotactic stimuli for macrophage recruitment into developing crescents.

Macrophages may also play a pivotal role in the initiation of glomerular fibrin deposition. Glomerular fibrin deposition is temporally associated with macrophage infiltration and enhanced expression of tissue factor in glomeruli (Tipping and Holdsworth 1986). Tissue factor is a glycoprotein, which, when expressed on the cell surface in association with phospholipids, is the major initiator of coagulation *in vivo*. Tissue factor binds and activates factor VII thus initiating the extrinsic coagulation pathway. Macrophages may initiate glomerular fibrin deposition via their ability to enhance tissue factor activity in glomeruli (Holdsworth and Tipping 1985). Glomerular macrophages themselves express high levels of tissue factor (Tipping *et al.* 1988*b*) and have the potential to enhance tissue factor expression on intrinsic glomerular cells by releasing pro-inflammatory cytokines, including IL-1 and TNFα (Tipping *et al.* 1991*b*).

Evidence from human crescentic glomerulonephritis also suggests an important role for fibrin as a mediator of injury. In patients with lupus nephritis, defibrination is associated with preservation of renal function and an improved clinical outcome (Pollak *et al.* 1982; Kant *et al.* 1985). Augmented glomerular tissue factor activity is associated with glomerular fibrin deposition and macrophage infiltration in severe proliferative forms of human glomerulonephritis (Neale *et al.* 1988 Tipping *et al.* 1988*a*;) demonstrating close parallels with observations in crescentic glomerulonephritis in rabbits.

The normal mechanisms of fibrin clearance are also severely disturbed in experimental crescentic glomerulonephritis. Production of plasminogen activators, urokinase (uPA) and tissue type plasminogen activator (tPA) by normal glomeruli usually provides a local fibrinolytic environment. However, in crescentic anti-GBM glomerulonephritis in rabbits, production of plasminogen activators in glomeruli is inhibited, whereas plasminogen activator inhibitor type 1 (PAI-1) production is enhanced (Malliaros *et al.* 1993). These changes are associated with glomerular macrophage infiltration, and are likely to be directed by macrophage-derived cytokines. Similar changes have been observed in crescentic glomerulonehphritis in humans (Rondeau *et al.* 1990).

The contribution of glomerular endothelial, mesangial, and epithelial cells to the initiation of glomerular fibrin deposition remains to be established. However, where severe local immunologically initiated glomerular injury occurs in the absence of macrophage infiltration, fibrin deposition is rarely observed (Holdsworth and Tipping 1985; Neale *et al.* 1988). Thus, the close association between macrophage infiltration, changes in glomerular expression of procoagulant and fibrinolytic molecules, and fibrin deposition, suggests that these mediators of inflammation may provide an important positive feedback loop resulting in severe glomerular injury and crescent formation.

Signals for inflammatory cell recruitment in crescentic glomerulonephritis

Despite its importance for glomerular neutrophil recruitment, complement does not appear to be an essential signal for recruitment of macrophages in glomerulonephritis (Holdsworth *et al.* 1981). Intact antibody, but not F(ab′)$_2$ fragments have been shown to induce glomerular macrophage recruitment, suggesting an important role for antibody Fc interaction with macrophage Fc receptors (Holdsworth 1983).

More recently, attention has focused on the role of CAMs in inflammatory cell recruitment in severe proliferative forms of glomerulonephritis. Monoclonal antibodies have been raised against key adhesion molecules which are expressed in activated endothelium or on circulating leucocytes. Up-regulation of adhesion molecules on the glomerular endothelium has been demonstrated in experimental models following immunoglobulin deposition and complement activation in glomeruli (Tipping *et al.* 1994*b*; Wuthrich 1992; Wuthrich *et al.* 1990), and enhanced expression of intercellular adhesion molecule-1 (ICAM-1) has been demonstrated in human glomerulonephritis (Bishop and Hall 1989; Lhotta *et al.*

1991). Monoclonal antibodies have been used to block the function of adhesion molecules *in vivo* in order to study their role in glomerulonephritis. Using these reagents in rat models of crescentic glomerulonephritis, inflammatory cell recruitment, glomerular injury and crescent formation have been prevented by antibodies to ICAM-1 and lymphocyte function-associated antigen-1 (LFA-1) (Kawasaki *et al.* 1993; Nishikawa *et al.* 1993). In heterologous phase anti-GBM glomerulonephritis, glomerular neutrophil recruitment and proteinuria were attenuated by antibodies to ICAM-1, LFA-1 (anti-CD11b and anti-CD18), and very late activation antigen-4 (VLA-4), but not by antibodies to endothelial leucocyte adhesion molecule-1 (ELAM-1 now known as E-selectin) (Mulligan *et al.* 1993). These studies suggest that expression of leucocyte adhesion molecules on glomerular endothelial cells may be an essential prerequisite to leucocyte recruitment and subsequent glomerular crescent formation.

T lymphocytes in crescentic glomerulonephritis

It is now widely recognized that accumulation of T cells in glomeruli is commonly observed in crescentic glomerulonephritis. In many patients with crescentic glomerulonephritis, immunoglobulin deposition is absent or sparse leading to their description as 'immune-negative' (Stilmant *et al.* 1979). In these cases, as well as in patients with abundant immunoglobulin deposition, T cells are observed in glomeruli. Immunohistological studies of T cells in glomerulonephritis have demonstrated a close association between their presence, glomerular accumulation of macrophages, and the appearance of crescents in human biopsies (Tipping *et al.* 1988*a*; Stachura *et al.* 1984*a,b*; Bolton *et al.* 1987; Nolasco *et al.* 1987). These data suggest that T cells are the major determinant of glomerular macrophage accumulation and crescent formation in human glomerulonephritis (for a review, see Tam and Pusey 1995).

Experimental data support the hypothesis that T cells play a pivotal role in glomerular crescent formation. Cell transfer studies have demonstrated that T cells sensitized to GBM can induce glomerular proliferation and primitive crescents in chickens in the absence of humoral immunity (Bolton and Tucker 1984; Bolton *et al.* 1980). Bhan *et al.* (1978) were able to induce glomerular macrophage recruitment by transfering sensitized T cells to naive rats with a planted (sensitizing) glomerular antigen. Depletion of CD8-positive cells with monoclonal antibodies before initiation of nephritis prevented renal injury, macrophage accumulation, and crescent formation in anti-GBM glomerulonephritis in rats, suggesting an important role for T cells or natural killer (NK) cells in this disease (Kawasaki *et al.* 1992). By depleting CD5- and CD4-positive T cells in a similar model of anti-GBM glomerulonephritis, an important role for T helper cells in glomerular crescent formation has been recently demonstrated in rats (Huang *et al.* 1994). In these studies, glomerular macrophage accumulation, proteinuria, and giant cell formation were reduced and renal function was protected by depletion of T helper cells, without altering the glomerular deposition of antibody or complement.

T lymphocytes have now been shown to be present in the more aggressive proliferative and crescentic forms of experimental and human glomerulonephritis. In many other inflammatory situations, they initiate chronic forms of injury by the mechanism of delayed-type hypersensitivity (DTH). In these situations, antigen-specific T cells elaborate a number of lymphokines which localize and activate macrophages, the key effectors of injury. T cells elaborating lymphokines have been observed in experimental glomerulonephritis (Boyce *et al.* 1986). T cells can also mediate cytotoxicity reactions, but this mechanism has not yet been demonstrated in glomerulonephritis.

Thus, studies so far point to the involvement of cell-mediated immunity akin to cutaneous DTH in the generation of crescents. The finding of T cells, macrophages, and augmented tissue factor in human proliferative glomerulonephritis in association with fibrin deposition, suggest that T cell-directed events may be pivotal in these severe forms of glomerulonephritis. The experimental evidence demonstrating an important functional role for T cells in glomerular macrophage recruitment, giant cell formation, and crescent formation, and the ability of transferred, sensitized T cells to induce primitive crescents in chickens strongly supports this hypothesis. The role of T cells in the initiation and amplification of glomerular crescent formation remains to be fully elucidated.

Human crescentic glomerulonephritis

Crescentic glomerulonephritis occurs in a variety of clinical settings, often as the renal manifestation of a systemic disease process (Table 2.1). For this reason patients with crescentic glomerulonephritis may be classified according to their underlying extrarenal disease. Major groups include infectious diseases, connective tissue diseases, vasculitis, and anti-GBM disease. Crescentic glomerulonephritis is also seen in a subgroup of idiopathic forms of glomerulonephritis.

Table 2.1   Clinical settings of crescentic glomerulonephritis (GN)

Infectious disease	*Autoimmune glomerular disease*
Postinfectious GN	Anti-GBM disease
Bacterial endocarditis	
Shunt nephritis	*Extrarenal diseases*
Occult sepsis/absesses	Malignancy
	Malignant hypertension
Vasculitis	Drug reactions
Wegener's granulomatosis	
Henoch–Schönlein purpura	*Idiopathic glomurulonephritis*
Microscopic polyarteritis	IgA disease
Cryoglobulinaemia	Membranoproliferative GN
	Hereditary nephritis
Connective tissue diseases	Membranous GN
Systemic lupus erythematosus (SLE)	
Relapsing polychondritis	
Scleroderma	

Finally, a number of less common disease processes are associated with crescentic glomerulonephritis. Thus a variety of immune-initiating signals have been documented in human crescentic glomerulonephritis. These include deposition of anti-GBM autoantibody and circulating immune complexes, *in situ* immune complex formation, and glomerular T cell localization.

Classification of crescentic glomerulonephritis according to the pattern of antibody deposition is now widely employed (see also Fig. 2.1):

Linear immunoglobulin deposition: anti-GBM antibody-associated glomerulonephritis.

Scanty immunoglobulin deposition: ANCA/vasculitis-associated glomerulonephritis.

Granular immunoglobulin deposition: immune complex-associated glomerulonephritis.

The increasing acceptance of this classification is in part because of the seemingly rational association between diagnosis, immunohistology, and immunopathogenetic mechanisms. However, closer inspection suggests that this view of this association may be somewhat simplistic.

Immunopathogenesis of crescent formation in human glomerulonephritis

Despite the widely varying immune responses associated with crescentic glomerulonephritis and the variety of immune-initiating signals within glomeruli, a common pattern of involvement of mediators of injury is observed. Fibrin, T cells, and macrophages are all commonly seen in crescentic glomerulonephritis despite the clinical setting or immunohistological category. The simultaneous colocalization of the essential effectors of DTH–T cells, macrophages expressing enhanced tissue factor activity, and fibrin—seen in all three categories of human crescentic glomerulonephritis cited above, provides evidence to suggest the participation of DTH-like mechanisms in crescent formation.

In a prospective study, human biopsies demonstrating glomerulonephritis with prominent fibrin deposition were compared with biopsies without demonstrable fibrin (Neale *et al.* 1988). Crescent formation was observed in most of the fibrin positive biopsies and they all showed a significant influx of macrophages and T cells in association with prominent glomerular tissue factor expression. Fibrin-negative biopsies were not crescentic and had few infiltrating T cells or macrophages; glomerular tissue factor expression was not enhanced. These data provide further evidence for the association of fibrin deposition and crescent formation with the mediators of DTH.

Anti-GBM antibody-associated crescentic glomerulonephritis

This form of glomerulonephritis is associated with the development of autoimmunity to a specific component of the non-collagenous domain of type IV collagen, which has been recently cloned (Turner *et al.* 1992). An immunogenetic susceptibiltiy to anti-GBM antibody-induced crescentic glomerulonephritis has been suggested by its strong association with expression of the HLA-DR2 antigen (Rees *et al.* 1978, 1984; Rees 1994). The potential for autoimmune responses to be initiated by hydrocarbon-induced damage releasing sequested neoantigens has been suggested (Heale *et al.* 1969; D'Apice *et al.* 1978) but conclusive evidence is not available. Experimentally, hydrocarbons have been shown to induce pulmonary vascular injury, which facilitates the binding of anti-basement membrane antibodies in the lung (Yamamoto and Wilson 1987).

Scanty or negative (pauci-immune)/ANCA-associated crescentic glomerulonephritis

In 1979, Stillmant *et al.* recognized that the largest group of patients with crescentic glomerulonephritis have few or no demonstrable deposits of immunoglobulin or complement and defined these as 'pauci-immune' crescentic glomerulonephritis (Stilmant *et al.* 1979). Pauci-immune ANCA-associated crescentic glomerulonephritis is often seen in patients who have evidence of extrarenal, often multi-system vasculitis (Hall *et al.* 1984; Davies *et al.* 1982). Although a spectrum of manifestations are reported, three entities are most often recognized: Wegener's granulomatosis (van der Woude *et al.* 1985), microscopic polyarteritis (Falk and Jennette 1988), and idiopathic crescentic pauci-immune glomerulonephritis (Jennette *et al.* 1989). These observations raised the likely possibility that pauci-immune glomerulonephritis was a form of small vessel necrotizing vasculitis affecting the glomerular capillary bed. The discovery that ANCA were associated with this subgroup of vasculitis (Hall *et al.* 1984; Davies *et al.* 1982) offered a serological marker and the potential for a unifying explanation of the immunopathogenesis of this form of crescentic nephritis.

ANCA have now been recognized to be directed to a variety of lysosomal neutrophil antigens. Two different antigen/antibody patterns have been defined in patients with this type of crescentic glomerulonephritis. These are defined by the pattern of immunofluorescence staining of neutrophils incubated with serum from vasculitic patients and have been designated c-ANCA (diffuse cytoplasmic staining due to PR3 reactivity) (van der Woude *et al.* 1985) and p-ANCA (a perinuclear pattern predominantly due to myeloperoxidase reactivity) (Falk and Jennette 1988). c-ANCA is strongly associated with Wegener's granulomatosis (over 90%) although it is also seen in up to 20% of patients with microscopic polyarteritis and idiopathic pauci-immune crescentic glomerulonephritis (Jennette *et al.* 1989). p-ANCA is rarely observed with Wegener's granulomatosis (less than 5%) but is commonly observed in microscopic polyarteritis and idiopathic crescentic pauci-immune glomerulonephritis (40–70%) (Jennette *et al.* 1989; Gross *et al.* 1993).

A number of experiments have been contrived to provide evidence for a pathogenetic role for ANCA in endothelial and glomerular injury. The first apparent difficulty with this proposition is the fact that the target antigens are cytoplasmic. However, cytokines have been shown to induce their membrane expression. The antigens have also been shown on the surface of circulating neutrophils in patients with Wegener's granulomatosis (Csernok *et al.* 1990). *In vitro*, ANCA can stimulate the respiratory burst in cytokine-primed neutrophils (Falk *et al.* 1990) and cause translocation of protein kinase C to the cell membrane supporting its putative role in neutrophil activation (Lai and Lockwood 1991).

The reasons for the development of autoimmunity to neutrophil cytoplasmic antigens and the mechanisms by which they localize to glomeruli are unknown. In human pauci-immune crescentic glomerulonephritis, macrophages, neutrophils, and T cells are present in glomerular lesions and immunoglobulin is absent (Brouwer *et al.* 1991). T cells reactive with PR3 can be demonstrated in the circulation of these patients (Mathieson *et al.* 1992). A number of hypotheses have been constructed to link ANCA with crescentic glomerulonephritis. These include the 'ANCA cytokine theory' which postulates that infection leads to increased circulating levels of cytokines that results in membrane expression of cytoplasmic antigens in primed neutrophils. Development of autoimmunity to these activated neutrophils leads to intravascular cytoclasis, allowing neutrophil products to bind to endothelial sites in the kidney where further autoimmune reactions produce crescentic glomerulonephritis.

An alternative view is that ANCA are an epiphenomenon secondary to the release of a previously sequestered antigen. It would, therefore, be expected in other situations leading to leucocytoclasis, such as infection. This view is supported by increasing numbers of reports of ANCA being associated with a variety of forms of infection, including pneumonia, tuberculosis, bacterial endocarditis, human immunodeficiency virus infection, and infection associated with cystic fibrosis (Davenport, 1992; Klaassen *et al.* 1992; Koderisch *et al.* 1990; Efthimiou *et al.* 1991). A possible middle-ground position would be to suggest that ANCA may perpetuate and exacerbate disease produced by some other mechanism.

Immune complex-associated crescentic glomerulonephritis

This form of human crescentic glomerulonephritis is associated with a long list of extrarenal diseases as well as idiopathic forms of glomerulonephritis. Immune complex formation and deposition is clearly established in SLE; however the evidence for an immune complex-initiated form of glomerular injury is not as strong in many other associated diseases. Cryoglobulinaemia represents a special case where true immune complexes (i.e. antibody-antigen complexes) as well as immunoglobulin aggregates (with similar phlogistic potential) are clearly associated with widespread vascular deposition and injury. Several forms of vasculitis (e.g. serum sickness and bacterial endocarditis) are likely to be induced by immune complex deposition.

Evolution of crescent formation and outcome

Knowledge of the evolution of crescents is based on examination of human biopies and studies in crescentic animal models. The most extensively studied models in this regard are anti-GBM antibody-initiated glomerulonephritis in rats, rabbits, and mice and chronic serum sickness in rabbits. In experimental models, crescents appear and resolve in a relatively synchronous manner. However, in a human biopsy, crescents may be seen in various stages of development. Despite this apparent difference, experimental models provide the best opportunity to study the sequential evolution of crescents.

Crescent formation progresses through a series of distinct stages leading to glomerulosclerosis or resolution with preservation of function. The factors that allow some crescents to resolve, whereas other glomeruli with histologically similar crescents progress to glomerulosclerosis are unknown. However, there appears to be a critical point, probably during the development of the cellular crescent, after which healing will invariably lead to scar formation and sclerosis.

Stages in evolution of crescents.

Evolution of crescents may be considered in a number of histologically distinct phases (see Fig. 2.4).

Glomerular hypercellularity

The initial stage of crescent formation involves an inflammatory response within the glomerular tuft resulting in intracapillary macrophage accumulation. Glomerular expression of procoagulant activity and plasminogen activator inhibitor type 1 (PAI-1) is enhanced, while tissue type plasminogen activator, urokinase plasminogen activator (Malliaros *et al* 1993) and tissue-factor pathway inhibitor is reduced. This establishes a procoagulant and antifibrinolytic environment within the glomerulus resulting in the initiation of local fibrin deposition. Deposition of collagen has been demonstrated in the renal cortex and interstitium at this time, prior to the appearance of fibrin in Bowman's space (Downer *et al.* 1988).

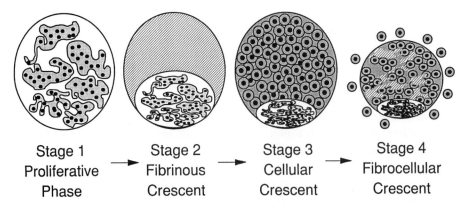

Stage 1	Stage 2	Stage 3	Stage 4
Proliferative	Fibrinous	Cellular	Fibrocellular
Phase	Crescent	Crescent	Crescent

Fig. 2.4 Evolution of glomerular crescents. Stage 1, infiltration of glomeruli by leucocytes. Stage 2, formation of a fibrinous crescent in Bowman's space. Stage 3, migration of macrophages into Bowman's space. Stage 4, collagen deposition produces a fibrocellular scar.

Fibrinous crescents

Deposition of fibrin in Bowman's space marks the next phase in crescent formation. It is uncertain whether this fibrin is formed within capillaries and leaks into Bowman's space or whether fibrinogen leaking across the GBM into Bowman's space is cleaved to fibrin and cross-linked *in situ*. In a number of types of non-crescentic glomerulonephritis, the presence of fibrinogen and fibrin degradation products in the urine demonstrates that circulating coagulation factors and fibrinogen can enter Bowman's space without forming a stable clot (Scott *et al.* 1986). This suggests that local changes in Bowman's space contribute to the deposition of stable cross-linked fibrin. Parietal epithelial cells lining Bowman's space have the potential to express tissue factor and PAI-1, thus promoting coagulation and inhibiting fibrin removal (Yambe *et al.* 1993; Bukovsky *et al.* 1992; Aya *et al.* 1992; Iwamoto *et al.* 1990). Their capacity to contribute to fibrin deposition in Bowman's space in crescentic glomerulonephritis has not been addressed.

Cellular crescents

After formation of fibrinous crescents, the next distinct phase of their evolution is the appearance of cells in Bowman's space. As previously discussed, both invasion by macrophages and proliferation of glomerular parietal epithelial cells contribute to the formation of cellular crescents. The migration of macrophages into fibrinous crescents may represent a critical point in their evolution, because of the capacity of macrophages to direct the subsequent sclerosis and scarring by their local production of cytokines and growth factors. Downer *et al.* (1988) have shown that renal cortical and glomerular collagen synthesis increases within 24 hours of T cell and macrophage accumulation in glomeruli. Macrophage accumulation in Bowman's space, but not in the glomerular tuft, is inhibited by defibrination, suggesting that fibrin is a critical signal for macrophage recruitment into crescents (Holdsworth *et al.* 1979). However, in a mouse model of anti-GBM glomerulonephritis, crescents were shown to be of epithelial cell origin but were not dependent on fibrin deposition in Bowman's space (Wheeler *et al.* 1993). The factors that lead to proliferation of parietal epithelial cells are unknown, but a role for macrophage-derived cytokines or growth factors is likely.

Fibrocellular crescents

After cellular infiltration has peaked, increased deposition of extracellular matrix becomes apparent, resulting in fibrocellular crescents with periglomerular fibrosis. In humans, the predominant matrix proteins are types IV and V collagen (Striker *et al.* 1984; Foellmer *et al.* 1986), suggesting that intrinsic glomerular cells are a major site of their production. Similarly, in anti-GBM glomerulonephritis in rabbits, Downer *et al.* (1988) found predominantly type IV collagen in glomeruli and crescents with minimal amounts of type III collagen, predominantly in the interstitium (this process is discussed in greater detail in Chapter 3).

Glomerulosclerosis

In the final stages of the evolution of crescents, glomeruli become completely sclerosed with ablation of the glomerular capillary bed and marked periglomerular and interstitial fibrosis.

Mechanisms of epithelial cell proliferation in crescents

Epithelial cell proliferation is often a prominent feature in human crescentic glomerulonephritis and appears to be associated with more advanced stages of crescent formation in experimental models. The factors responsible for epithelial cell proliferation during crescent formation remain uncertain. In rabbits, fibrin deposition in Bowman's space has been shown to be necessary preliminary event leading to macrophage recruitment and subsequent development of a cellular crescent (Naish *et al.* 1975).

There has been considerable recent interest in the potential role of growth factors in crescent formation because of their ability to regulate cellular proliferation and repair. A number of growth factors either produced by infiltrating monocytes or by intrinsic glomerular cells may contribute to epithelial cell proliferation. Epidermal derived growth factor (EGF) can stimulate glomerular epithelial cell proliferation when cells are grown on a matrix of type I or IV collagen (Floege *et al.* 1993*b*; Cybusky *et al.* 1990). *In vitro*, rat glomerular epithelial cells express receptors for basic fibroblast growth factor (bFGF) and proliferate in its presence (Tukeuchi *et al.* 1992). Basic FGF is also mitogenic for normal mesangial cells *in vitro* (Floege *et al.* 1992). However, bFGF did not induce glomerular epithelial cell proliferation when infused into normal rats or rats given a subnephritogenic dose of anti-Thy-1 antibody (Floege *et al.* 1993*a*).

Glomerular epithelial cells express receptors for platelet-derived growth factor (PDGF), but do not proliferate in response to PDGF *in vitro* (Floege *et al.* 1993*b*). *In vivo*, infusion of PDGF in normal rats or rats given anti-Thy-1 antibody, resulted in mesangial cell proliferation but proliferation of glomerular epithelial cells was not observed (Floege *et al.* 1993*a*).

Extracellular matrix turnover and its regulation

Excessive accumulation of extracellular matrix (predominantly collagens, proteoglycans, fibronectin, and laminin) is a prominent feature of glomerulosclerosis and may develop over a matter of days to years. Both intrinsic glomerular cells and infiltrating cells may influence the glomerular accumulation of extracellular matrix. Mesangial and epithelial cells can produce both normal and pathological extracellular matrix, and molecules which may regulate its turnover (Bruijn *et al.* 1994; Davies *et al.* 1992). Infiltrating monocytes may also produce extracellular matrix and have the capacity to influence its synthesis by intrinsic glomerular cells.

Some insight into the molecular signals regulating matrix turnover and the development of glomerulosclerosis has been gained from observations in transgenic mice. Transgenic mice expressing excessive levels of growth hormone (GH) or growth hormone releasing factor (GHRF) develop mesangial cell proliferation which leads to glomerulosclerosis (Dui *et al.* 1988; Quaife *et al.* 1989). This effect may be mediated in part by insulin-like growth factor-1 (IGF-1) which can stimulate proteoglycan synthesis by microvascular endothelial cells (Sedor 1992). IGF-1 can also act synergistically with GH and glucocorticoids to stimulate fibroblast proliferation (Sedor 1992). However, animals transgenic for IGF-1 develop mild glomerular hypertrophy without glomerulosclerosis, suggesting that GH may act independently of IGF-1 (Dui *et al.* 1990). IL-6 is present in the glomeruli of humans and animals with mesangial proliferative glomerulonephritis and its expression has been suggested to correlate with the degree of mesangial proliferation (Hirano *et al.* 1990; Horii *et al.* 1989). Transgenic mice with very high circulating levels of IL-6 spontaneously develop mesangial proliferative glomerulonephritis, implying a causative role for IL-6 in this disease (Suematsu *et al.* 1989). Transgenic mice selectively expressing high levels of transforming growth factor-β (TGFβ) intrarenally also develop glomerulosclerosis (Isaka *et al.* 1993).

Thy-1.1 is a mesangial cell antigen which is the target antigen in the anti-Thy-1 model of mesangial proliferative glomerulonephritis in rats. This model has been used extensively to study glomerular matrix accumulation. Recently, mice over-expressing a human hybrid Thy-1.1 have been shown to develop glomerulosclerosis (Kollias *et al.* 1987). The functional role of Thy-1.1 in mesangial cells and the mechanism by which its over-expression leads to glomerulosclerosis is unknown. Mice carrying the SV-40 virus and expressing the SV-40 T antigen also develop some glomerulosclerosis (MacKay *et al.* 1987). This was thought to result from dysregulation of genes controlling growth and suggests that glomerulosclerosis may occur through loss of normal growth regulatory mechanisms.

Matrix metalloproteinases (MMPs) are key molecules in the regulation of extracellular matrix turnover. These enzymes are secreted as zymogens and their activity can be regulated by changes in their production or activation, or changes in their inhibitors, such as tissue inhibitors of matrix metalloproteinase (TIMPs). Plasmin has the potential to be an important activator of MMPs and thus the regulation of activation of plasmin may have important consequences for extracellular matrix turnover. The role of plasmin has been studied indirectly in transgenic mice over-expressing PAI-1, an important inhibitor of the plasminogen activators (Carmeliet *et al.* 1993). These mice did not develop significant renal disease during their growth and development. However, studies of the outcome of glomerulonephritis in PAI-1 transgenic mice have not yet been reported.

Cytokines and growth factors can influence the production of extracellular matrix and the expression of molecules regulating its turnover. IL-1 and TNFα stimulate production of matrix metalloproteinases (MMPs) and tissue inhibitors of MMPs (TIMPs) by macrophages and resident glomerular cells (Davies *et al.* 1992; Goshowaki *et al.* 1988). They also stimulate IL-6 production which can up-regulate TIMPs, which may feed back to reduce the catabolic effects of IL-1 and TNFα (Davies *et al.* 1992).

Transforming growth factor-β (TGFβ) is the growth factor which has been most extensively studied in crescentic glomerulonephritis and glomerulosclerosis. TGFβ is a widely distributed growth factor, capable of up-regulating its own activity. It is secreted in a latent form and can be activated to a 25 KDa homodimer *in vitro* by plasmin, cathepsin D, and acid treatment. TGFβ has been demonstrated to influence the synthesis of extracellular matrix proteins by intrinsic glomerular cells (Bruijn *et al.* 1994). It stimulates epithelial and mesangial cells, *in vitro*, to produce the proteoglycans decorin and biglycan, which are abundant in the extracellular matrix of sclerotic glomeruli (Border *et al.* 1990a). TGFβ also stimulates production of extracellular matrix proteins—collagen IV, fibronectin, and, to a lesser extent, laminin—by glomerular epithelial cells (Nakamura *et al.* 1992). It upregulates expression of the α5, β1-integrin (the fibronectin receptor) in cultured rat glomeruli, in association with increased deposition of fibronectin in the extracellular matrix (Kagami *et al.* 1993).

The involvement of TGFβ in extracellular matrix accumulation and glomerulosclerosis has been most extensively studied in the anti-Thy-1 model of mesangial proliferative glomerulonephritis. In this model, antibody-initiated complement-dependent mesangial lysis results in leucocyte infiltration, mesangial proliferation, and increased proteoglycan (predominantly decorin and biglycan) deposition in the mesangial matrix (Border *et al.* 1990a). Increased glomerular PAI-1 expression and deposition in the extracellular matrix is also observed (Tomooka *et al.* 1992). This accumulation of mesangial matrix is significantly reduced by administration of a neutralizing anti-TGFβ antibody (Border *et al.* 1990b) and by administration of decorin, which binds and inhibits TGFβ (Border *et al.* 1992). Repeated doses of anti-Thy-1 antibody result in persistently elevated TGFβ in association with progressive interstitial fibrosis and glomerulosclerosis (Yamamoto *et al.* 1994).

TGFβ stimulates glomerular production of PAI-1 and TIMPs and reduces the expression of stromolysin (Edwards *et al.* 1987; Matri *et al.* 1994). These changes favour increased deposition of extracellular matrix. Increased glomerular TGFβ activity (capable of stimulating collagen production by cultured mesangial cells) and increased TGFβ mRNA has been demonstrated in crescentic anti-GBM glomerulonephritis in rabbits (Coimbra *et al.* 1991). Increased TGFβ expresssion is associated with increased glomerular mesangial matrix deposition in a rat model of diabetic nephropathy (Yamamoto *et al.* 1993). Increased expression of TGFβ has also been demonstrated in human glomerulonephritis (Yoshioka *et al.* 1993).

Expression of TIMP mRNA in normal glomeruli and increased levels in sclerotic glomeruli of patients with renal carcinoma has been demonstrated using competitive PCR, supporting a role for TIMP in glomerulosclerosis in humans (Carome *et al.* 1993). TGFβ and TIMP mRNA are up-regulated in association with glomerulosclerosis in purinomycin aminonucleoside nephrosis in rats (Jones *et al.* 1991) and TGFβ has been shown to up regulate TIMP production in cultured rat mesangial cells (Matri *et al.* 1994). Thus, human and experimental evidence suggests that TGFβ may play an important role in the development of glomerulosclerosis by both increasing proteoglycan production and inhibiting its removal.

Extrarenal influences on progression of glomerular injury and crescents

In human disease, renal function often continues to decline and glomerulosclerosis develops even when the acute glomerular insult seems to be over. A number of factors have been identified with the potential to perpetuate this decline in renal function. These include hypertension, hyperlipidaemia, low grade persistence of underlying disease, steroid therapy, hyperparathyroidism, hyperphosphataemia, and hyperfiltration in remaining glomeruli (El Nahas 1992). Dietary protein restriction has been shown to reduce the rate of decline of renal function in rodents, but whether it is similarly effective in man is uncertain. In the anti-Thy-1 model of glomerulonephritis in rats, protein restriction reduced TGFβ production by nephritic glomeruli and substantially decreased cellular matrix accumulation (Yamamoto *et al.* 1993). The mechanisms by which hypertension, hyperlipidaemia, and steroid therapy lead to glomerulosclerosis and progressive loss of renal function are unknown.

References

Abbott, F., Ryan, J.J., Ceska, M., Matsushima, K., Sarraf, C.E., and Rees, A.J. (1991). Interleukin-1 beta stimulates human mesangial cells to synthesize and release interleukins-6 and -8. *Kidney International*, **40**, 597–605.

Andrews, B.S., Eisenberg, R.A., Theofilopoulos, A.N., Izui, S., Wilson, C.B., McConahey, P.J. *et al.* (1978). Spontaneous murine lupus-like syndromes. Clinical and immunopathological manifestations in several strains. *Journal of Experimental Medicine*, **148**, 1198–1215.

Aya, N., Yoshioka, K., Murakami, K., Hino, S., Okada, K., Matsuo, O., and Maki, S. (1992). Tissue-type plasminogen activator and its inhibitor in human glomerulonephritis. *Journal of Pathology*, **166**, 289–95.

Banks, K.L. (1967). Anti-glomerular basement membrane antibody in horses. *American Journal of Pathology*, **94**, 443–6.

Bhan, A.K., Schneeberger, E.E., Collins, A.B., and McCluskey, R.T. (1978). Evidence for a pathogenic role of a cell-mediated immune mechanism in experimental glomerulonephritis. *Journal of Experimental Medicine*, **148**, 246–60.

Bishop, G.A. and Hall, B.M. (1989). Expression of leucocyte and lymphocyte adhesion molecules in the human kidney. *Kidney International*, **36**, 1078–85.

Bolton, W.K. and Sturgill, B.C. (1989). Proliferative glomerulonephritis. Postinfectious, non-infectious and crescentic forms. In *Renal pathology with clinical and functional correlations*, (ed. C.C. Tischer and B.M. Brenner), pp. 156–95. Lippincott, Philadelphia.

Bolton, W.K., Tucker, F.L., and Sturgill, B.C. (1980). Experimental autoimmune glomerulonephritis in chickens. *Journal of Clinical and Laboratory Immunology*, **3**, 179–84.

Bolton, W.K., Tucker, F.L., and Sturgill, B.C. (1984). New avian model of experimental glomerulonephritis consistent with mediation by cellular immunity Nonhumorally mediated glomerulonephritis in chickens. *Journal of Clinical Investigation*, **73**, 1263–76.

Bolton, W.K., Innes, D.J., Jr., Sturgill, B.C., and Kaiser, D.L. (1987). T-cells and macrophages in rapidly progressive glomerulonephritis: clinicopathologic correlations. *Kidney International*, **32**, 869–76.

Border, W.A., Kamil, F.S., Ward, H.J., and Cohen, A.H. (1981). Antigenic charge as a determinant of immune complex localization in the rat glomerulus. *Laboratory Investigation*, **40**, 429–42.

Border, W.A., Okuda, S., Languino, L.R., and Ruoslahti, E. (1990*a*). Transforming growth factor-beta regulates production of proteoglycans by mesangial cells. *Kidney International*, **37**, 689–695.

Border, W.A., Okuda, S., Languino, L.R., Sporn, M.B., and Ruoslahti, E. (1990*b*). Suppression of experimental glomerulonephritis by antiserum against transforming growth factor beta 1. *Nature*, **346**, 371–4.

Border, W.A., Noble, N.A., Yamamoto, T., Harper, J.R., Yamaguchi, Y., Pierschbacher, M.D. *et al.* (1992). Natural inhibitor of transforming growth factor-beta protects against scarring in experimental kidney disease. *Nature*, **360**, 361–4.

Boyce, N.W. and Holdsworth, S.R. (1985). Anti-glomerular basement membrane antibody-induced experimental glomerulonephritis: evidence for dose-dependent, direct antibody and complement-induced, cell-independent injury. *Journal of Immunology*, **135**, 3918–21.

Boyce, N.W., Tipping, P.G., and Holdsworth, S.R. (1986). Lymphokine (MIF) production by glomerular T-lymphocytes in experimental glomerulonephritis. *Kidney International*, **30**, 673–7.

Boyce, N.W., Holdsworth, S.R., Dijkstra, C.D., and Atkins, R.C. (1987). Quantitation of intraglomerular mononuclear phagocytes in experimental glomerulonephritis in the rat using specific monoclonal antibodies. *Pathology*, **19**, 290–3.

Briggs, J.D., Kwaan, H.C., and Potter, E.V. (1969). The role of fibrinogen in renal disease: III. Fibrinolytic and anticoagulant treatment of nephrotoxic serum nephritis. *Laboratory and Clinical Medicine*, **74**, 724–51.

Brouwer, E, Cohen Tervaert, J.W., Weening, J.J., and Kallenberg, C.G.M. (1991). Immunohistology of renal biopsies in Wegener's granulomatosis (WG): clues to its pathogenesis. *Kidney International*, **39**, 1055–6 (abstract).

Brown, Z., Sirieter, R.M., Chensue, S.W., Ceska, M., Lindley, I., *et al.* (1991). Cytokine-activated human mesangial cells generate the neutrophil chemoattractant, interleukin 8. *Kidney International*, **40**, 86–90.

Bruijn, J.A., Roos, A., de Geus, B., and de Heer, E. (1994). Transforming growth factor-beta and the glomerular extracellular matrix in renal pathology. *Journal of Laboratory and Clinical Medicine*, **123**, 34–47.

Bukovsky, A., Labarrere, C.A., Haag, B., Carter, C., and Faulk, W.P. (1992). Tissue factor in normal and transplanted human kidneys. *Transplantation*, **54**, 644–50.

Carmeliet, P., Stassen, J.M., Schoonjans, L., Ream, B., van den Oord, J.J., De Mol, M., *et al.* (1993). Plasminogen activator inhibitor-1 gene-deficient mice: II. Effects on hemostasis, thrombosis, and thrombolysis. *Journal of Clinical Investigation*, **92**, 2756–60.

Carome, M.A., Striker, L.J., Peten, E.P., Moore, J., Yang, C.W., Stetler-Stevenson, W.G., *et al.* (1993). Human glomeruli express TIMP-1 mRNA and TIMP-2 protein and mRNA. *American Journal of Physiology*, **264**, F923–9.

Cattell, V. and Jamieson, S.W. (1978). The origin of glomerular crescents in experimental nephrotoxic serum nephritis in the rabbit. *Laboratory Investigation*, 39, 584–90.

Cochrane, C.G., Unanue, E.R., and Dixon, F.J. (1965). A role of polymorphonuclear leukocytes and complement in nephrotoxic nephritis. *Journal of Experimental Medicine*, 122, 99–116.

Coimbra, T., Wiggins, R., Noh, J.W., Merritt, S., and Phan, S.H., (1991). Transforming growth factor-beta production in anti-glomerular basement membrane disease in the rabbit. *American Journal of Pathology*, 138, 223–34.

Cotran, R. (1987). New roles for the endothelium in inflammation and immunity. *American Journal of Pathology*, 129, 407–13.

Couser, W.G. (1986). In situ formation of immune complexes and the role of complement activation in glomerulonephritis. *Clinical Immunology and Allergy*, 6, 287–36.

Csernok, E., Ludemann, J., Gross, W.L. and Bainton, D.F. (1990). Ultrastructural localization of proteinase 3, the target antigen of anti-cytoplasmic antibodies circulating in Wegener's granulomatosis. *American Journal of Pathology*, 137, 1113–20.

Cybulsky, A.V., Bonventre, J.V., and Quigg, R.J. (1990). Extracellular matrix regulates proliferation and phospholipid turnover in glomerular epithelial cells. *American Journal of Physiology*, 359, F326–37.

D'Apice, A.J.F., Kincaid-Smith, P., and Becker, G.J. (1978). Goodpasture's syndrome in identical twins. *Annals of Internal Medicine*, 88, 61.

Davenport, A. (1992). 'False positive' perinuclear and cytoplasmic anti-neutrophil cytoplasmic antibody results leading to misdiagnosis of Wegener's granulomatosis and/or microscopic polyarteritis. *Clinical Nephrology*, 37, 124–30.

Davies, D.J., Moran, J.E., Niall, J.F., and Ryan, G.B. (1982). Segmental necrotizing glomerulonephritis with anti-neutrophil antibody: possible arbovirus aetiology. *British Medical Journal*, 285, 606.

Davies, M., Martin, J., Thomas, G.J., and Lovett, D.H. (1992). Proteinases and glomerular matrix turnover. *Kidney International*, 41, 671–8.

Dixon, F.J., Feldman, J.D., and Vazquez, J.J. (1961). Experimental glomerulonephritis: the pathogenesis of a laboratory model resembling the spectrum of human glomerulonephritis. *Journal of Experimental Medicine*, 113, 399.

Downer, G., Phan, S.H. and Wiggins, R.C. (1988). Analysis of renal fibrosis in a rabbit model of crescentic nephritis. *Journal of Clinical Investigation*, 82, 998–1006.

Drake, C.G. and Kotzin, B.L. (1992). Genetic and immunological mechanisms in the pathogenesis of systemic lupus erythematosus *Current Opinion in Immunology*, 4, 733–40.

Druet, E., Sapin, C., Gunther, E., Feingold, N., and Druet, P. (1977). Mercuric chloride-induced anti-glomerular basement membrane antibodies in the rat. *European Journal of Immunology*, 7, 348–51.

Dui, T., Striker, L.J., Quaife, C., Palmiter, F.G., Behringer, R., Binster, R. *et al.* (1988). Progressive glomerulosclerosis develops in mice chronically expressing growth hormone releasing factor but not in those expressing insulin like growth factor-1. *American Journal of Pathology*, 131, 398–403.

Dui, T., Striker, L.J., Gisbons, C.C., Agoda, L.Y., Brinster, R.L., and Striker, G.E. (1990). Glomerular lesions in mice transgenic for growth hormone and insulin-like growth factor-1. *American Journal of Pathology*, 137, 541–52.

Edwards, D.R., Murphy, G., Reynolds, J.J., Whitham, S.E., Docherty, A.J., Angel, P., *et al.* (1987). Transforming growth factor beta modulates the expression of collagenase and metalloproteinase inhibitor. *EMBO Journal*, 6, 1899–1904.

Efthimiou, J., Spickett, G., Lane, D., and Thompson, A. (1991). Antineutrophil cytoplasmic antibodies, cystic fibrosis, and infection. *Lancet*, **337**, 1037–8. (letter).

El Nahas, A.M. (1992). Mechanisms of progression and consequences of nephron reduction. In *Oxford textbook of clinical nephrology*, (ed. J.S. Cameron, A.M. Davison, A. Davison, J.P. Grunfeld, D. Kerr, and E. Ritz), pp. 1195–1227. Oxford University Press.

Falk, R.J. and Jennette, J.C. (1988). Anti-neutrophil cytoplasmic autoantibodies with specificity for myeloperoxidase in patients with systemic vasculitis and idiopathic necrotizing and crescentic glomerulonephritis. *New England Journal of Medicine*, **318**, 1651–7.

Falk, R.J., Terrell, R.S., Charles, L.A., and Jennette, J.C. (1990). Anti-neutrophil cytoplasmic autoantibodies induce neutrophils to degranulate and produce oxygen radicals in vitro. *Proceedings of the National Academy of Science USA*, **87**, 4115–19.

Floege, J., Eng, E., Lindner, V., Young, A., Reidy, M.A., and Johnson, R.J. (1992). Rat glomerular mesangial cells synthesize basic FGF. Release, upregulated synthesis and mitogenicity in mesangial proliferative glomerulonephritis. *Journal of Clinical Investigation*, **90**, 2362–9.

Floege, J., Eng, F., Young, B.A., Alpers, C.E., Burrett, T.B., Bowen-Pope, D.F. *et al.* (1993a). Infusion of platelet-derived growth factor or basic fibroblast growth factor induces selective glomerular mesangial cell proliferation and matrix accumulation in rats. *Journal of Clinical Investigation*, **92**, 2952–2962.

Floege, J., Johnson, R.J., Alpers, C.E., Fatemi-Nainie, S., Richardson, C.A., Gordon, K. *et al.* (1993b). Visceral glomerular epithelial cells can proliferate in vivo and synthesize platelet-derived growth factor B-chain. *American Journal of Pathology*, **142**, 637–50.

Foellmer, H.G., Sterzel, R.B., and Kashgarian, M. (1986). Progressive glomerular sclerosis in experimental antiglomerular basement membrane glomerulonephritis. *American Journal of Kidney Diseases*, **7**, 5–11.

Glassock, R.J., Adler, S.G., Ward, H.J., and Cohen, A.H. (1991). Primary glomerular disease. In *The kidney*, (ed. B.M. Brenner and F.C. Rector), pp. 1182–1368. Saunders, Philadephia.

Golbus, S.M. and Wilson, C.B. (1979). Experimental glomerulonephritis induced by in situ formation of immune complexes in glomerular capillary wall. *Kidney International*, **16**, 148–57.

Goshowaki, H., Suto, T., Mari, Y., Yamashita, K., Hayatiawa, T., and Nagase, H. (1988). Human recombinant interleukin-1 alpha mediated stimulation of procollagenase production and suppression of biosynthesis of tissue inhibitor of metalloproteinases in rabbit uterine cervical fibroblasts. *FEBS Letters*, **234**, 326–30.

Groggel, G.C., Adler, S., Rennke, H.G., Couser, W.G., and Salant, D.J. (1983). Role of the terminal complement pathway in experimental membranous nephropathy in the rabbit. *Journal of Clinical Investigation*, **72**, 1948–57.

Groggel, G.C., Salant, D.J., Darby, C., Rennke, H.G., and Couser, W.G. (1985). Role of terminal complement pathway in the heterologous phase of antiglomerular basement membrane nephritis. *Kidney International*, **27**, 643–51.

Gross, W.L., Schmitt, W.H., and Csernok, E. (1993). ANCA and associated diseases: immunodiagnostic and pathogenetic aspects. *Clinical and Experimental Immunology*, **91**, 1–12.

Hall, B., Wadham, B., Wood, C.J., Ashton, V., and Adam, W.R. (1984). Vasculitis and glomerulonephritis: a subgroup with an antineutrophil cytoplasmic antibody. *Australia and New Zealand Journal of Medicine*, **14**, 277–8.

Hancock, W.W. and Atkins, R.C. (1984). Cellular composition of crescents in human rapidly progressive glomerular nephritis, identified using monoclonal antibodies. *American Journal of Nephrology*, 3, 177–82.

Heale, W.F., Mathieson, A.M., and Niall, J.F. (1969). Lung haemorrhage and nephritis (Goodpasture's syndrome). *Medical Journal of Australia*, 2, 355–7.

Heymann, W., Hackel, D.B., Harwood, S., Wilson, S.G.F., and Hunter, J.L.P. (1959). Production of the nephrotic syndrome in rats by Freund's adjuvant and rat kidney suspension. *Proceedings of The Society of Experimental Biology and Medicine*, 100, 66.

Hirano, T., Akira, S., Taga, T., and Kishimoto, T. (1990). Biological and clinical aspects of interleukin 6. *Immunology Today*, 11, 443–9.

Holdsworth, S.R. (1983). Fc dependence of macrophage accumulation and subsequent injury in experimental glomerulonephritis. *Journal of Immunology*, 130, 735–9.

Holdsworth, S.R. and Tipping, P.G. (1985). Macrophage-induced glomerular fibrin deposition in experimental glomerulonephritis in the rabbit. *Journal of Clinical Investigation*, 76, 1367–74.

Holdsworth, S.R., Thomson, N.M., Glasgow, E.F., and Atkins, R.C. (1979). The effect of defibrination on the participation of the macrophage in nephrotoxic nephritis. Studies using glomerular culture. *Clinical and Experimental Immunology*, 37, 38–44.

Holdsworth, S.R., Allen, D.E., Thomson, N.M., Glasgow, E.F., and Atkins, R.C. (1980a). Histochemistry of glomerular cells in animal models of crescentic glomerulonephritis. *Pathology*, 339, 346.

Holdsworth, S.R., Neale, T.J., and Wilson, C.B. (1980b). The participation of macrophages and monocytes in experimental immune complex glomerulonephritis. *Clinical Immunopathology*, 15, 510–24.

Holdsworth, S.R., Neale, T.J., and Wilson, C.B. (1981). Abrogation of macrophage dependent injury in experimental glomerulonephritis in the rabbit. Use of a specific anti-macrophage serum. *Journal of Clinical Investigation*, 68, 689–98.

Holzman, L.B. and Wiggins, R.C. (1991). Consequences of glomerular injury. Glomerular crescent formation. *Seminars in Nephrology*, 11, 346–53.

Hooke, D.H., Hancock, W.W., Gee, D.C., Kraft, N., and Atkins, R.C. (1984). Monoclonal antibody analysis of glomerular hypercellularity in human glomerulonephritis. *Clinical Nephrology*, 22, 163–8.

Horii, Y., Muraguchi, A., Iwano, M., Matsuda, T., Hirayama, T., Yamada, H. *et al.* (1989). Involvement of IL-6 in mesangial proliferative glomerulonephritis. *Journal of Immunology*, 143, 3949–55.

Huang, X.R., Holdsworth, S.R., and Tipping, P.G. (1994). Evidence for delayed type hypersensitivity mechanisms in glomerular crescent formation. *Kidney International*, 46, 69–78.

Humair, L., Kwaan, H.C., and Potter, E.V. (1969). The role of fibrinogen in renal disease. II: Effect of anticoagulants and urokinase on experimental disease in mice. *Laboratory and Clinical Medicine*, 74, 724–51.

Isaka, Y., Fujiwara, Y., Ueda, N., Kaneda, Y., Kamada, T., and Imai, E. (1993). Glomerulosclerosis induced by in vivo transfection of transforming growth factor-beta or platelet-derived growth factor gene into the rat kidney. *Journal of Clinical Investigation*, 92, 2597–601.

Iwamoto, T., Nakashima, Y., and Sueishi, K. (1990). Secretion of plasminogen activator and its inhibitor by glomerular epithelial cells. *Kidney International*, 37, 1466–76.

Jennette, J.C., Wilkman, A.S., and Falk, R.J. (1989). Anti-neutrophil cytoplasmic auto-antibody-associated glomerulonephritis and vasculitis. *American Journal of Pathology*, 135, 921–30.

Jones, C.L., Buch, S., Post, M., McCulloch, L., Liu, E., and Eddy, A.A. (1991). Pathogenesis of interstitial fibrosis in chronic purine aminonucleoside nephrosis. *Kidney International*, **40**, 1020–31.

Kagami, S., Border, W.A., Ruoslahti, E., and Noble, N.A. (1993). Coordinated expression of beta 1 integrins and transforming growth factor-beta-induced matrix proteins in glomerulonephritis *Laboratory Investigation*, **69**, 68–76.

Kant, K.S., Pollack, V.E., Dosekun, A., Glas-Greenwalt, P., Weiss, M.A., and Glueck, H.I. (1985). Lupus nephritis with thrombosis and abnormal fibrinolysis: Effect of Ancrod. *Journal of Laboratory and Clinical Medicine*, **105**, 77–8.

Kawasaki, K., Yaoita, E., Yamamoto, T., and Kihara, I. (1992). Depletion of CD8 positive cells in nephrotoxic serum nephritis of WKY rats. *Kidney International*, **41**, 1517–26.

Kawasaki, K., Yaoita, E., Yamamoto, T., Tamatani, T., Miyasaka, M., and Kihara, I. (1993). Antibodies against intercellular adhesion molecule-1 and lymphocyte function-associated antigen-1 prevent glomerular injury in rat experimental crescentic glomerulonephritis. *Journal of Immunology*, **150**, 1074–83.

Klaassen, R.J.L., Goldschmeding R., Dolman, K. *et al.* (1992). Anti-neutrophil cytoplasmic autoantibodies in patients with symptomatic HIV infection. *Clinical and Experimental Immunology*, **87**, 24–30.

Koderisch, J., Andrassy, K., and Rassmussen, N. *et al.* (1990). 'False positive' anti-neutrophil cytoplasmic antibodies in HIV infection. *Lancet*, **335**, 1227–8.

Kollias, G., Evans, D.J., Ritter, M., Beech, J., Morris, R., and Grosveld, F. (1987). Ectopic expression of Thy-1 in the kidneys of transgenic mice induces functional and proliferative abnormalities. *Cell*, **51**, 21–31.

Kondo, Y., Shigematsu, H., and Kobayashi, Y. (1972). Cellular aspects of rabbit Masugi nephritis:II. Progressive glomerular hypercellularity in crescent formation. *Laboratory Investigation*, **27**, 620–31.

Kusner, D.J., Luebbers, E.L., Nowinski, R.J., Konieczkowski, M., King, C.H., and Sedor, J.R. (1991). Cytokine- and LPS-induced synthesis of interleukin-8 from human mesangial cells. *Kidney International*, **39**, 1240–8.

Lai, K.N. and Lockwood, C.M. (1991). The effect of anti-neutrophil cytoplasm autoantibodies on the signal transduction in human neutrophils. *Clinical and Experimental Immunology*, **85**, 396–401.

Lake, R.A., Morgan, A., Henderson, B., and Staines, N.A. (1985). A key role for fibronectin in the sequential binding of native dsDNA and monoclonal anti-DNA antibodies to components of the extracellular matrix: its possible significance in glomerulonephritis. *Immunology*, **54**, 389–95.

Lerner, R.A., Glassock, R.J., and Dixon, F.J. (1967). The role of anti-glomerular basement membrane antibody in the pathogenesis of human glomerulonephritis. *Journal of Experimental Medicine*, **126**, 989–1004.

Lhotta, K., Neumayer, H.P., Joannidis, M., Geissler, D., and Konig, P. (1991). Renal expression of intercellular adhesion molecule-1 in different forms of glomerulonephritis. *Clinical Science*, **81**, 477–81.

Li, P.K., Burns, A.P., So, A.K., Pusey, C.D., Feehally, J., and Rees, A.J. (1991). The DQw7 allele at the HLA-DQB locus is associated with susceptibility to IgA nephropathy in Caucasians. *Kidney International*, **39**, 961–5.

MacKay, K., Striker, L.J., Pinkert, C.A., Brinster, R.L., and Striker, G.E. (1987). Glomerulosclerosis and renal cysts in mice transgenic for the early region of SV40. *Kidney International*, **32**, 827–37.

Magil, A. (1985). Histogenesis of glomerular crescents. Immunohistochemical demonstration of cytokeratin in crescent cells. *American Journal of Pathology*, **120**, 222–9.

Magil, A.B. and Wadsworth, L.D. (1981). Monocytes in human glomerulonephritis. An electronmicroscopic study. *Laboratory Investigation*, **45**, 77–81.

Magil, A.B. and Wadsworth, L.D. (1982). Monocyte involvement in glomerular crescents. A histochemical and ultrastructural study. *Laboratory Investigation*, **45**, 160–6.

Malliaros, J., Holdsworth, S.R., Wojta, J., Erlich, J., and Tipping, P.G. (1993). Glomerular fibrinolytic activity in anti-GBM glomerulonephritis in rabbits. *Kidney International*, **44**, 557–64.

Mathieson, P.W., Lockwood, C.M., and Oliveira, D.B. (1992). T and B cell responses to neutrophil cytoplasmic antigens in systemic vasculitis. *Clinical Immunology and Immunopathology*, **63**, 135–41.

Matri, H., Lee, L., Kashgarian, M., and Lovett, D.H. (1994). Transforming growth factor-beta modulates the expression of collagenase and metalloproteinase inhibitor. *American Journal of Pathology*, **144**, 82–94.

Mulligan, M.S., Johnson, K.J., Todd, R.F., Issekutz, T.B., Miyasaka, M., Tamatani, T. *et al.* (1993). Requirement for leukocyte adhesion molecules in nephrotoxic nephritis. *Journal of Clinical Investigation*, **91**, 577–87.

Naish, P.F., Evans, D.J., and Peters, DK. (1975). The effects of defibrination with Ancrod in experimental allergic glomerular injury. *Clinical and Experimental Immunology*, **20**, 303–9.

Nakamura, T., Miller, D., Ruoslahti, E., and Border, W.A. (1992). Production of extracellular matrix by glomerular epithelial cells is regulated by transforming growth factor-beta 1. *Kidney International*, **41**, 1213–21.

Neale, T.J., Tipping, P.G., Carson, S.D., and Holdsworth, S.R. (1988). Participation of cell mediated immunity in deposition of fibrin in glomerulonephritis. *Lancet*, **ii**, 421–4.

Nishikawa, K., Guo, Y.J., Miyasaka, M., Tamatani, T., Collins, A.B., Sy, M.S. *et al.* (1993). Antibodies to intercellular adhesion molecule 1/lymphocyte function-associated antigen 1 prevent crescent formation in rat autoimmune glomerulonephritis. *Journal of Experimental Medicine*, **177**, 667–77.

Nolasco, F.E., Cameron, J.S., Hartley, B., Coelho, A., Hildreth, G., and Reuben, R. (1987). Intraglomerular T cells and monocytes in nephritis: study with monoclonal antibodies. *Kidney International*, **31**, 1160–6.

Pollak, V.E., Glueck, H.E., Weiss, M.A., Lebron-Berges, A., and Miller, M.A. (1982). Defibrination with Ancrod in glomerulonephritis. Effect on clinical and histologic findings and on blood coagulation. *American Journal of Nephrology*, **2**, 195–207.

Quaife, C.J., Mathews, L.S., Pinkert, C.A., Hammer, R.E., Brinster, R.L., and Palmiter, R.D. (1989). Histopathology associated with elevated levels of growth hormone and insulin-like growth factor I in transgenic mice. *Endocrinology*, **124**, 40–8.

Rees, A.J. (1984). The HLA complex and susceptibility to glomerulonephritis. *Plasma Therapy*, **4**, 455–71.

Rees, A.J. (1994). The immunogenetics of glomerulonephritis. *Kidney International*, **45**, 377–83.

Rees, A.J., Peters, D.K., and Compston, D.A. (1978). Strong association between HLA-DRw2 and antibody-mediated Goodpasture's syndrome. *Lancet*, **1**, 966–8.

Rees, A.J., Peters, D.K., Amos, N., Welsh, K.I., and Batchelor, J.R. (1984). The influence of HLA-linked genes on the severity of anti-GBM antibody-mediated nephritis. *Kidney International*, **26**, 445–50.

Rondeau, E., Mougenot, B., Lacave, R., Peraldi, M.N., Kruithof, E.K., and Sraer, J.D. (1990). Plasminogen activator inhibitor 1 in renal fibrin deposits of human nephropathies. *Clinical Nephrology*, **33**, 55–60.

Sapin, G., Druet, E., and Druet, P. (1977). Induction of anti-glomerular basement membrane antibodies in the Brown-Norway rat by mercuric chloride. *Clinical and Experimental Immunology*, **28**, 173–9.

Savage, C., Gaskin, G., Pusey, C.D., and Pearson, J.D. (1993). Myeloperoxidase binds to vascular endothelial cells, is recognized by ANCA and can enhance complement dependent cytotoxicity. In *ANCA associated vasculitides: immunodiagnostic and pathogenetic value of antineutrophil cytoplasmic antibodies*, (ed. W.L. Gross). Plenum, London.

Savage, C.O.S. (1994). The endothelial cell:active participant or innocent bystander in primary vasculitis. *Clinical and Experimental Immunology*, **93**, 4–6.

Schiffer, M.S. and Michael, A.F. (1978). Renal cell turnover studied by Y chromosome (Y body) staining of the transplanted human kidney. *Journal of Laboratory and Clinical Medicine*, **92**, 841–8.

Scott, W.L., Francis, C.W., Knutson, D.W., and Marder, V.J. (1986). Specific identification of urinary fibrinogen, fibrinogen degradation products, and cross-linked fibrin degradation products in renal diseases and after renal allotransplantation. *Journal of Laboratory and Clinical Medicine*, **107**, 534–43.

Sedor, J.R. (1992). Cytokines and growth factors in renal injury. *Seminars in Nephrology*, **12**, 428–440.

Spencer, S.J., Burns, A., Gaskin, G., Pusey, C.D., and Rees, A.J. (1992). HLA class II specificities in vasculitis with antibodies to neutrophil cytoplasmic antigens. *Kidney International*, **41**, 1059–63.

Stachura, I., Si, L., Madan, E., and Whiteside, T. (1984*a*). Mononuclear cell subsets in human renal disease. Enumeration in tissue sections with monoclonal antibodies. *Clinical Immunology and Immunopathology*, **30**, 362–73.

Stachura, I., Si, L., and Whiteside, T.L. (1984*b*). Mononuclear-cell subsets in human idiopathic crescentic glomerulonephritis (ICGN): analysis in tissue sections with monoclonal antibodies. *Journal of Clinical Immunology*, **4**, 202–8.

Steblay, R.W. (1962). Glomerulonephritis induced in sheep by injection of heterologous glomerular basement membrane and Freund's complete adjuvant. *Journal of Experimental Medicine*, **116**, 253–72.

Steinglen, B., Thoenes, G., and Gunther, E. (1978). Genetic control of susceptibility to autologous immune complex glomerulonephritis in inbred rat strains. *Clinical and Experimental Immunology*, **33**, 88–94.

Stilmant, M.M., Bolton, K.W., Sturgill, B.C., Schmidt, G.W., and Couser, W.G. (1979). Crescentic glomerulonephritis without immune deposits. Clinicopathological features. *Kidney International*, **15**, 184–95.

Striker, G.E., Mannik, M., and Tung, M.Y. (1979). Role of marrow derived monocytes and mesangial cells in removal of immune complexes from renal glomeruli. *Journal of Experimental Medicine*, **149**, 127–36.

Striker, L.J., Killen, P.D., Chi, E., and Striker, G.E. (1984) The composition of glomerulosclerosis. *Laboratory Investigation*, **51**, 181–92.

Suematsu, S., Matsuda, T., Aozasa, K., Akira, S., Nakano, N., Ohno, S. *et al.* (1989). IgG1 plasmacytosis in interleukin 6 transgenic mice. *Proceedings of the National Academy of Science USA*, **86**, 7547–51.

Tam, F.W.K. and Pusey, C.D. (1995). The role of T lymphocytes in extracapillary glomerulonephritis. *J Nephrol*, **8**, 305–16

Thompson, N.M., Simpson, I.J., and Peters, D.K. (1975*a*). A quantitative evaluation of anticoagulants in experimental nephrotoxic nephritis. *Clinical and Experimental Immunology*, **19**, 301–8.

Thomson, N.M., Simpson, I.J., Evans, D.S., and Peters, D.K. (1975*b*). Defibrination with ancrod in experimental chronic immune-complex nephritis. *Clinical and Experimental Immunology*, **20**, 527–35.

Tipping, P.G. and Holdsworth, S.R. (1986). The participation of macrophages, glomerular procoagulant activity, and factor VIII in glomerular fibrin deposition. Studies on anti-GBM antibody-induced glomerulonephritis in rabbits. *American Journal of Pathology*, **124**, 10–17.

Tipping, P.G., Thomson, N.M., and Holdsworth, S.R. (1986). A comparison of fibrinolytic and defibrinating agents in established experimental glomerulonephritis. *British Journal of Experimental Pathology*, **67**, 48–91.

Tipping, P.G., Dowling, J.P., and Holdsworth, S.R. (1988*a*). Glomerular procoagulant activity in human proliferative glomerulonephritis. *Journal of Clinical Investigation*, **81**, 119–25.

Tipping, P.G., Lowe, M.G., and Holdsworth, S.R. (1988*b*). Glomerular macrophages express augmented procoagulant activity in experimental fibrin-related glomerulonephritis in rabbits. *Journal of Clinical Investigation*, **82**, 1253–9.

Tipping, P.G., Boyce, N.W., and Holdsworth, S.R. (1989). Relative contributions of chemo-attractant and terminal components of complement to anti-glomerular basement membrane (GBM) glomerulonephritis. *Clinical and Experimental Immunology*, **78**, 444–8.

Tipping, P.G., Leong, T.W., and Holdsworth, S.R. (1991*a*). Tumor necrosis factor production by glomerular macrophages in anti-glomerular basement membrane glomerulonephritis in rabbits. *Laboratory Investigation*, **65**, 272–9.

Tipping, P.G., Lowe, M.G., and Holdsworth, S.R. (1991*b*). Glomerular interleukin 1 production is dependent on macrophage infiltration in anti-GBM glomerulonephritis. *Kidney International*, **39**, 103–10.

Tipping, P.G., Cornthwaite, L., and Holdsworth, S.R. (1994). Beta 2 integrin independent neutrophil recruitment and injury in anti-GBM glomerulonephritis in rabbits. *Immunology and Cell Biology*, **72**, 471–9.

Tipping, P.G., Huang, X.R., Berndt, M.C., and Holdsworth, S.R. (1994*b*). A role for P selectin in complement independent, neutrophil mediated glomerular injury. *Kidney International*, **46**, 79–88.

Tomooka, S., Border, W.A., Marshall, B.C., and Noble, N.A. (1992). Glomerular matrix accumulation is linked to inhibition of the plasmin protease system. *Kidney International*, **42**, 1462–9.

Takeuchi, A., Yoshizawa, N., Yamamoto, M., Sawasaki, Y., Oda, T., Senoo, A. *et al.* (1992). Basic fibroblast growth factor promotes proliferation of rat glomerular visceral epithelial cells in vitro. *American Journal of Pathology*, **141**, 107–16.

Turner, N., Mason, P.J., Brown, R., Fox, M., Povey, S., Rees, A. *et al.* (1992). Molecular cloning of the human Goodpasture antigen demonstrates it to be the α 3 chain of type IV collagen. *Journal of Clinical Investigation*, **89**, 592–601.

Van der Woude, F.J., Rasmussen, N., Lobatto, S., Wiik, A., Permin, H., van Es, L.A. *et al.* (1985). Autoantibodies against neutrophils and monocytes: tool for diagnosis and marker of disease activity in Wegener's granulomatosis. *Lancet*, **i**, 425–9.

West, C.D., Ruley, E.J., Forristal, J., and Davis, N.C. (1973). Mechanisms of hypocomplementemia in glomerulonephritis. *Kidney International*, **3**, 116–25.

Wheeler, J., Robertson, H., Morley, A.R., and Appleton, D.R. (1993). Anti-glomerular basement membrane glomerulonephritis (anti-GBM GN) in the mouse: BrdU-labelling indices and histological damage. *International Journal of Experimental Pathology*, **74**, 9–19.

Wilson, C.B. (1979). Immune reactions with antigens in or of the glomerulus. In *Immunopathology*, (ed. F. Migrom and B. Albini), pp. 126–31. Basel, Karger.

Wilson, C.B. (1991). The renal response to immunologic injury. In *The kidney*, (ed. B.M. Brenner and F.C. Rector), pp. 1062–181. Philadelphia, Saunders.

Wuthrich, R.P., Jevnikar, A.M., Takei, F., Glimcher, L.H., and Kelley, V.E. (1990). Intercellular adhesion molecule-1 (ICAM-1) expression is upregulated in autommune murine lupus nephritis. *American Journal of Pathology*, **136**, 441–50.

Wuthrich, R.P. (1992). Intercellular adhesion molecules and vascular cell adhesion molecule-1 and the kidney [editorial]. *Journal of the American Society of Nephrology*, **3**, 1201–11.

Yamamoto, T. and Wilson, C.B. (1987). Binding of anti-basement membrane antibody to alveolar basement membrane after intratracheal gasoline instillation in rabbits. *American Journal of Pathology*, **126**, 497–505.

Yamamoto, T., Nakamura, T., Noble, N.A., Ruoslahti, E., and Border, W.A. (1993). Expression of transforming growth factor beta is elevated in human and experimental diabetic nephropathy. *Proceedings of the National Academy of Science USA*, **90**, 1814–18.

Yamamoto, T., Noble, A., Miller, D.E., and Border, W.A. (1994). Sustained expression of TGFβ1 underlies development of progressive kidney fibrosis. *Kidney International*, **45**, 916–27.

Yambe, H., Yoshikawa, S., and Ohsawa, H. *et al.* (1993). Tissue factor production by cultured rat glomerular epithelial cells. *Nephrology Dialysis Transplantation*, **8**, 519–23.

Yoshioka, K, Takemura, T., Musahami, K., Okada, M., Hino, S., Miyamoto, H., and Maki, S. (1993). Transforming growth factor-beta protein and mRNA in glomeruli in normal and diseased human kidneys. *Laboratory Investigation*, **68**, 154–63.

Zoja, C., Corna, D., Macconi, D., Zilio, P., Bertani, T., and Remuzzi, G. (1990). Tissue plasminogen activator therapy of rabbit nephrotoxic nephritis. *Laboratory Investigation*, **62**, 34–40.

Zoja, C., Wang, J.M., Bettoni, S., Sironi, M., Renzi, D., Chiaffarino, F. *et al.* (1991). Interleukin-1 beta and tumor necrosis factor-alpha induce gene expression and production of leukocyte chemotactic factors, colony-stimulating factors, and interleukin-6 in human mesangial cells. *American Journal of Pathology*, **138**, 991–1003.

3

Rapidly progressive glomerulonephritis: resolution and scarring

Roger C. Wiggins

Scarring takes place in glomeruli and interstitium in patients with the clinical syndrome of rapidly progressive glomerulonephritis (RPGN). The extent of scarring determines outcome, and depends on the balance of pro-and anti-sclerotic forces at particular sites and at particular times during the inflammatory event. In this chapter, two factors affecting this balance will be emphasized: (1) the importance of maintenance of the normal architecture of the kidney (the barrier hypothesis); and (2) the identification of collagen-producing cells in the interstitial compartment and the communication between inflamed glomeruli and these interstitial cells (glomerulointerstitial signals).

Scarring in the interstitial compartment is the best indicator of outcome in many forms of progressive renal disease, even when the primary injury appears to be in the glomerulus (Risdon *et al.* 1966; Schainuck *et al.* 1970; Bohle *et al.* 1979; Wehrmann *et al.* 1989). Interstitial inflammation and scarring are also an important component of crescentic nephritis. Therefore, any model of progression and scarring must take into account the relationship between the glomerulus and interstitial compartments. Based upon experimental work and previous reports from other investigators (Silva *et al.* 1984; Southwest Pediatric Nephrology Study Group, SPNSG 1985; Striker *et al.* 1984; Boucher *et al.* 1987), a model will be suggested that provides a framework for the analysis of the scarring process in the kidney.

The stages of glomerular inflammation in RPGN (the barrier hypothesis)

The stages passed through by a glomerulus en route to sclerosis in crescentic nephritis have previously been described (Holzman and Wiggins 1991). The importance of the integrity of Bowman's capsule in determining outcome has also been emphasized (Silva *et al.* 1984; Striker *et al.* 1984; SPNSG 1985; Boucher *et al.* 1987). There are therefore two barriers that must be breached for major glomerular inflammation to escape into the interstitial compartment (Fig. 3.1). These barriers are the glomerular capillary wall (barrier I) and Bowman's capsule (barrier II). According to whether one or both barriers are breached, and

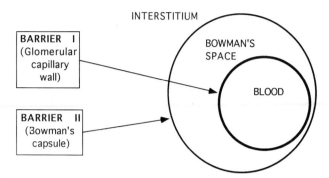

Fig. 3.1 Diagrammatic illustration of the two major barriers to movement of mediators and cells between glomerulus and interstitium. Barrier I is the glomerular capillary wall defended by endothelial cells on its inner aspect and by visceral glomerular epithelial cells (podocytes) on its outer aspect. Barrier II is Bowman's capsule defended by parietal glomerular epithelial cells on its inner aspect.

whether the holes allow mediators or cells to pass through, glomerular inflammation can be conveniently subdivided as is illustrated diagrammatically in Fig. 3.2. Three major stages can be defined:

Stage 1. Glomerular inflammatory cells (platelets, neutrophils, monocytes, T cells) remain within the capillary lumen. No crescent is formed and substantial recovery of normal structure and function occurs. Poststreptococcal glomerulonephritis would be a typical example (Fig. 3.2B).

Stage 2. The glomerular capillary wall is breached allowing blood components to leak into Bowman's space. A proteinaceous clot (containing fibrin) forms and occupies Bowman's space (Fig. 3.2C). Cells accumulate in Bowman's space from the blood compartment (macrophages) or divide *de novo* (epithelial cells) in response to growth factors produced by macrophages in Bowman's space. These accumulating cells occupy and may fill Bowman's space, having the two-dimensional appearance of a crescent (Fig. 3.2D). The 'cellular crescent' may interfere with glomerular function but it is still a potentially reversible lesion. This sequence of events is seen in antineutrophil cytoplasmic antibody (ANCA)-associated vasculitis and other conditions causing crescent formation.

Stage 3. Bowman's capsule is breached, allowing inflammatory mediators including cytokines and lipid factors, to leak directly out of the glomerulus through holes in Bowman's capsule (Fig. 3.2E) and activate cells in the interstitial compartment. Chemotactic factors attract cells to accumulate in the periglomerular region and, if the holes in Bowman's capsule are large enough, to migrate into the glomerulus through these holes (Fig. 3.2F and Fig. 3.3). These cells can include macrophages, T cells and fibroblasts (Silva *et al.* 1984; SPNSG 1985; Striker *et al.* 1984; Boucher *et al.* 1987; Holzman and Wiggins 1991; Downer

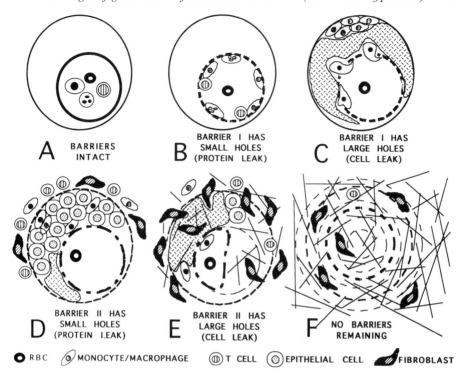

A   BARRIERS INTACT

B   BARRIER I HAS SMALL HOLES (PROTEIN LEAK)

C   BARRIER I HAS LARGE HOLES (CELL LEAK)

D   BARRIER II HAS SMALL HOLES (PROTEIN LEAK)

E   BARRIER II HAS LARGE HOLES (CELL LEAK)

F   NO BARRIERS REMAINING

● RBC   ⊘ MONOCYTE/MACROPHAGE   ⦷ T CELL   ⊚ EPITHELIAL CELL   ◤ FIBROBLAST

Fig. 3.2 Diagrammatic illustration of the stages of progression of glomerular inflammation. (A) A normal glomerulus with blood cells coursing through the glomerular capillary not in contact with the wall, and no holes present in either barrier I or II. (B) Inflammation of the glomerular capillary wall provoked, for example, by immune complexes deposited on the filter wall. Inflammatory cells accumulate, cytokines are released, adhesion proteins are expressed, cells adhere and become activated. They release proteases and oxidants resulting in damage to the glomerular filter so that protein and some red cells leak into Bowman's space. (C) Inflammatory cell-induced injury to the glomerular capillary wall has resulted in monocyte accumulation, conversion of monocytes to macrophages under the influence of activated T cells, migration of macrophages out of the capillaries into Bowman's space where they may form small cellular 'crescents' and where they produce procoagulant molecules that trigger the accumulation of a proteinaceous clot (cast) containing fibrin and fibronectin within Bowman's space. (D) Activated macrophages within Bowman's space release growth factors causing glomerular epithelial cells to divide and accumulate in Bowman's space. Cell division may be facilitated by the fibrin/fibronectin matrix in Bowman's space. At the same time, small holes appear in Bowman's capsule, allowing mediators to leak out into the periglomerular interstitium. These mediators attract and activate periglomerular cells. (E) As a consequence of communication between activated cells on both sides of Bowman's capsule, larger holes are formed and cells move in and out of the glomerulus through these holes. Fibroblasts become activated, move into the glomerulus, and begin to lay down interstitial collagen. (F) Collagen accumulates in and around the glomerulus leading to permanent obliteration of glomerular structures. (From Atkins *et al.* 1976; Cattell and Jamieson 1978; Lan *et al.* 1992.)

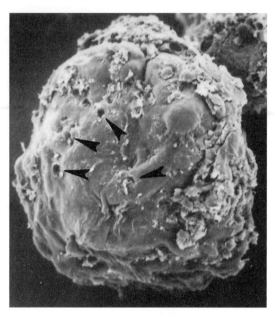

Fig. 3.3 Scanning electron micrograph of an isolated rabbit glomerulus with Bowman's capsule in place from an animal with anti-GBM disease (day 7) showing holes in Bowman's capsule (arrowheads) through which mediators and cells could move between the glomerulus and interstitial compartments.

et al. 1988; Merritt *et al.* 1990; Wiggins *et al.* 1993). Fibroblast-like cells lay down the interstitial collagens which constitute the fibrous scar, which ultimately seals the fate of that glomerulus. Anti-GBM disease probably results in glomerular scarring by this mechanism.

According to the barrier hypothesis, barriers may become leaky to mediators (small holes) and cells (large holes). Outcome is largely dependent on the barrier breached, the size and number of the holes, and the proportion of glomeruli affected. These factors reflect the severity of the inflammatory insult. Furthermore, in an individual, the clinical syndrome will depend on whether all glomeruli are at the same stage of crescent formation (synchronous), or whether they are at many different stages (asynchronous) as is illustrated in Fig. 3.4.

A crescent can also be considered as a granuloma-like reaction to an inflammatory stimulus. Like a granuloma, the formation of a crescent involves the production of growth and chemotactic factors leading to cell division and concentric cell accumulation, and subsequently to scarring. The role of T cells and macrophages in driving this process and the inflammatory mechanisms involved are discussed in detail in Chapter 2. Crescent formation with or without subsequent scarring of the glomerulus may function as a protective mechanism which prevents loss of large amounts of blood and protein into the urine from the very large inflamed glomerular surface area.

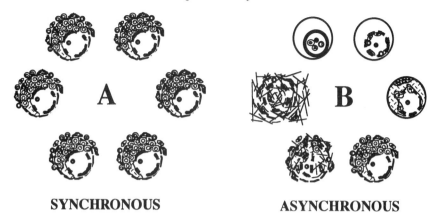

SYNCHRONOUS   **ASYNCHRONOUS**

Fig. 3.4 Diagrammatic illustration of patterns of glomerular involvement. Glomeruli may all be at the same stage of crescent formation (synchronous) (A), or they may be at different stages of crescent formation (asynchronous) (B). Synchronous disease often presents early and, if recognized and treated rapidly, may be susceptible to therapy. Asynchronous disease may present late.

The prosclerotic forces

An accelerated model of anti-GBM disease in the rabbit has been used to analyse the prosclerotic events in a model of crescentic nephritis. This model, like human anti-GBM disease, develops progressive scarring in the glomerulus and interstitium. The time course of events in the model have been extensively characterized with respect to cell dynamics, functional changes, the coagulation system, fibronectin metabolism and collagen synthesis (Wiggins *et al.* 1985, 1993; Downer *et al..* 1988; Merritt *et al.* 1990; McClurkin *et al.* 1990; Eldredge *et al.* 1991). Some points relevant to the scarring process in crescentic nephritis in man will be emphasized.

The time course of collagen synthesis and accumulation is rapid

Figure 3.5 shows that collagen synthesis (steady state $\alpha 1(I)$ procollagen mRNA levels and measured collagen synthetic rate) is increased by day 4 of the model before serum creatinine has begun to rise (Holzman and Wiggins 1991). By the time serum creatinine is increased at day 7, collagen synthetic rate is maximal and hydroxyproline is beginning to accumulate. Hydroxyproline continues to accumulate over the subsequent 7 days. Masson trichrome-stainable collagen is delayed behind hydroxyproline accumulation. The time between reduction in GFR and significant scarring detectable histologically by Masson trichrome is about 14 days. In spite of continued progression of scarring, the serum creatinine falls as oedema and inflammation decrease in the renal cortex.

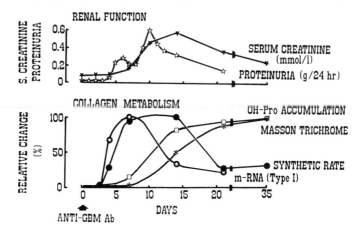

Fig. 3.5 Data from rabbit model of anti-GBM disease showing the relationship between renal function and collagen metabolism. Note that collagen synthesis (mRNA levels and collagen synthetic rate) is increased before the serum creatinine has begun to rise, and is maximal within 7 days of the first rise of serum creatinine. Hydroxyproline accumulation and detection of Masson trichrome-stainable cross-linked matrix follows within 7 days of the increased collagen synthetic rate. Thus, the time between the increased serum creatinine and accumulated matrix is about 14 days. This model is synchronous and therefore indicates a time frame for a single glomerulus which may not reflect the time frame for all glomeruli in a population. The time frame for human glomeruli is likely to be similar. The conclusion from this type of analysis is that the time course of crescent formation and scarring is similar to that of wound healing (i.e. it is rapid, taking 10–14 days).

Collagen synthesis is extraglomerular when inflammation is intraglomerular at early time points

In the anti-GBM model we measured steady state relative α1(I) procollagen mRNA synthesis in isolated glomeruli and in whole renal cortex during progression of crescent formation. We found that although inflammation was intraglomerular by day 4 of the model, collagen synthesis was predominantly extraglomerular (increased in whole renal cortex but not in isolated glomeruli) at this time (Fig. 3.6) (Merritt *et al.* 1990). Therefore, we concluded that factor(s) were being produced within glomeruli that were driving collagen synthesis by unidentified cells in the extraglomerular renal cortex (glomerulointerstitial signals). We set out to identify the target cells and the mediator(s) involved.

Identification of cells responsible for producing interstitial collagen in the renal cortex

To identify type I (interstitial) collagen producing cells in the renal cortex, we elected to use *in situ* hybridization (Wiggins *et al.* 1993). The 3′ end of rabbit α2(I) procollagen was cloned using a PCR approach from reverse transcribed

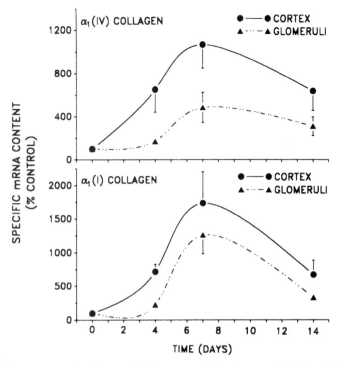

Fig. 3.6 Time course of collagen mRNA accumulation in a model of anti-GBM disease in the rabbit. By day 4 when renal cortical collagen mRNAs were increased, glomerular collagen mRNAs were not significantly different from normal. At this time increased inflammatory cells were present in glomeruli, but not in the interstitium. Therefore, signals must be passing from inflamed glomeruli to cells in the interstitial compartment at this time. Inflammatory cells also accumulate in the periglomerular region (probably in response to mediators leaking through holes in Bowman's capsule) and at later times throughout the interstitium.

RNA purified from a rabbit with anti-GBM disease. Following subcloning into Bluescript vector, sense and antisense riboprobe templates were prepared. The antisense probe hybridized with day 7 rabbit RNA but not with control rabbit renal cortical RNA on Northern blot (Fig. 3.7). Similarly, the antisense probe hybridized with day 7 renal cortex, whereas the sense probe did not (Fig. 3.8).

When we analysed the time course of $\alpha2(I)$ procollagen *in situ* hybridization, we found that the earliest hybridization (day 4) occurred to cells in the perivascular cuff of adventitial tissue surrounding arteries and veins (Figs 3.9A, B). At day 14, widespread hybridization to cells in the periglomerular and interstitial compartments was present (Fig. 3.10). Some glomeruli contained cells that were positive for $\alpha2(I)$ procollagen mRNA, particularly in the fibrin-containing matrix in Bowman's space. At this time point in the model we have previously shown that Bowman's capsule is disrupted (Eldredge *et al.* 1991; and Fig. 3.3); therefore these cells could have gained access to glomeruli from the interstitial compartment. By

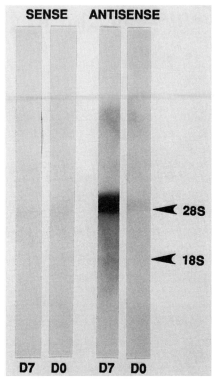

Fig. 3.7 Northern blot of RNA from renal cortex of control and day 7 rabbits with anti-GBM disease hybridized with [^{32}P]-sense and [^{32}P]-antisense α2(I) procollagen ribo-probes. Note that the antisense probe did not detect a signal in normal renal cortex, indicating the low level of synthesis of type I collagen present under normal conditions. In contrast, at day 7 a very intense signal corresponding to the expected size of the α2(I) procollagen transcript was detected. No hybridization with the sense probe was detected at either time point. We conclude that α2(I) procollagen synthesis increases from a very low baseline to high levels in renal cortex during anti-GBM disease in the rabbit, and that the probes and conditions used should allow specific *in situ* hybridization.

days 10–14 many cells in the glomeruli as well as in the periglomerular and interstitial compartments hybridized with the α2(I) procollagen riboprobe. These conclusions were substantiated by quantitation of silver grains under conditions where sections from different time points were mounted on the same slide to allow direct comparisons (Wiggins *et al.* 1993). The potential importance of holes in Bowman's capsule and the relationship between these holes and the appearance of interstitial collagens within Bowman's space has previously been emphasized (Wehrmann *et al.* 1989; Silva *et al.* 1984; SPNSG 1985; Striker *et al.* 1984; Boucher *et al.* 1987; Eldredge *et al.* 1991; Lan *et al.* 1992).

We conclude from this analysis that the earliest cells to begin to make collagen in response to glomerular inflammation are the fibroblast-like cells in the

Antisense   Sense

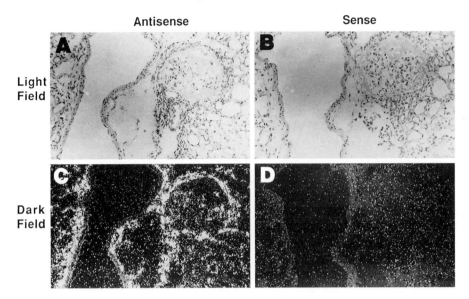

Fig. 3.8 *In situ* hybridization using sections of day 7 renal cortex hybridized with [^{35}S]-sense and [^{35}S]-antisense probes and detected by autoradiography. Adjacent sections were used as shown in the upper panels stained with H & E. Background silver grains are seen in the dark-field photomicrographs of the sense probe (D). In contrast, intense clumps of silver grains are seen around vessels and glomeruli with the antisense probe (C). These results were quantitated by grain-counting (Wiggins *et al.* 1993). This result confirms the specificity of the *in situ* hybridization.

perivascular adventitium (Wiggins *et al.* 1993). We have called these cells vascular adventitial cells (VACs). This result is not surprising, since type I collagen is normally present in this compartment (perivascular 'cuff') of the kidney. In fact, this is the only site at which type I collagen is present in the normal renal cortex with the exception of the capsule. These type I collagen-producing cells (VACs) normally accompany the vasculature down to the level of the arteriole and venule as it arborizes into and out of the renal cortex. These cells are therefore well placed to participate in scarring processes in the renal cortex wherever it occurs.

We speculate that during inflammatory renal injury, VACs migrate out of their perivascular 'hotel' in response to chemotactic signals from the glomerulus. We further speculate that under normal conditions, VACs might leave their home site and patrol the interstitial compartment. Thus, we could look on this population as a defence system that could be activated to divide, chemotax, and produce interstitial matrix under the influence of signals produced from any site in the cortex. We also suggest that similar systems exist in other organs, such as liver and lung, where VACs may also play a key role in the scarring process.

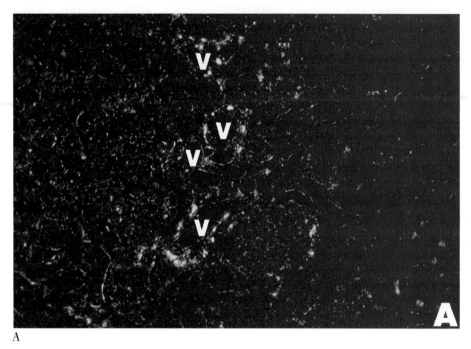

A

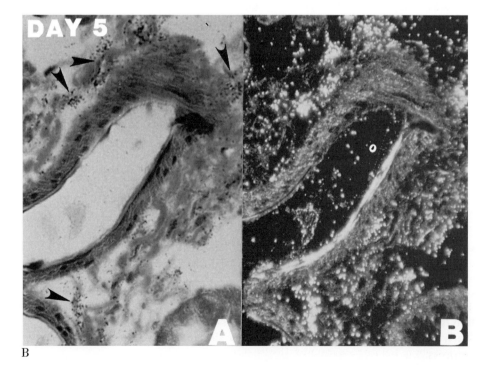

B

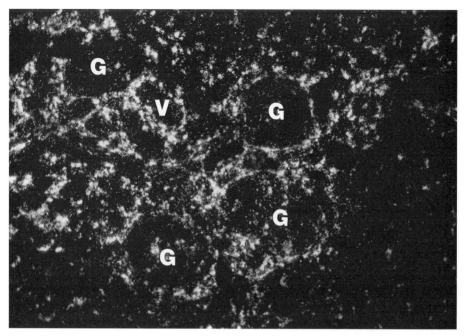

Fig. 3.10 Photomicrograph of *in situ* hybridization (dark field ×100) from a day 14 animal (α2(I) procollagen antisense riboprobe). Silver grains are present in the periglomerular and perivascular regions as well as more diffusely throughout the interstitium and within Bowman's space of some glomeruli. At lower right is the medulla which is demarcated by the absence of α2(I) procollagen-producing cells (V, vessel; G, glomerulus).

Mediators driving collagen synthesis

We have looked for factors produced by inflamed glomeruli and renal cortex that drive cultured cells to produce collagen. The major factor identified was transforming growth factor-β (TGFβ) (Coimbra *et al.* 1991). This cytokine was shown to be released by normal isolated glomeruli, but in the latent form. Inflamed glomeruli and renal cortex produce more TGFβ, and the TGFβ that is

---

Fig. 3.9 (A) Dark-field photomicrograph (×100) showing silver grain distribution from a section of renal cortex from a day 5 animal hybridized using the α2(I) procollagen riboprobe. Clumps of silver grains are limited to cells in the perivascular regions. There are single background silver grains throughout the section and streaks of non-specific silver staining of basement membranes (V, vessel). (B) The photomicrographs (×400) from a day 5 animal show part of an artery photographed under light field (left panel) or dark field (right panel). The silver grains overlying cells in the perivascular cuff of the vessel are clearly seen (arrowheads). Thus, at early time points the cells producing α2(I) procollagen are in the perivascular area. (From Wiggins *et al.* 1993.)

produced is in the active form. Our results support the conclusion that TGFβ may play an important role in driving collagen synthesis in this model, as has been emphasized in another model by Border and colleagues (1990).

Chemotaxin(s) for fibroblasts produced by glomeruli

We looked for factors produced by inflamed glomeruli which would be chemotactic for fibroblasts. The major chemotaxins identified in preliminary experiments are fibronectin fragments (Phan *et al.* 1992). Fibronectin accumulates in glomeruli from plasma early during glomerular injury in the model (Goyal and Wiggins 1991). As the cellular crescent begins to form in glomeruli, fibronectin is synthesized by cells within the crescent. The fibronectin released by isolated glomeruli at this time is largely fragmented (80%), indicating that fibronectin is rapidly turning over during this time (Goyal and Wiggins 1991). These data support the concept that fibronectin may play an important chemotactic role for fibroblasts in the model, attracting these cells into glomeruli where they participate in the glomerular scarring process. Fibronectin fragments have been previously shown to be chemotactic for fibroblasts (Postlethwaite 1981).

Pathways for glomerulointerstitial signals

There are several possible pathways by which signals could pass from the glomerulus to cells in the interstitial compartment, and the signalling system could sequentially use more than one product. These pathways include: (1) passage with the glomerular filtrate down the proximal tubule to be reabsorbed, possibly modified within the tubules, as has been suggested by Thomas and Schreiner (1993), and then to gain access to interstitial cells; (2) passage out of the glomerulus via the efferent arteriole and then to contact endothelium, cross the peritubular capillary walls, and gain access to interstitial cells; (3) movement out of the glomerulus in lymph which flows through the glomerular stalk and thence to interstitial cells; (4) leakage through Bowman's capsule directly via holes caused by macrophage, T cell (Lan *et al.* 1992), or fibroblast products which damage parietal epithelial cells and the basement membrane of Bowman's capsule. Each of these pathways may be relevant under particular conditions. Given the frequently seen accumulation of cells in the immediate periglomerular region, the commonly seen periglomerular scarring, and the fact that holes can be directly seen in Bowman's capsule (See Fig. 3.3), we favour the 'holes' hypothesis as an important pathway by which mediators gain direct access to the interstitial compartment. This pathway could also account for pathophysiological features of the nephritic syndrome seen in acute glomerulonephritis (salt and water retention).

Overview of the prosclerotic pathways (glomerulointerstitial signals)

Figure 3.11 shows in diagrammatic form the series of interactions we suggest plays a role in the scarring process during severe glomerular inflammation. We

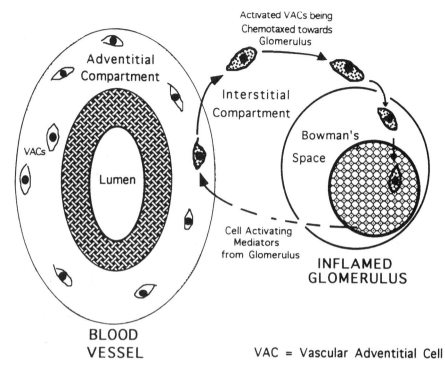

Fig. 3.11 Diagrammatic illustration of a proposed sequence of events whereby signals pass directly from the glomerulus through holes in Bowman's capsule to activate periglomerular fibroblast-like cells (VACs). In response to these signals, VACs migrate into the interstitial space, divide, and move towards the glomerulus. They accumulate in the periglomerular region where they lay down collagen to cause periglomerular scarring. If large holes are present in Bowman's capsule, these cells gain access to Bowman's space and the glomerulus where they lay down collagen to cause permanent scarring (fibrotic crescents) and loss of that glomerulus (glomerulosclerosis). Our data support the hypotheses that TGFβ is an important mediator promoting collagen synthesis and that fibronectin fragments are important chemotaxins for fibroblasts.

suggest that the perivascular compartment of the renal cortex, and the vascular adventitial cells in particular, may be important players in the scarring process. Further studies are required to understand how this cell type is regulated under normal conditions and to devise methods to modify its behaviour.

Antisclerotic forces

Very few data are available on this topic. In a general sense, prostaglandin E_2 (PGE$_2$) produced within the renal cortex would be expected to maintain fibroblasts and other inflammatory cells in a down-regulated state. Inhibition of PGE$_2$ production would be expected to result in amplification of prosclerotic forces. Whether this is an important factor remains to be determined.

Collagenolytic metalloproteinase enzymes and their inhibition by TIMPs (tissue inhibitors of metalloproteinase) probably play an important role in removing collagen, particularly at early stages of synthesis prior to cross-linking. The importance of the balance between collagenases and TIMPs at various stages of crescent formation *in vivo* has yet to be defined.

Strategies for the future

Crescentic nephritis leading to end-stage renal disease is probably more common than is currently recognized. As has been emphasized, previously conventional therapies are effective in most cases of rapidly progressive glomerulonephritis, *provided they are used in time* (Holzman and Wiggins 1991). Therefore, the single most important aspect of management of these patients is timely diagnosis and therapeutic intervention. The front-line physician must be trained to recognize the condition and refer the patient to the nephrologist early. The nephrologist must confirm the diagnosis immediately by renal biopsy, and start treatment urgently. Strategies that buy time by slowing up the fibrotic process (e.g. by the use of glucocorticoids or colchicine) or increasing collagenolysis may prove to be useful adjuncts to other forms of therapy. Meanwhile we need to understand better where and how collagens are made in the kidney and how the cells that produce them are regulated, so that we can learn how to swing the balance from pro-to anti-sclerosis in our patients with rapidly progressive glomerulonephritis and other forms of inflammatory renal disease.

References

Atkins, R.C., Holdsworth, S.R., Glasgow, E.F., and Matthews, F.E. (1976). The macrophage in human rapidly progressive glomerulonephritis. *Lancet*, **1**, 830.

Bohle, A., Christ, H., Grund, K.E., and Mackensen, S. (1979). The role of the interstitium of the renal cortex in renal disease. *Contributions to Nephrology*, **16**, 109–14.

Border, W.A., Okuda, S., Languino, L.R., Sporn, M.B., and Rouslahti, E. (1990). Suppression of experimental glomerulonephritis by antiserum against TGF-β1. *Nature*, **346**, 371–4.

Boucher, A., Droz, D., Adafer, E., and Noel, L.H. (1987). Relationship between the integrity of Bowman's capsule and the composition of cellular crescents in human crescentic nephritis. *Laboratory Investigation*, **56**, 526–33.

Cattell, V. and Jamieson, S.W. (1978). The origin of glomerular crescents in experimental nephrotoxic serum nephritis in the rabbit. *Laboratory Investigation*, **39**, 584–90.

Coimbra, T., Wiggins, R., Noh, J.W., Merritt, S., and Phan, S.H. (1991). Transforming growth factor-β production in anti-glomerular basement membrane disease in the rabbit. *American Journal of Pathology*, **138**, 223–4.

Downer, G., Phan, S.H., and Wiggins, R.C. (1988). Analysis of renal fibrosis in rabbit model of crescentic nephritis. *Journal of Clinical Investigation*, **82**, 998–1006.

Eldredge, C., Merritt, S., Goyal, M., Kulaga, H., Kindt, T.J., and Wiggins, R. (1991). Analysis of T cells and MHC class I and class II mRNA and protein content and distribution in anti-GBM disease in the rabbit. *American Journal of Pathology*, **139**, 1021–35.

Goyal, M. and Wiggins R. (1991). Fibronectin mRNA and protein accumulation and breakdown in rabbit anti-glomerular basement membrane disease. *Journal of the American Society of Nephrology*, **1**, 1334–42.

Holzman, L.B., and Wiggins, R.C. (1991). Glomerular crescent formation. *Seminars in Nephrology*, **11**, 346–53.

Lan, H.Y., Nikolic-Paterson, J., and Atkins, R.C. (1992). Involvement of activated periglomerular leukocytes in the rupture of Bowman's capsule and glomerular crescent progression in experimental glomerulonephritis. *Laboratory Investigation*, **67**, 743–51.

McClurkin, C., Phan, S.H., Hsu, C.H., Patel, S.R., Spicker, J.K., Kshirsagar, A.M. *et al.* (1990). Moderate protection of renal function and reduction of fibrosis by colchicine in a model of anti-GBM disease in the rabbit. *Journal of the American Society of Nephrology*, **1**, 257–65.

Merritt, S.E., Killen, P.D., Phan, S.H., and Wiggins, R.C. (1990). Analysis of α1(I) procollagen, α1(IV) collagen, and β-actin mRNA in glomerulus and cortex of rabbits with experimental anti-glomerular basement membrane disease: Evidence for early extraglomerular collagen biosynthesis. *Laboratory Investigation*, **63**, 762–8.

Phan, S.H., Wolber, F., and Wiggins, R. (1992). Fibronectin is the major fibroblast chemotactin in crescentic nephritis. *Journal of the American Society of Nephrology*, **3**, 610 abstract.

Postlethwaite, A.E., Keski-Oja, J., Balian, G., and Kang, A.H. (1981). Induction of fibroblast chemotaxis by fibronectin. Localization of the chemotactic region to a 140 000-molecular weight non-gelatin-binding fragment. *Journal of Experimental Medicine*, **153**, 494–9.

Risdon, R.A., Sloper, J.C., and DeWardener, H.E. (1966). Relationship between renal function and histological changes found in renal biopsy specimens from patients with persistent glomerular nephritis. *Lancet*, **ii**, 363–6.

Schainuck, L.I., Striker, G.E., Luther, R.E., and Benditt, E.P. (1970). Structural-functional correlations in renal disease: II. The correlations. *Human Pathology*, **1**, 631–41.

Silva, F.G., Hoyer, J.R., and Pirani, C.L. (1984). Sequential studies of glomerular crescent formation in rats with antiglomerular basement membrane-induced glomerulonephritis and the role of coagulation factors. *Laboratory Investigation*, **51**, 404–15.

SPNSG (Southwest Pediatric Nephrology Study Group) (1985). A clinico-pathologic study of crescentic glomerulonephritis in 50 children. A report of the Southwest Pediatric Nephrology Study Group. *Kidney International*, **27**, 450–8.

Striker, L.M.M., Killen, P.D., Chi, E., and Striker, G.E. (1984). The composition of glomerulosclerosis: I. Studies in focal sclerosis, crescentic glomerulonephritis, and membranoproliferative glomerulonephritis. *Laboratory Investigation*, **51**, 181–92.

Thomas, M., and Schreiner, G. (1993). The contribution of proteinuria to progressive renal injury; consequences of tubular uptake of fatty acid-bearing albumin. *American Journal of Nephrology*, **13**, 385–8.

Wehrmann, M., Bohle, A., Bogenschutz, O., Eissele, R., Freislederer, A., Ohlschlegel, C. *et al.* (1989). Long-term prognosis of chronic idiopathic membranous glomerulonephritis. An analysis of 334 cases with particular regard to tubulointerstitial changes. *Clinical Nephrology*, **31**, 67–76.

Wiggins, R.C., Glatfelter, A., and Brukman, J. (1985). Procoagulant activity in glomeruli and urine of rabbits with nephrotoxic nephritis. *Laboratory Investigation*, **53**, 156–65.

Wiggins, R., Goyal, M., Merritt. S., and Killen, P.D. (1993). Vascular adventitial cell expression of collagen I messenger ribonucleic acid in anti-glomerular basement membrane antibody-induced crescentic nephritis in the rabbit. *Laboratory Investigation*, **68**, 557–65.

4

Pathology of rapidly progressive glomerulonephritis

Franco Ferrario and Maria Pia Rastaldi

Rapidly progressive glomerulonephritis (RPGN) is the name given to a syndrome characterized clinically by an acute rapid deterioration of renal function, and morphologically by widespread formation of circumferential extracapillary proliferation, generally involving more than 50% of glomeruli (Neild *et al.* 1983; Baldwin *et al.* 1987; Couser 1988). Many types of glomerulonephritis can present with crescent formation and renal failure, including both primary glomerular diseases and systemic diseases with glomerular involvement. Consequently, definition of RPGN has been difficult and the terminology and classification criteria have varied over the years, as a result of different approaches to the disease based on mainly clinical, pathological, or immunological components.

Crescents were first described by Langhans more than 100 years ago, but in 1914 Volhard and Fahr provided the classic description of 'crescentic glomerulonephritis' in autopsy specimens. They described a picture of glomerular destruction with the tuft totally surrounded by cells filling Bowman's capsule. Lölein, in 1910, preferred a clinical definition, calling this type of glomerulonephritis a 'stormy course' because of the renal failure that led to death. Ellis (1942) also approached the problem from a clinical point of view, introducing the term 'rapidly progressive glomerulonephritis', and subsequently this disease has also been called 'acute anuric' or 'acute oliguric' (Alwall *et al.* 1958; Brun *et al.* 1958; Berlyne and Baker 1964; Harrison *et al.* 1964) or 'malignant' glomerulonephritis (Hamburger 1956).

In 1948, Davson *et al.* introduced a new important morphological element. They described a group of patients with widespread crescent formation associated with fibrinoid necrosis of the glomerular tufts and systemic symptoms suggestive of vasculitis involving small arteries. The term 'necrotizing crescentic glomerulonephritis' became widely accepted, mainly to indicate primary renal vasculitis (Wegener's granulomatosis, microscopic polyarteritis), and this topic has been discussed thoroughly during the past few years (Serra *et al.* 1984; Furlong *et al.* 1987; Adu *et al.* 1987; Bindi *et al.* 1993; Jennette *et al.* 1994; Pettersson *et al.* 1995). Despite this historical background to the terminology, we think that the morphologically defined name 'crescentic glomerulonephritis' is more appropriate, in order to emphasize the histological aspect of these disorders (Heptinstall 1992).

It is now clear that 'crescents' are, in fact, a superimposed feature, found in many forms of nephritis with different pathogenetic and probably morphogenetic mechanisms, and that they are only a unifying feature in a clinically heterogeneous group of diseases. There is no agreement concerning the percentage of glomeruli that need to be involved before the term 'crescentic glomerulonephritis' can be used. It varies from 20% of glomeruli involved (Stilmant *et al.* 1979; Cohen *et al.* 1981; Heptinstall 1992), to 60% (Neild *et al.* 1983; McLeish *et al.* 1978), to more than 80% (Withworth *et al.* 1976; Morrin *et al.* 1978). In many disorders classified within the group of 'rapidly progressive glomerulonephritis', some patients present with morphological evidence of crescents in a relatively small percentage of glomeruli. It is worth emphasizing that clinical (Rees *et al.* 1977; Gill *et al.* 1977; Juncos *et al.* 1979; Fairley *et al.* 1987) and experimental (Wilson and Dixon 1986) studies have shown that glomerular inflammation can evolve very rapidly, and that an individual with crescents in 20% of glomeruli one day can have them in 80% only three days later.

Frequent discrepancies between the degree of renal failure at time of renal biopsy and the extent of extracapillary lesions have been reported in many recent studies (Ronco *et al.* 1983; Adu *et al.* 1987; Gans *et al.* 1993; Pettersson *et al.* 1995). In our experience, in a large cohort of 231 cases of primary renal vasculitis studied by the Italian Group of Renal Immunopathology, many patients with marked acute renal failure surprisingly showed only focal forms of necrotizing crescentic lesions (< 50% crescents). In contrast, some cases with only mild renal insufficiency or normal renal function showed massive and diffuse necrotizing crescentic glomerulonephritis (> 50% crescents). This suggests that morphological criteria are more appropriate than clinical parameters to define the various types of crescentic glomerulonephritis, and that renal biopsy is crucial for their diagnosis and management.

Many different classifications of crescentic or rapidly progressive glomerulonephritis were proposed during the 1970s and 1980s, based on clinical, morphological, immunohistological, and serological criteria. The classification which is still the most acceptable, because it is based on possible pathogenetic mechanisms as defined by immunohistological patterns, was proposed by Couser in 1988 (Table 4.1). This classification recognized three subgroups: (1) linear deposition of antibody along the glomerular basement membrane (GBM), an expression of anti-glomerular basement membrane disease; (2) none or scanty non-specific immune deposits, suggesting the possibility of cell-mediated mechanisms; and (3) granular immune deposits along the capillary wall, probably due to deposition of immune complexes.

Morphological features

The pathognomonic characteristic of RPGN on light microscopy is the presence of crescents within Bowman's space. It is not clear what definition should be used to differentiate between tuft adhesion, with a mild capsular reaction, and true crescents. The majority of authors require two or three layers of cells to be present when using the term 'crescentic nephritis' (Neild *et al.* 1983). Extracapillary proliferation can occupy a small segment (usually less than 50%)

Table 4.1 Immunopathogenetic classification of rapidly progressive glomerulonephritis

I. Anti-GBM antibody	**II. No immune deposits**	**III. Immune complex**
With lung haemorrhage (Goodpasture's syndrome)	*Vasculitis*	*Postinfectious*
Without lung haemorrhage	Microscopic polyarteritis	Poststreptococcal
Complicating membranous nephropathy	Wegener's granulomatosis	Visceral abscess
	Hypersensitivity vaculitides	Other
		Collagen–vascular disease
	'Idiopathic'	Lupus nephritis
	(renal-limited vasculitis)	Henoch–Schönlein purpura
		Mixed cryoglobulinaemia
		Primary renal diseases
		IgA nephropathy
		Membranoproliferative glomerulonephritis
		Idiopathic

of Bowman's space, when it is referred to as a 'segmental crescent'. In other cases, the accumulation of cells is massive, largely filling Bowman's space, and the contradictory term 'circumferential crescent' has been employed.

Morphological features of crescentic glomerulonephritis are heterogeneous, and this histological variability is frequently correlated with different alterations of the glomerular tuft and/or with the type and extent of interstitial involvement, mainly due to inflammatory cell infiltration. In some cases, the circumferential cellular crescent evenly fills a great part of Bowman's space with multiple layers of 'epithelial' cells (Fig. 4.1). The glomerular tuft can be hypercellular, comprising proliferating intrinsic glomerular cells and also infiltrating leucocytes (Fig. 4.1). Sometimes, the glomerular tuft is extremely compressed, making it difficult to evaluate precisely the underlying glomerular alterations (Fig. 4.2). There may be interstitial leucocyte infiltration, but periglomerular localization of the infiltrates is usually absent or mild, and rupture of Bowman's capsule is very rare. This type of intracapillary proliferative crescentic glomerulonephritis is more common in immune complex-mediated primary glomerulonephritis (Rees and Cameron 1992; Heptinstall 1992; Atkins and Thomson 1993).

In many other cases, the crescents are less uniformly distributed within Bowman's space, and strictly related to necrosis of the glomerular tuft, making

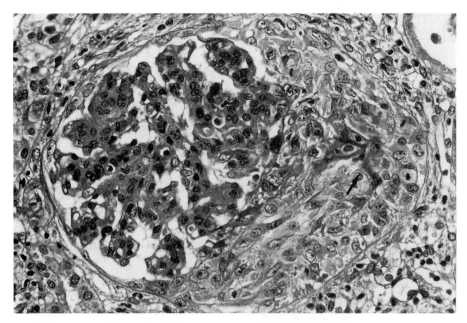

Fig. 4.1 A circumferential cellular crescent evenly fills Bowman's space. The glomerular tuft shows hypercellularity, mainly comprising proliferating intrinsic glomerular cells. Some deposits of fibrin in the context of the crescent are evident (arrow) (Masson trichrome, ×250).

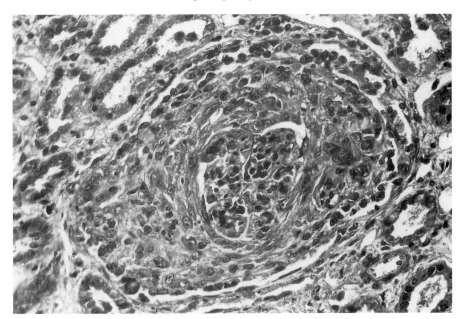

Fig. 4.2 A large circumferential crescent totally surrounds a glomerular tuft that appears to be extremely compressed, making precise evaluation of the underlying glomerular alterations difficult. There is no interstitial periglomerular leucocyte infiltration and Bowman's capsule is preserved (Masson trichrome, ×250).

precise differentiation between intracapillary and extracapillary lesions difficult (Fig. 4.3). Areas in which capillary walls are disrupted are frequently seen in these cases (Fig. 4.4) and interstitial leucocyte infiltration is often extensive, containing large numbers of monocytes/macrophages as well as lymphocytes (Hooke *et al.* 1987; Nolasco *et al.* 1987; Boucher *et al.* 1987; Rastaldi *et al.* 1996). Periglomerular localization of the infiltrates is common and often associated with segmental or massive rupture of Bowman's capsule (Fig. 4.5). The breaks in Bowman's capsule create a fusion of crescentic cells with the periglomerular infiltrate, making it extremely difficult to differentiate between the two lesions, and consequently to evaluate clearly the cells involved in the pathological process (Boucher *et al.* 1987). Necrotizing crescentic glomerulonephritis with intense periglomerular infiltrates has mainly been described in patients with ANCA-associated vasculitis and anti-GBM disease (Balow 1985; Cameron 1991; Jennette 1991; Heptinstall 1992; Ferrario *et al.* 1994). When the periglomerular inflammatory infiltration is massive, a granuloma-like reaction (sometimes with giant cells) is evident (Fig. 4.6). This picture is not pathognomonic of Wegener's granulomatosis, since it is also described in microscopic polyarteritis and anti-GBM disease (Hoffman *et al.* 1992; Bindi *et al.* 1993). Occasionally, large numbers of eosinophils are seen, and this feature suggests a diagnosis of Churg–Strauss syndrome (Lanham *et al.* 1984; Clutterbuck *et al.* 1990).

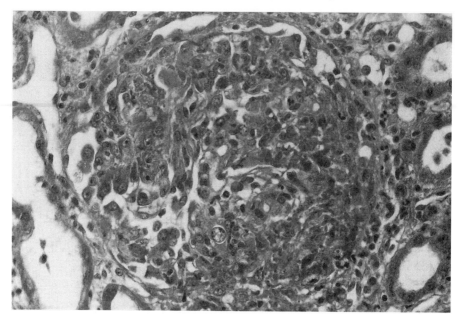

Fig. 4.3 A glomerulus with a crescent non-homogeneously distributed in Bowman's space, and strictly connected with necrotizing areas of the glomerular tuft. A precise differentiation between intra- and extra-capillary lesions is quite difficult (Masson trichrome, ×250).

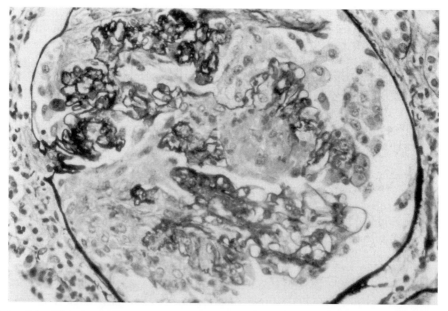

Fig. 4.4 The glomerulus presents vast areas of capillary wall disruption at the site of tuft necrosis (silver stain, ×250).

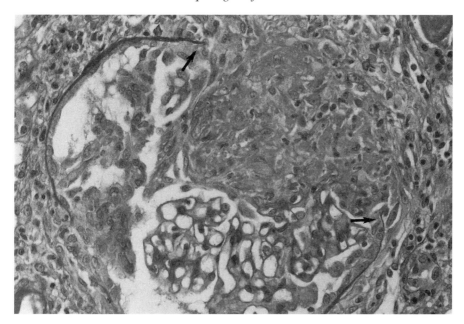

Fig. 4.5 A massive rupture of Bowman's capsule (arrows), creating fusion between crescentic cells and an intense periglomerular leucocyte infiltration (PAS, ×250).

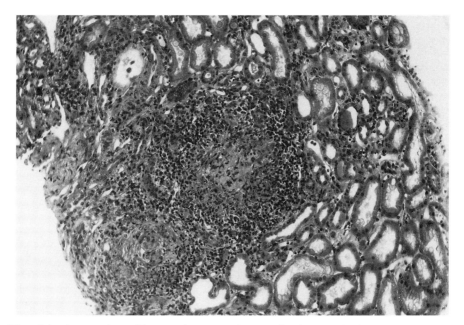

Fig. 4.6 A granuloma-like reaction around a totally destroyed glomerulus (Masson trichrome, ×100).

Regardless of different morphological characteristics, the early cellular crescents become fibrocellular and fibrous with the passage of time (Figs 4.7, 4.8). The origin of the collagen that appears and eventually replaces the original cellular crescent is not clear. In some cases, the collagen, especially type IV, is the product of glomerular cells. In other cases, type III collagen is present, particularly when there are breaks in Bowman's capsule, suggesting that interstitial cells have grown into the crescent (Striker *et al.* 1984; Yoshioka *et al.* 1989). Cells with the characteristics of fibroblasts have been described (Silva *et al.* 1984) and myofibroblasts have recently been identified, but their origin is still a matter for discussion (El Nahas *et al.* 1996).

The nature of the glomerular immune aggregates in crescent glomerulonephritis, as detected by immunofluorescence, depends on the underlying type of glomerulonephritis and will be discussed later. Fibrin is always found in cellular crescents, and its pattern of distribution is variable in the different morphological pictures previously described. Fibrin can be intensely and evenly stained in circumferential crescents whereas the tuft appears to be totally negative (Fig. 4.9). This picture is common in proliferative forms of crescentic glomerulonephritis. In segmental necrotizing forms, fibrin can be restricted to delineated areas of intracapillary necrosis (Fig. 4.10), whereas in the diffuse necrotizing forms it occupies most of the glomerular tuft and Bowman's space with a non-homogeneous pattern (Fig. 4.11). In cases with large ruptures of Bowman's capsule, fibrin stains can also be positive in periglomerular interstitial areas (Fig. 4.12).

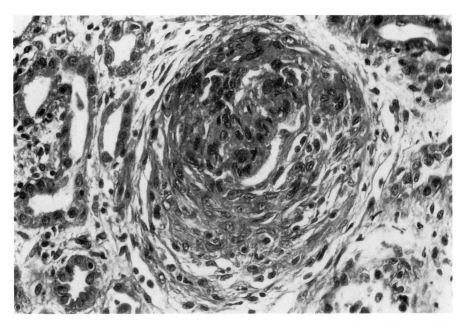

Fig. 4.7 With the passage of time, the crescent appears to be fibrocellular, and the glomerular tuft is compressed (Masson trichrome, ×250).

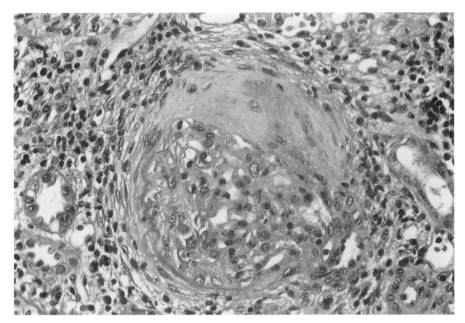

Fig. 4.8 A late stage of crescentic glomerulonephritis, characterized by a totally fibrotic crescent (Masson trichrome, ×250).

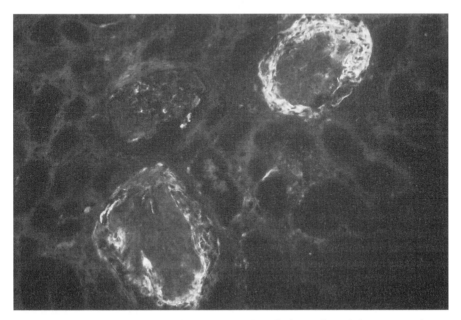

Fig. 4.9 Immunofluorescence: fibrinogen stain of circumferential crescents in two glomeruli, with a totally negative tuft (fluorescein–conjugated antifibrinogen antiserum, ×100).

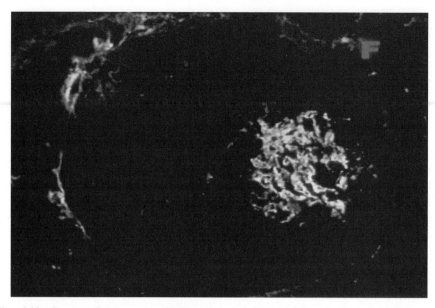

Fig. 4.10 Immunofluorescence: fibrinogen intensely positive only in a well-delineated area of the glomerular tuft, corresponding to an area of segmental intracapillary necrosis (flluorescein-conjugated antifibrinogen antiserum, ×250).

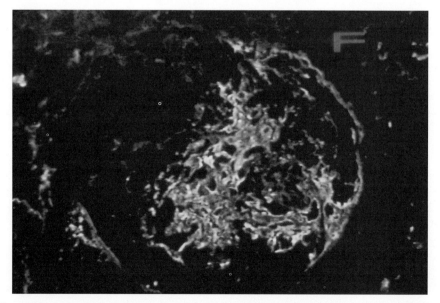

Fig. 4.11 Immunofluorescence: non-homogeneous fibrinogen stain occupies most of the glomerular tuft and Bowman's space in diffuse necrotizing glomerulonephritis (fluorescein-conjugated antifibrinogen antiserum, ×250).

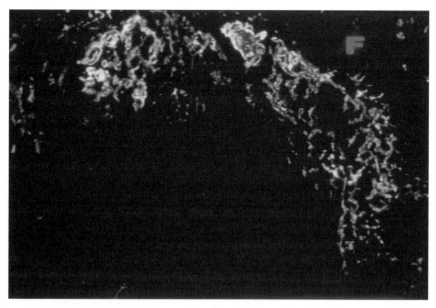

Fig. 4.12 Immunofluorescence: a case with large ruptures of Bowman's capsule, observed by light microscopy. Fibrinogen is also positive in periglomerular interstitial areas (fluorescein-conjugated antifibrinogen antiserum, ×250).

Electron microscopy has been used to evaluate the deposits in crescentic glomerulonephritis and to identify the nature of the cells within the crescent. The characteristics and the location of deposits vary considerably, depending on the underlying nephritis, and will be discussed individually. Regardless of the presence or absence of deposits, electron microscopy can provide further information about the different types of lesion associated with crescent formation. Crescents can be composed mainly of epithelial cells, in which mitotic figures are frequent (Bacani *et al.* 1968; Morita *et al.* 1973; Bohman *et al.* 1974; Bonsib 1988) (Fig. 4.13). A break of the GBM can sometimes be seen clearly, with evident fibrin deposition in the crescent (Burkholder 1969; Stejskal *et al.* 1973) (Fig. 4. 14). When Bowman's capsule has been disrupted, it becomes difficult to distinguish between intraglomerular and extraglomerular cells, and many inflammatory cells are found (D'Agati *et al.* 1986) (Fig. 4.15). Collapse and wrinkling of the capillary wall are frequently observed (Bonsib 1988) (Fig. 4.15).

Mechanisms of crescent formation

The cellular composition of glomerular crescents and the mechanisms underlying crescent formation have been studied extensively by many investigators, but are still incompletely understood. Initial studies, both of human and experimental glomerulonephritis, suggested that epithelial cells predominated. For example, in

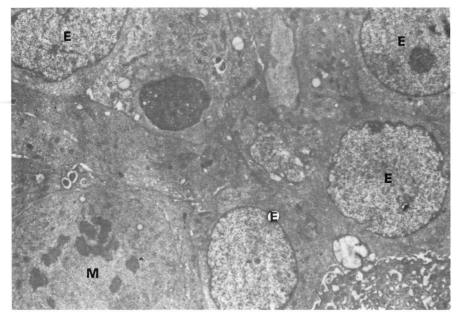

Fig. 4.13 Electron micrograph: a crescent mainly composed of epithelial cells (E). A mitotic figure can be recognized (lead citrate–uranyl acetate, ×2800). (Courtesy of Dr E. Schiaffino, Department of Pathology, S. Carlo Hospital, Milan.)

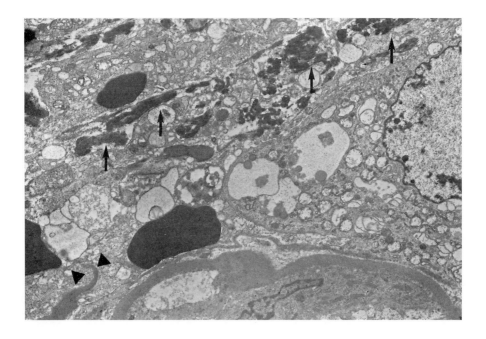

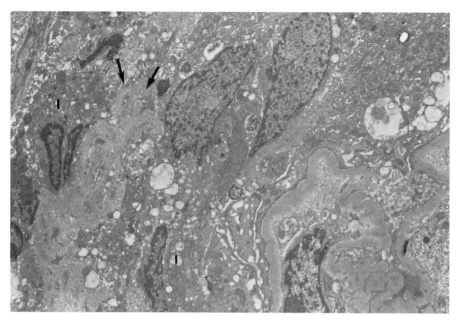

Fig. 4.15 Electron micrograph: Bowman's capsule disrupted and destroyed (arrow). Many inflammatory cells (I) are present. A capillary wall has collapsed and is wrinkled (lead citrate–uranyl acetate, ×2800). (Courtesy of Dr E. Schiaffino, Department of Pathology, S. Carlo Hospital, Milan.)

1973, Morita *et al.* studied 36 human renal biopsies by light and electron microscopy and concluded that crescent cells were epithelial in origin, being parietal in most cases but visceral in others. They noted the presence of breaks in the GBM by electron microscopy and hypothesized that leakage of fibrinogen and red blood cells might accelerate crescent formation. They also observed occasional phagocytic cells in the crescent but attributed this to metaplastic change of the epithelial cells. These results were confirmed by Min *et al.* (1979) by electron microscopy using serial sections of human renal biopsies. In 1978, Cattell and Jamieson reached similar conclusions in studies of an experimental model of nephrotoxic serum nephritis in the rabbit. However, in 1976, Atkins and coworkers cultured isolated glomeruli from patients with RPGN and demonstrated an increased number of monocytes-macrophages, which was the first evidence for an important role of mononuclear leucocytes in the extracapillary proliferative

Fig. 4.14 Electron micrograph: a cellular crescent containing epithelial cells (E), massive fibrin deposits (arrows), and a break in the glomerular basement membrane (arrow heads) (lead citrate–uranyl acetate, ×2800). (Courtesy of Dr E. Schiaffino, Department of Pathology, S. Carlo Hospital, Milan.)

lesions. Subsequent studies, of both human (Ferrario *et al.* 1985) and experimental (Holdsworth *et al.* 1980; Clarke *et al.* 1983) glomerulonephritis, showed the prevailing presence of monocytes-macrophages in the crescents by electron microscopy and by histochemistry. Magil and Wadsworth (1982), in a histochemical and electron microscopic study of human renal biopsies, observed a difference between crescents in anti-GBM disease, in which monocytes-macrophages were prevalent, and cases of immune complex glomerulonephritis, characterized by epithelial crescent formation.

The availability of monoclonal antibodies directed against epithelial cells and leucocytes allowed more precise identification of the crescent cells. Many authors (Yoshioka *et al.* 1987; Müller *et al.* 1988) have demonstrated immunohistochemically the presence of both epithelial cells and monocytes in crescents, but there is still debate about the different percentages in which they are found. Hancock and Atkins (1984) reported that macrophages predominated in cellular crescents, but that polymorphs and epithelial cells were also present. They also observed that the number of macrophages decreased when the crescents became fibrotic. Other authors (Jennette and Hipp 1985; Harrison and Macdonald 1986; Guettier *et al.* 1986) found that epithelial cells were more frequent than macrophages. These discrepancies were explained by Boucher *et al.* (1987), who observed that monocytes prevailed in the crescent when there was a rupture of Bowman's capsule, whereas epithelial cells were in the majority when the integrity of Bowman's capsule was preserved.

With an immunoperoxidase streptavidin-biotin method, we have studied the intraglomerular positivity for total leucocytes, monocytes-macrophages, cytokeratins, and the adhesion molecule VCAM-1, in frozen serial sections of 46 human renal biopsies from patients with different types of RPGN. Of the adhesion molecules, we selected VCAM-1 because it had been suggested that monocytes might be recruited preferentially by interaction between the β1-integrin VLA-4 and VCAM-1 (Cattell 1994). Two groups of patients could be identified on the basis of immunohistochemical features. The first was characterised by large numbers of leucocytes, especially monocytes-macrophages, in the crescents (Fig. 4.16), with few cells being positive for cytokeratins (Fig. 4.17). In these biopsies, VCAM-1 (which is found on epithelial cells of Bowman's capsule in normal kidneys but not cells within the tuft) was markedly positive, not only in the crescents, but also in well-delineated areas of the tuft, in close proximity to the extracapillary proliferation (Fig. 4.18). These areas corresponded exactly with the necrotizing lesions seen by light microscopy and with the segmental fibrinogen deposition observed by immunofluorescence. In many of these cases, there was considerable periglomerular leucocytic infiltration, which made it impossible to distinguish intra- from extra-capillary infiltrating leucocytes (Fig. 4.19), The second group had minimal intraglomerular leucocyte infiltration (Fig. 4.20), and almost all cells in the crescent were positive for cytokeratins (Fig. 4.21). VCAM-1 was completely negative in the tuft and was only found on the extracapillary proliferating cells (Fig. 4.22). Significant periglomerular leucocyte infiltration was observed only rarely. We could not detect necrotizing glomerular lesions by light

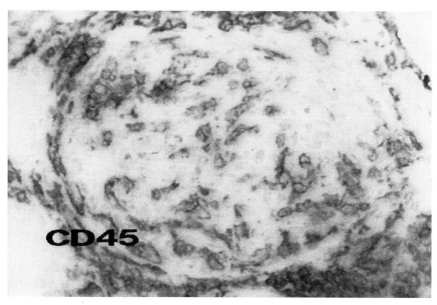

Fig. 4.16 Mechanisms of crescent formation. A large number of leucocytes (CD45+ cells) infiltrate the glomerulus, both the tuft and the crescent. Periglomerular leucocytes also present (immunoperoxidase-conjugated anti-CD45 antibody, ×250).

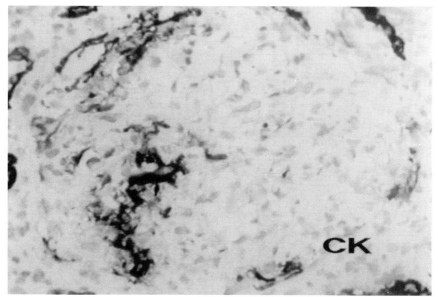

Fig. 4.17 Mechanisms of crescent formation. Staining for cytokeratins shows only a few positive cells in the crescent (immunoperoxidase-conjugated anti-cytokeratin antibody, ×250).

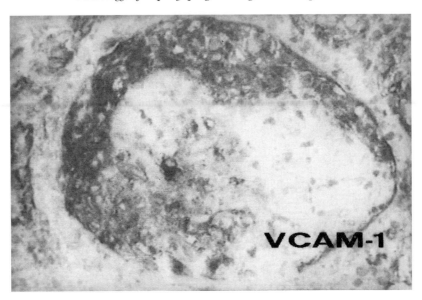

Fig. 4.18 Mechanisms of crescent formation. The markedly positive adhesion molecule VCAM-1 is not only in the crescent, but is also in a well-delineated area of the tuft (immunoperoxidase-conjugated anti-VCAM-1 antibody, ×250).

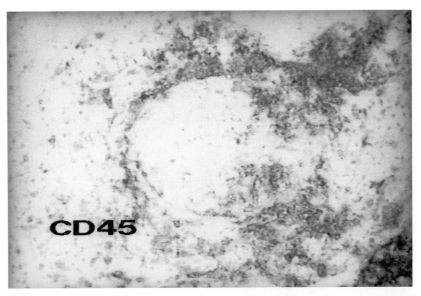

Fig. 4.19 Mechanisms of crescent formation. Significant intraglomerular and periglomerular leucocyte (CD45+ cells) infiltration. Precise delineation of the intra-glomerular area is not possible (immunoperoxidase-conjugated anti-CD45 antibody, ×100).

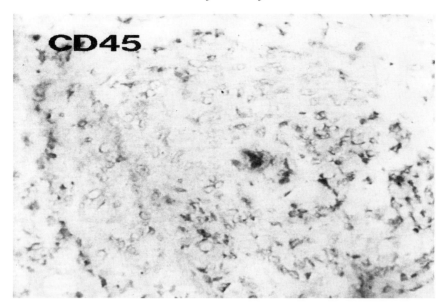

Fig. 4.20 Mechanisms of crescent formation. There are very few leucocytes (CD45+ cells) in the glomerulus (immunoperoxidase-conjugated anti-CD45 antibody, ×250).

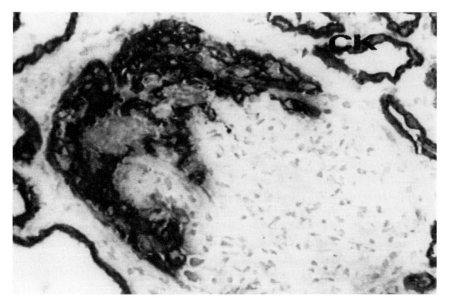

Fig. 4.21 Mechanisms of crescent formation. Positivity for cytokeratins in the crescent, staining almost all the crescent cells (immunoperoxidase-conjugated anticytokeratin antibody, ×250).

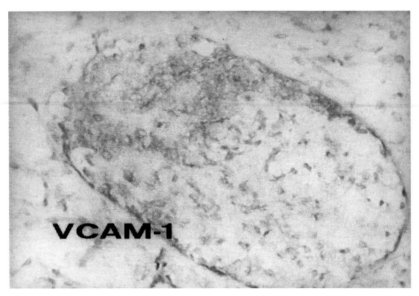

Fig. 4.22 Mechanisms of crescent formation. The glomerulus stains slightly for adhesion molecule VCAM-1, which lines the crescent cells and is completely negative in the tuft (immunoperoxidase-conjugated anti-VCAM-1 antibody, ×250).

microscopy, whereas intraglomerular proliferation was seen frequently. Immunofluorescence demonstrated fibrinogen positivity only in the crescents.

It is possible to hypothesize that two different mechanisms are responsible for the formation of crescents in glomerular disease, which might also explain the discrepancies in different studies. The presence of necrosis of the capillary wall can induce a marked inflammatory reaction, with the recruitment of a large number of leucocytes, especially monocytes, not only into Bowman's space but also, as demonstrated in an experimental model of crescentic glomerulonephritis (Lan *et al.* 1991), through the hilus of the glomerulus into the interstitium with a characteristic periglomerular localization. This strong inflammatory reaction might also result in the rupture of Bowman's capsule, confirming, in our opinion, the observations of Boucher *et al.* in 1987. These lesions, as noted by Rees and Cameron (1992), are mainly observed in anti-GBM disease, renal vasculitis, Henoch–Schönlein purpura, and lupus nephritis. On the other hand, in the absence of obvious necrosis, but with prevalent intraglomerular proliferation, small gaps in the GBM, as demonstrated by Bonsib in 1985, can allow extravasation of fibrin and inflammatory cells into Bowman's space that trigger proliferation of the parietal epithelial cells of Bowman's capsule, without severe damage to its integrity. In these circumstances, crescents are composed mainly of epithelial parietal cells, although some leucocytes may also be found. This type of lesion is more frequently observed in acute or chronic immune complex proliferative glomerulonephritis, such as acute poststreptococcal glomerulonephritis, membranoproliferative glomerulonephritis, and the so-called 'idiopathic' forms (Rees and Cameron 1992; Heptinstall 1992; Atkins and Thomson 1993).

Anti-glomerular basement membrane antibody disease

The morphological characteristics, using light microscopy, reveal a wide spectrum of lesions, although the most typical feature is the presence of necrotizing crescentic glomerulonephritis. The glomeruli may appear normal or have only a small increase in mesangial cellularity in some cases, despite the presence of widespread and clear linear staining of IgG along the glomerular capillaries (McPhaul and Mullins 1976; Saraf *et al.* 1978; Bailey *et al.* 1989; Glassock *et al.* 1991). However, the majority of cases have variable degrees of necrotizing crescentic lesions, ranging from focal and segmental to massive and diffuse (Figs 4.23, 4.24). In these cases, the remnant parts of uninvolved tufts usually show mesangial proliferation, and an increased number of intracapillary leucocytes. These are mainly monocytes, but T lymphocytes are also frequently present (Stachura *et al.* 1984; Ferrario *et al.* 1985; Bolton *et al.* 1987; Nolasco *et al.* 1987). Interstitial inflammation is common and mainly periglomerular, with local or massive destruction of Bowman's capsule. About 50% of cases have multinucleated giant cells in the crescent or in the adjacent periglomerular infiltrate, giving a picture of granulomatous glomerulonephritis (Kaslowsky *et al.* 1976;

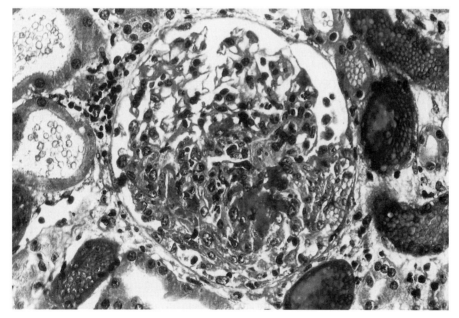

Fig. 4.23 Anti-glomerular basement membrane antibody disease. Focal and segmental necrotizing glomerulonephritis: the glomerulus shows a localized area of tuft necrosis surrounded by a segmental crescent (Masson trichrome, ×250).

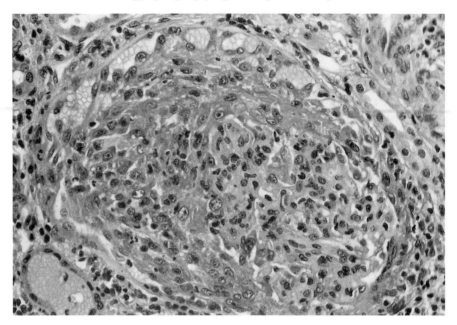

Fig. 4.24 Anti-glomerular basement membrane antibody disease. Diffuse necrotizing glomerulonephritis: the glomerulus presents more extensive intraglomerular necrosis and a large circumferential crescent. The glomerular tuft also shows some mesangial proliferation and an increased number of intracapillary leucocytes (Masson trichrome, ×250).

Bathena *et al.* 1987) (Fig. 4.25). Tubular atrophy and interstitial fibro–oedema are common and usually correlate with the degree of glomerular involvement. Vascular lesions are uncommon, but some authors have documented the presence of necrotizing arteritis of small vessels (Wahls *et al.* 1987; Dean *et al.* 1991) and, more rarely, an expression of thrombotic microangiopathy (Stave and Croker 1984).

The pathognomic feature of this form of nephritis is undoubtedly the immunohistological pattern of linear staining with anti-IgG serum along all glomerular capillary basement membranes (Wilson and Dixon 1973; McPhaul and Mullins 1976; Briggs *et al.* 1979; Salant 1987; Glassock *et al.* 1991) (Fig. 4.26). Anti-IgG is frequently the only positive antiserum, but a combination of linear deposits of IgG and C3 is also described (Teague *et al.* 1978; Savage *et al.* 1986). Isolated reports have described linear deposits of IgA (Border *et al.* 1979; Gris *et al.* 1991) or IgM (Wilson 1991) instead of IgG. In well-preserved glomeruli, the linear deposits outline the entire tuft (Fig. 4.26), but in glomeruli extensively destroyed by necrotizing extracapillary lesions only small segments of basement membrane may remain, so that linear patterns may be segmental (Fig. 4.27). When crescent formation is extensive, the glomerular tuft may be totally collapsed, with crumpled and corrugated basement membrane which makes it difficult to discern a clear linear pattern (Fig. 4.28). The presence

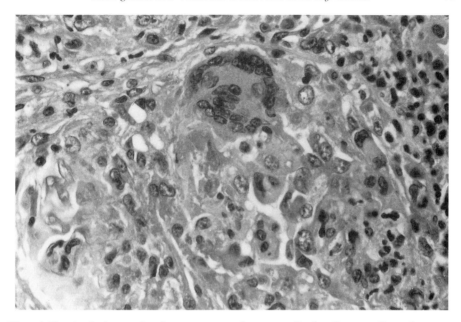

Fig. 4.25 Anti-glomerular basement membrane antibody disease. Granulomatous glomerulonephritis: a multinucleated giant cell in the crescent (PAS, ×400).

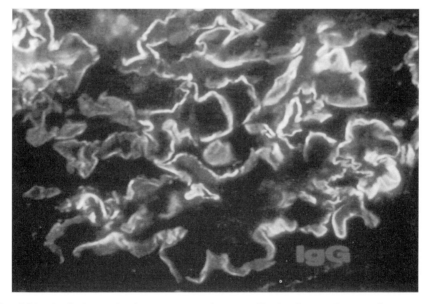

Fig. 4.26 Anti-glomerular basement membrane antibody disease. Immunofluorescence: the typical linear staining of IgG along glomerular capillaries (fluorescein-conjugated anti-IgG antiserum, ×400).

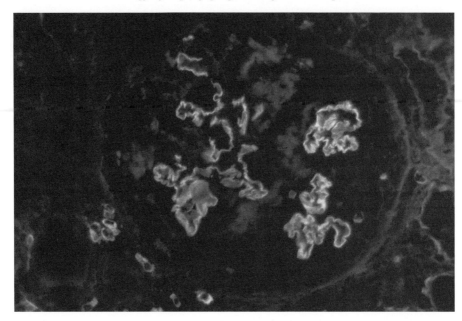

Fig. 4.27 Anti-glomerular basement membrane antibody disease. Immunofluorescence: in a glomerulus extensively destroyed by necrotizing extracapillary lesions only small segments of the basement membrane show linear staining (fluorescein-conjugated anti-IgG antiserum, ×250).

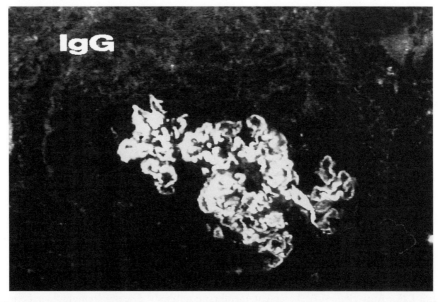

Fig. 4.28 Anti-glomerular basement membrane antibody disease. Immunofluorescence: with an extensive circumferential crescent, the glomerular tuft appears totally collapsed, with crumpled and corrugated basement membrane, making it difficult to discern a clear linear pattern (fluorescein-conjugated anti-IgG antiserum, ×250).

of linear deposits of IgG along Bowman's capsule has frequently been reported (Wilson and Dixon 1979; Glassock *et al.* 1991; Heptinstall 1992). These can entirely encircle the glomerulus or be interrupted by rupture of Bowman's capsule when there is extensive crescent formation. Focal or diffuse linear staining of the tubular basement membrane is present in many cases (McCluskey *et al.* 1974; Andres *et al.* 1978; Border *et al.* 1979). As in other forms of necrotizing crescentic glomerulonephritis, fibrin is present within the necrotic tuft and the crescents. Both linear and granular staining may occasionally occur, suggesting that anti-GBM and immune complex mechanisms can operate simultaneously (Agodoa *et al.* 1976; Pasternack *et al.* 1978; Richman *et al.* 1981; Pettersson *et al.* 1984).

By electron microscopy, the only distinctive feature is the presence of slightly widened and lucent subendothelial zones of the laminae rarae internae of capillary walls, an ultrastructural expression of the site of binding of anti-glomerular basement membrane antibody (Poskitt 1970; Briggs *et al.* 1979). The glomerular features are the same as those of other forms of necrotizing crescentic glomerulonephritis described earlier in this chapter.

Anti-GBM disease may manifest either as a combination of glomerulonephritis and pulmonary haemorrhage (Goodpasture's syndrome) or as glomerulonephritis alone. It is of interest that renal symptoms and renal morphological lesions are identical in cases of lung haemorrhage and in the renal-limited form. In our experience of 16 cases with anti-GBM disease, the 8 patients with lung haemorrhage showed the same histological alterations as the cases without lung haemorrhage, and comparable renal syndromes, mainly rapidly progressive glomerulonephritis.

Renal microscopic vasculitis (ANCA-associated)

The topic of systemic vasculitis is vast and we will focus our attention on the so-called 'ANCA-associated microscopic vasculitis', characterized by necrotizing extracapillary lesions and a rapidly progressive course. The current classifications of renal vasculitis, based on a mixture of histological, clinical, and, more recently, immunological features are incomplete and still confusing. Since the first descriptions (Davson *et al.* 1948; Zeek 1953), and also in more recent attempts at classification (Cameron 1988; Jennette *et al.* 1994), the morphological approach to differentiating different forms of vasculitis is mainly based on the type and size of the vessels involved. The presence of necrotizing lesions in large, medium, or small vessels differentiated classic polyarteritis nodosa from the 'small vessel vasculitis' group (Wegener's granulomatosis, microscopic polyarteritis, and 'idiopathic' necrotizing glomerulonephritis). In fact, the frequency of histologically identifiable arteritis in renal specimens is relatively low, ranging from about 10% to 30% (Serra *et al.* 1984; Savage *et al.* 1985; Adu *et al.* 1987; Wilkowsky *et al.* 1989; Gans *et al.* 1993). Moreover, simultaneous involvement of small- and medium-sized arteries led some authors to describe an 'overlap syndrome', adding further to the confusion in terminology (Fauci 1978; Ronco *et al.* 1983; Balow 1985). The presence of necrotizing glomerulonephritis in the majority of patients influenced many authors to consider the involvement of vessels smaller than arteries, especially glomerular capillaries (capillaritis), as an expression of renal vasculitis (Cameron 1988; Heptinstall 1992; Ferrario *et al.* 1993; Jennette and Falk 1994). A recent Chapel Hill consensus conference on nomenclature of systemic vasculitides concluded that the presence or absence of necrosis in glomerular capillaries, or involvement of capillaries at other sites, should be the differentiating characteristic for polyarteritis nodosa and microscopic polyarteritis (polyangiitis) (Jennette *et al.* 1994).

The discovery of antineutrophil cytoplasmic antibodies (ANCA) and their prevalent association with necrotizing glomerulonephritis allowed a more precise classification of these disorders, and the term 'ANCA-associated renal vasculitis' is now widely accepted (Falk and Jennette 1988; Nölle *et al.* 1989; Cohen Tervaert *et al.* 1990; Sinico *et al.* 1994) (Table 4.2). The majority of previous reports and our personal experience in a large cohort of 231 patients with renal vasculitis, evaluated in a multi-centre study of the Italian Renal Immunopathology Group, clearly demonstrated that histological lesions in the kidney are similar, irrespective of differences in the degree of systemic involvement (Adu *et al.* 1987; Cameron 1988; Pettersson and Heigl 1992; Gans *et al.* 1993; Jennette *et al.* 1994). Wegener's granulomatosis, microscopic polyarteritis, and 'idiopathic' necrotizing glomerulonephritis should therefore be considered as a single pathological condition with different organ involvement. Those patients with only constitutional symptoms, previously defined as 'idiopathic' necrotizing glomerulonephritis, must be considered to have a renal-limited variant of microscopic polyarteritis, as also confirmed by the positivity of ANCA with the same patterns (Ferrario *et al.* 1994).

Two major glomerular lesions are characteristic of ANCA-associated renal vasculitis: necrosis of the tuft and extracapillary proliferation, with wide variability in intensity and degree. Necrosis can be the only lesion present, and is probably an expression of an early phase of the disease (Savage *et al.* 1985; Croker *et al.* 1987; Cameron 1988; Bindi *et al.* 1993) (Fig. 4.29). In about one-third of cases,

---

Table 4.2   ANCA-associated renal vasculitis: clinical definitions

1. *Wegener's granulomatosis*
Necrotizing glomerulonephritis
Clinical symptoms of systemic vasculitis (fever, arthralgia, myalgia, purpura, pulmonary symptoms)
Prominent upper respiratory tract involvement

2. *Microscopic polyarteritis*
Necrotizing glomerulonephritis
Clinical symptoms of systemic vasculitis (fever, arthralgia, myalgia, purpura, pulmonary symptoms)

3. *'Idiopathic' necrotizing glomerulonephritis (renal-limited vasculitis)*
Necrotizing glomerulonephritis without convincing clinical symptoms of systemic vasculitis

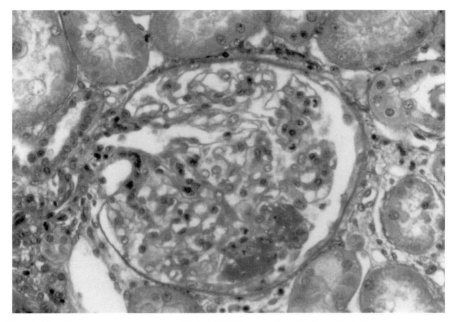

Fig. 4.29 Renal microscopic vasculitis (ANCA-associated). A well-delineated segmental area of tuft necrosis is the only evident lesion (Masson trichrome, ×250).

the picture is characterized by typical focal and segmental necrotizing extracapillary glomerulonephritis (Fig. 4.30). Massive tuft necrosis with diffuse, non-homogeneous circumferential crescents can also be observed (Fig. 4.31). Mesangial proliferation, mesangial matrix expansion, and endocapillary infiltration are usually mild, and undamaged glomeruli and non-necrotic parts of the glomerular tuft often appear to be normal (Heptinstall 1992) (Fig. 4.30). This is of great importance when differentiating vasculitides from the other necrotizing forms of nephritis, characterized by variable but frequently important intracapillary proliferation (systemic lupus erythematosus, Henoch-Schönlein purpura, infective endocarditis).

Most of the glomeruli are sclerotic at presentation in about 15–20% of cases (Bindi *et al.* 1993; Gans *et al.* 1993). The segmental sclerotic lesions are quite specific, and are characterized by well-delineated areas of sclerosis with adhesion to Bowman's capsule and no lesions in the remnant part of the tuft (Fig. 4.32). This alteration represents a late stage of repair of previous necrotic areas, confirmed by the simultaneous presence in the same biopsy of necrotic and sclerotic lesions (Serra *et al.* 1984; Bindi *et al.* 1993; Gans *et al.* 1993) (Fig. 4.33). In our experience, typical sclerotic lesions were found in 10 repeat biopsies of cases who showed focal necrotizing glomerulonephritis in the first biopsy. The frequent occurrence of relapses in systemic vasculitis is well known (Gordon *et al.* 1993) and the diagnosis of active arteritis is fundamental for management of patients with sclerotic lesions.

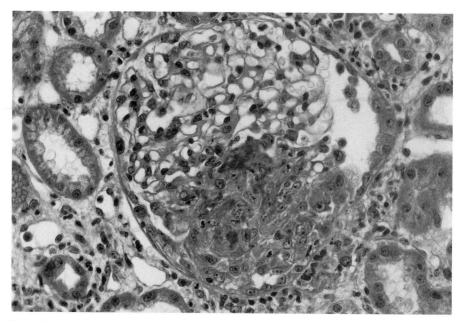

Fig. 4.30 Renal microscopic vasculitis (ANCA-associated). A typical segmental necrotizing extracapillary lesion. The remaining part of the tuft is normal (Masson trichrome, ×250).

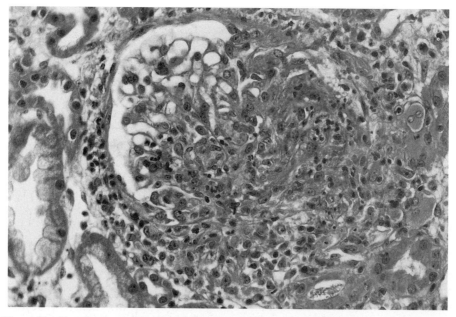

Fig. 4.31 Renal microscopic vasculitis (ANCA-associated). Massive tuft necrosis with a non-homogeneous circumferential crescent, a typical expression of diffuse necrotizing extracapillary glomerulonephritis (H&E, ×250).

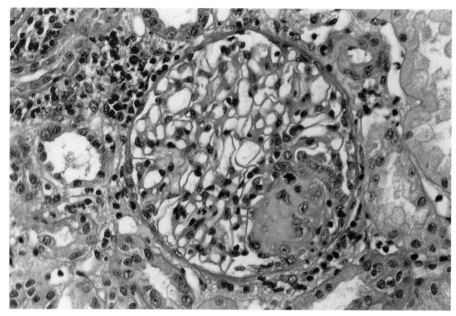

Fig. 4.32 Renal microscopic vasculitis (ANCA-associated). The glomerulus shows a well-delineated round area of sclerosis with adhesion to Bowman's capsule, and no lesions in the tuft remnant. This histological alteration may represent a late stage of repair of a previous segmental necrotic lesion (Masson trichrome, ×250).

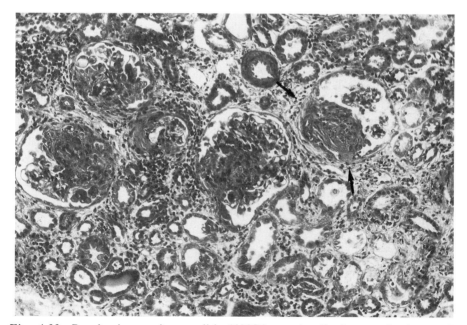

Fig. 4.33 Renal microscopic vasculitis (ANCA-associated). A case of microscopic polyarteritis, with three glomeruli with active necrotizing extracapillary lesions, plus a glomerulus that shows a segmental area of sclerosis (arrow) (Masson trichrome, ×100).

Interstitial leucocyte infiltrates are another important feature of renal vasculitis, and their intensity and extent usually correlate with the severity of the glomerular lesions (Jennette 1991; Adu *et al.* 1987; Rastaldi *et al.* 1996). The infiltrates are mainly composed of T lymphocytes and monocytes (Rastaldi *et al.* 1996). The leucocyte infiltration is sometimes intense, with periglomerular accentuation and concomitant rupture of Bowman's capsule, making it difficult to distinguish between glomerular and interstitial lesions (Boucher *et al.* 1987; Ferrario *et al.* 1993; Rastaldi *et al.* 1996) (Fig. 4.34). In some cases, there is a granuloma-like reaction around recognizable glomeruli, characterized by total destruction of glomeruli with circumferential accumulation of epitheloid cells and sometimes giant cells (Wilkowsky *et al.* 1989; Hoffman *et al.* 1992; Bindi *et al.* 1993) (Fig. 4.35). True interstitial granulomata, defined as an accumulation of epithelioid cells with or without giant cells, but without glomerular remnants, is very rare (Heptinstall 1992) (Fig. 4.36). The granulomatous reaction around glomeruli is not specific for Wegener's granulomatosis (Bindi *et al.* 1993) and was also seen in 17% of cases of microscopic polyarteritis and 7% of the renal-limited variant in our experience of 231 cases. In contrast, true interstitial granulomata have been described only in cases with Wegener's granulomatosis and can be of diagnostic value (Ronco *et al.* 1983; Heptinstall 1992). The crucial problem is the precise morphological criteria that distinguish between a granulomatous reaction around

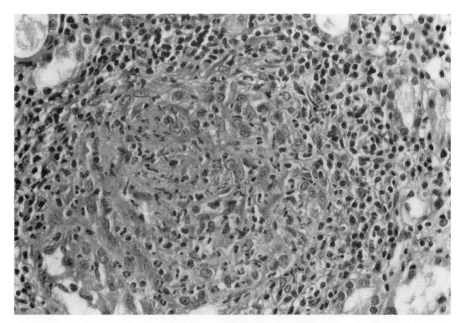

Fig. 4.34 Renal microscopic vasculitis (ANCA-associated). Massive periglomerular leucocyte infiltration. Bowman's capsule totally destroyed, making precise differentiation between intraglomerular necrotizing extracapillary lesions and interstitial leucocytes difficult (H&E, ×250).

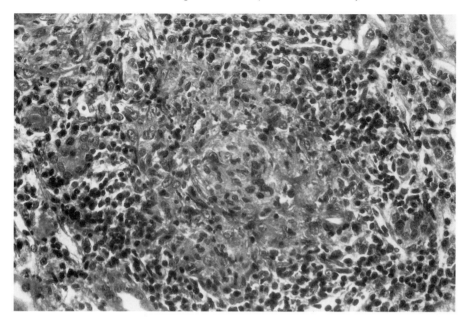

Fig. 4.35 Renal microscopic vasculitis (ANCA-associated). A granulomatous reaction around a recognizable glomerular structure (H&E, ×250).

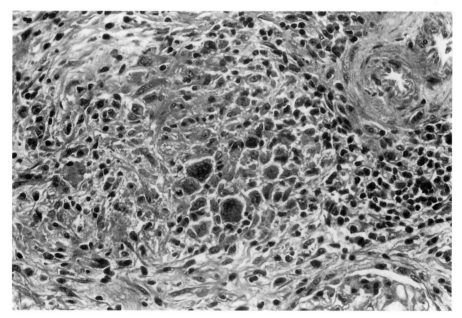

Fig. 4.36 Renal microscopic vasculitis (ANCA-associated). A case of Wegener's granulomatosis with an interstitial granuloma, defined as an accumulation of epithelioid and giant cells without glomerular remnants (H&E, ×250).

glomeruli and true interstitial granulomata, when the underlying structure is unrecognizable. Massive infiltrates and granulomatous reactions characterized by a prevalence of eosinophils, correlated with clinical symptoms of asthma, fever, and eosinophilia, suggest a diagnosis of Churg–Strauss syndrome (Chumbley *et al.* 1977; Lanham *et al.* 1984; Clutterbuck *et al.* 1990). Tubular alterations and interstitial fibro-oedema are frequent features in all renal vasculitides and usually correlate with the intensity of glomerular alterations.

The absence or the presence of only a few scattered glomerular immune deposits is described by the majority of authors as typical of ANCA-associated renal vasculitis, and the term 'pauci-immune' necrotizing glomerulonephritis is now widely accepted (Stilmant *et al.* 1979; Jennette 1991; Bindi *et al.* 1993; Gans *et al.* 1993; Pettersson *et al.* 1995). Nevertheless, other authors have described an immunohistological picture characterized by the presence of mesangial or parietal deposits (Ronco *et al.* 1983; Savage *et al.* 1985; Croker *et al.* 1987; Wilkowsky *et al.* 1989) and, in our experience, about two-thirds of patients with renal vasculitis have variable degrees of mesangial/parietal deposits of immunoglobulin and complement (Fig. 4.37). These apparently contradictory results could be the consequence of differences in interpretation of immunohistological preparations and one may ask how 'pauci' the deposits need be to remain insignificant. Another explanation is that the detectable immunoglobulins and complement

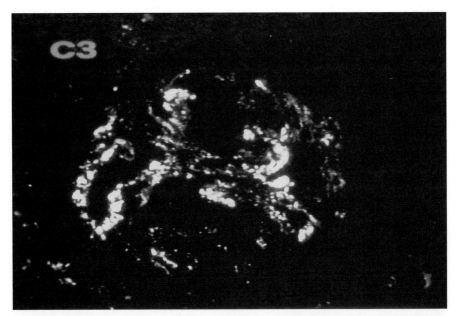

Fig. 4.37 Renal microscopic vasculitis (ANCA-associated). Immunofluorescence: a glomerulus with some mesangial and parietal deposits of C3, non-homogeneously distributed in the glomerular tuft. Deposition of C3 on the afferent arteriole (fluorescein-conjugated anti-C3 antiserum, ×250).

may be due to non-specific trapping of circulating proteins in damaged glomerular capillary walls. Nevertheless, negative or ill-defined immunofluorescence findings are very helpful in distinguishing between vasculitis and other forms of necrotizing glomerulonephritis (anti-GBM disease, SLE, Henoch–Schönlein purpura, infective endocarditis). By contrast, fibrin is always present in active renal vasculitis, with variable deposition in glomerular tufts and crescents, as previously described.

There are relatively few reports dealing with the glomerular ultrastructural changes in renal vasculitis (Bohman *et al.* 1974; Serra *et al.* 1984; D'Agati *et al.* 1986), and in particular a detailed examination of arteritic lesions is conspicuously lacking (D'Agati *et al.* 1986). However, ultrastructural examination confirms the rarity of electron-dense deposits and those present can be located in subendothelial, intramembranous, or mesangial positions (Serra *et al.* 1984; D'Agati *et al.* 1986) (Fig. 4.38). Cellular crescents are characterized by a great number of inflammatory cells (Fig. 4.38). A clear interruption of Bowman's capsule is frequently detected, making precise differentiation between glomerular and interstitial lesions difficult (Fig. 4.39).

Most authors agree that the prognosis of renal vasculitis has improved during the past decade, probably due to earlier diagnosis and therapeutic intervention, and the use of more aggressive treatment (Coward *et al.* 1986; Fuiano *et al.*

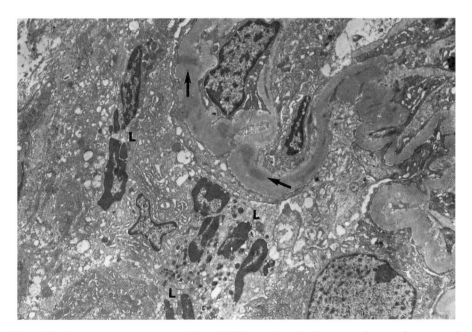

Fig. 4.38 Renal microscopic vasculitis (ANCA-associated). Electron micrograph: scattered and small intramembranous electron-dense deposits are evident (arrow). Prevailing leucocytes (L) in the crescent (lead citrate-uranyl acetate, ×2800). (Courtesy of Dr E. Schiaffino, Department of Pathology, S. Carlo Hospital, Milan.)

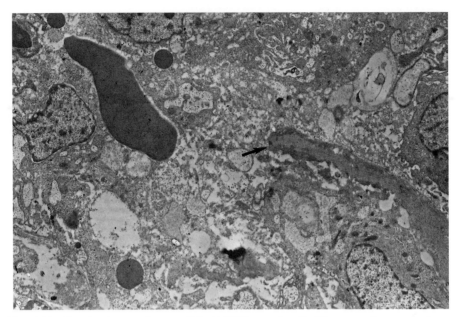

Fig. 4.39 Renal microscopic vasculitis (ANCA-associated). Electron micrograph: inter-ruption of Bowman's capsule (arrow), making it difficult to differentiate precisely between glomerular and interstitial lesions (lead citrate-uranyl acetate, ×2800). (Courtesy of Dr E. Schiaffino, Department of Pathology, S. Carlo Hospital, Milan.)

1988; Pusey *et al.* 1991; Gans *et al.* 1993; Bindi *et al.* 1993). Resolution of active lesions after early treatment is widely recognized (Adu *et al.* 1987; Hoffman *et al.* 1990; Pettersson and Heigl 1992; Nachman *et al.* 1996) and in our experience of repeat biopsies, the total disappearance of necrotizing lesions and interstitial infiltrates is impressive. Therefore, we agree with many authors (Adu *et al.* 1987; Bindi *et al.* 1993; Gans *et al.* 1993) that renal biopsy provides important inform-ation about the activity of renal vasculitis and is crucial for the therapeutic management of patients with these diseases (Ferrario *et al.* 1996).

Immune complex-associated glomerulonephritis

Postinfective glomerulonephritis

Poststreptococcal glomerulonephritis

It is often stated that poststreptococcal glomerulonephritis can occasionally be complicated by the presence of glomerular crescents (Gill *et al.* 1977; Fairley *et al.* 1987). These crescentic forms are highly variable, ranging from cases with focal and segmental lesions to those characterized by diffuse and circumferential crescents. The histological evidence of intracapillary proliferation and/or exuda-tion, the immunofluorescence pattern, with granular positivity of IgG and C3, and the electron microscopic evidence of subepithelial deposits (humps) are very useful for differential diagnosis of these forms of nephritis (Heptinstall 1992).

Other postinfective glomerulonephritis

Many systemic infectious diseases (infective endocarditis, infected atrio-ventricular shunts, visceral abscesses, Legionella, syphilis, leprosy, etc.) may be complicated by a crescentic glomerulonephritis, sometimes severe (Rees and Cameron 1992 and see Chapter 9). For example, during the course of infective endocarditis, renal biopsy can reveal the picture of a focal and segmental necrotizing glomerulonephritis (Heptinstall 1992).

Glomerulonephritis secondary to systemic diseases

Systemic lupus erythematosus (see also Chapter 8)

Histological changes in systemic lupus erythematosus (SLE) vary considerably from case to case, ranging from minimal to widespread glomerular proliferation, with variable degrees of mesangial and/or parietal immune deposits (Baldwin *et al.* 1977; Appel *et al.* 1978). Extensive extracapillary proliferation and the rapidly progressive glomerulonephritis syndrome has been reported infrequently (Glassock 1978; Cameron *et al.* 1979). Nevertheless, necrotizing crescentic lesions are found frequently in SLE, mostly in diffuse proliferative glomerulonephritis, but also in focal and segmental forms, and sometimes in the proliferative subvariant of membranous glomerulonephritis (Pollak and Pirani 1969; Appel *et al.* 1978) (Figs 4.40, 4.41). Many other glomerular lesions, quite typical of SLE nephritis, have value for differential diagnosis. Lupus nephritis is characterized by mesangial proliferation, mesangial matrix expansion, and variable degrees of endocapillary leucocyte infiltration. These are well-defined mesangial and parietal deposits, frequently massive, with typical 'wire loop' lesions, and in many cases, intracapillary hyaline thrombi (Hill 1992).

Moreover, immunohistological features in SLE, both the distribution of the deposits and positivity for different antisera, are fundamental for differential diagnosis from other forms of necrotizing crescentic glomerulonephritis. The patterns of deposition are variable, ranging from pure mesangial in focal forms to widespread mesangio-parietal in diffuse forms, but the deposits are always very intense and brilliant. IgG and complement C3 deposits are nearly always present, followed by C1q, which usually stains very intensely (Hill 1992). Fibrinogen is positive in necrotic areas of the glomerular tuft and in crescents. Electron microscopy is useful in evaluating more precisely deposits that are located on different sides of glomerular structures.

Henoch–Schönlein purpura

This is another well-known form of systemic vasculitis with necrotizing crescentic lesions by light microscopy and typical IgA deposition by immunofluorescence. The morphological characteristics, by light microscopy, are extremely

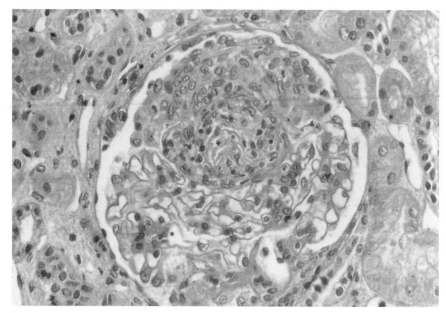

Fig. 4.40 Systemic lupus erythematosus. Focal and segmental form: glomerulus with a segmental area of intracapillary proliferation, exudation and karyorrhexis, surrounded by cellular crescent formation. Remnant of the tuft with some degree of mesangial proliferation (H&E, ×250).

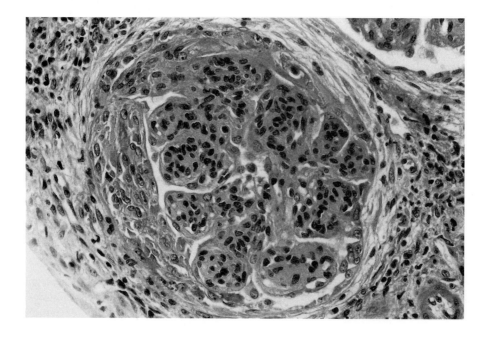

variable, ranging from minimal lesions to mild, moderate, or marked mesangial proliferation, and very different percentages of glomeruli also have segmental or diffuse necrotizing crescentic lesions (Meadow *et al.* 1972; Levy *et al.* 1976; Sinniah *et al.* 1978; Cameron 1984; Fogazzi *et al.* 1989). A true diffuse crescentic glomerulonephritis with a rapidly progressive course has been described, but this is unusual (Mota-Hernandez *et al.* 1975; Sinniah *et al.* 1978; Levy *et al.* 1979). In a recent study, by the Italian Group of Renal Immunopathology, of a series of 219 cases of Henoch–Schönlein nephritis in adults and children, none of the patients had more than 70% of crescents. The great majority of patients show a typical picture of focal and segmental necrotizing glomerulonephritis, similar to that already described for renal vasculitis (Fig. 4.42). Variable degrees of mesangial proliferation and mesangial matrix expansion in glomeruli not involved in crescent formation, or in non-necrotic parts of the glomerular tuft, are other common pictures (Fig. 4.42). Mild to marked interstitial leucocyte infiltration is frequently present, with a tendency to periglomerular localization, especially in cases with more marked crescentic lesions.

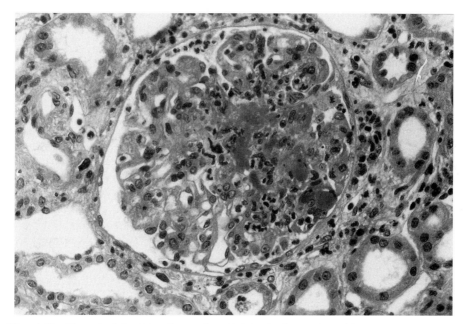

Fig. 4.42 Henoch–Schönlein glomerulonephritis. A glomerulus with a segmental necrotizing lesion; the remnant of the tuft shows important mesangial proliferation and segmental thickening of the 'double contour' basement membranes (Masson trichrome, ×250).

Fig. 4.41 Systemic lupus erythematosus. Diffuse intra-extracapillary form: glomerulus with a circumferential cellular crescent; the glomerular tuft is intensely hypercellular with diffuse thickening of the basement membranes (Masson trichrome, ×250).

Immunohistochemical studies show positivity for VCAM-1 in delineated areas of the glomerular tuft, and accumulation of leucocytes around glomeruli affected by crescent formation. By definition, immunofluorescence is characterized by mesangial and/or parietal deposition of IgA, together with IgG and C3 in a variable percentage of cases. Fibrin is positive in segmental areas of tuft necrosis and extracapillary proliferation.

Essential mixed cryoglobulinaemia

Renal involvement is frequent in this condition, especially in type II essential mixed cryoglobulinaemia (EMC), and is characterized by a peculiar picture of membranoproliferative exudative glomerulonephritis (Monga *et al.* 1976; Ferrario *et al.* 1986). The glomeruli show intense hypercellularity, mainly due to massive infiltration of monocytes, diffuse thickening of basement membranes with a 'double contour' appearance, and frequent presence of intraluminal thrombi totally filling the capillary lumen (Ferrario *et al.* 1985). In addition, there is an acute vasculitis of small- and medium-sized arteries in at least one-third of the patients (Gorevic *et al.* 1980; D'Amico *et al.* 1989). In our experience of 100 cases of EMC with renal involvement, small focal and segmental crescents were present in a minority of patients; however, diffuse circumferential crescents were never seen.

Primary glomerulonephritis

Berger's disease (IgA nephropathy)

Diffuse crescentic glomerulonephritis with a rapidly progressive course has been described in both adults and children, but only in a small percentage of patients (< 10%) (D'Amico *et al.* 1981; Abuelo *et al.* 1984; Levy *et al.* 1985; Welch *et al.* 1988). However, in about a third of patients, the presence of small segmental crescents has been reported by the majority of authors (Shigematsu *et al.* 1982; Bennett and Kincaid-Smith 1983; Abe *et al.* 1986; Katafuchi *et al.* 1994). The percentage of glomeruli involved is generally low (20–40% of glomeruli) but many data, including those from repeat biopsies, strongly suggest that extracapillary lesions are important in the progression of the disease, by repeated formation and accumulation of these lesions (Abe *et al.* 1986; Katafuchi *et al.* 1994). In some of these patients, segmental areas of intracapillary necrosis co-exist with crescents (Fig. 4.43). In the immunohistochemical study of a selected population of 54 patients with Berger's glomerulonephritis, half with features of intracapillary necrosis, we found strong positivity for VCAM-1 in well-delineated areas of the tuft, surrounded by accumulation of monocytes/macrophages, only in the 26 cases with necrotizing crescentic lesions, whereas there were no such features in the 28 cases with pure mesangial glomerulonephritis. The two groups also differed with regard to the presence and intensity of periglomerular leucocyte infiltration. Increased numbers of glomerular and interstitial monocytes were also reported by Li *et al.* (1990) in five cases of crescentic IgA nephritis, with fewer cells in 18 non-crescentic cases. By immunofluorescence, in addition to the

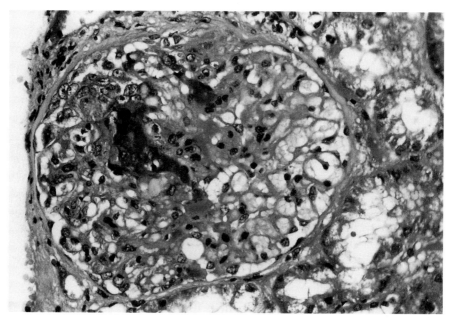

Fig. 4.43 Berger's disease. A segmental area of tuft necrosis with a small extracapillary reaction (Masson trichrome, ×250).

obvious presence of IgA deposits, fibrinogen is strongly positive in segmental areas of glomerular necrosis.

The morphological and immunohistochemical similarities of both necrotizing forms of Henoch–Schönlein purpura and segmental forms of renal vasculitis suggest that, in Berger's disease, it is also possible to find cases with 'capillaritis' associated with mesangial proliferative lesions (Ferrario *et al.* 1995). The relationship between Henoch–Schönlein nephritis and primary IgA nephropathy is now widely recognized (Meadow and Scott 1985; Clarkson 1987; Waldo 1988; Levy *et al.* 1989; Montoliou *et al.* 1990). In the multi-centre study of 219 cases of Henoch–Schönlein nephritis, performed by the Italian Group of Renal Immunopathology, 8.5% of patients were initially considered to have primary IgA nephropathy but developed systemic symptoms, such as purpura, after only a mean one-year follow-up period.

Membranous glomerulonephritis

There have been sporadic reports of membranous nephropathy evolving into acute crescentic rapidly progressive glomerulonephritis (Nicholson *et al.* 1975; Moorthy *et al.* 1975; Kurky *et al.* 1984; Abreo *et al.* 1986; Koethe *et al.* 1986). Interestingly, three cases had anti-GBM disease concomitantly (Kurky *et al.* 1984). For all the cases reported, the morphological picture was similar to that of the previously described extracapillary forms. Obviously, the thickening of the basement membrane and typical subepithelial deposits are of diagnostic value.

Membranoproliferative glomerulonephritis

Fifteen to twenty per cent of cases of membranoproliferative glomerulonephritis, both type I (subendothelial deposits) and type II (dense deposit disease), can present with some crescents. Diffuse circumferential crescentic glomerulonephritis with more than 60% of crescents is a rare occurrence (McCoy *et al.* 1975; Kleinknecht *et al.* 1980; Cameron *et al.* 1983; Korzets *et al.* 1987). In a recent multi-centre study by the Italian Group of Renal Immunopathology, of 368 cases of primary membranoproliferative glomerulonephritis (329 cases of type I and 39 cases of type II) there was a diffuse crescentic form in only 8 cases (2%).

The morphological picture is characterized by a typical circumferential crescent homogeneously filling Bowman's space and by well-recognizable membranoproliferative alterations of the glomerular tuft, both with the classic and the more nodular pattern (Figs 4.44, 4.45). Immunofluorescence is important for differential diagnosis from other forms of crescentic glomerulonephritis, showing typical diffuse and intense mesangioparietal deposits of C3 in the majority of cases, followed by IgG and rarely IgM. Fibrinogen is positive in crescents but negative in the glomerular tuft. Electron microscopy is useful for the more clear detection of mesangial and parietal subendothelial deposits and is frequently diagnostic for type II membranoproliferative forms with typical dense intramembranous deposits.

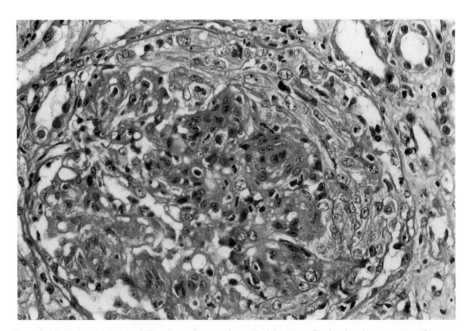

Fig. 4.44 Membranoproliferative glomerulonephritis type I. A classic pattern of membranoproliferative glomerulonephritis surrounded by a circumferential crescent. No intracapillary necrotizing areas (Masson trichrome, ×250).

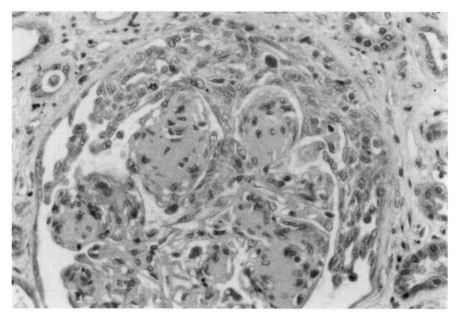

Fig. 4.45 Membranoproliferative glomerulonephritis type I. Nodular pattern of membranoproliferative glomerulonephritis. Glomerular alterations and the circumferential crescent are clearly delineated (Masson trichrome, ×250).

'Idiopathic' rapidly progressive glomerulonephritis

The term 'idiopathic' rapidly progressive glomerulonephritis has been used interchangeably, sometimes describing crescentic glomerulonephritis with no systemic involvement (Cohen *et al.* 1981; Glassock 1985), or immune complex-mediated forms without evidence of a clear primary glomerulopathy (Beirne *et al.* 1977; Heptinstall 1992), or, more recently, 'pauci-immune' necrotizing crescentic nephritis with no evidence of systemic vasculitis (Couser 1988; Jennette and Falk 1994). In fact, as described earlier, many patients, with 'idiopathic' immunofluorescence-negative, crescentic glomerulonephritis have features in common with patients whose morphological picture is that of vasculitis, and may actually be considered to have a pauci-symptomatic variant of systemic vasculitis confined primarily to the glomerular capillaries (Velosa 1987; Cameron 1988; Bindi *et al.* 1993; Jennette and Falk 1994; Pettersson *et al.* 1995).

What is still debated is whether all patients previously classified as 'idiopathic' RPGN are in fact patients with renal limited vasculitis. Couser (1988) stated that '*not all patients with idiopathic RPGN demonstrated focal necrotizing glomerular lesions and the possibility that other non-vasculitic disease mechanisms are included in this category cannot be excluded.*' We carried out a critical re-evaluation of 41 patients, clinically and morphologically classified as having 'idiopathic' crescentic glomerulonephritis because they had no evidence of systemic disease, no anti-GBM nephritis, and no clearly defined glomerulopathy (Ferrario *et al.* 1994). We

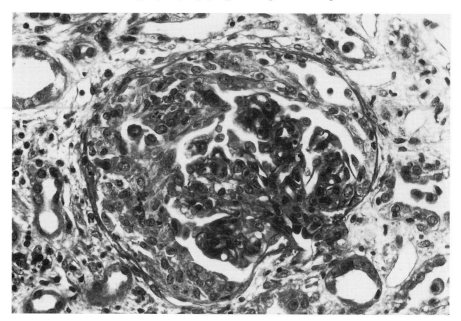

Fig. 4.46 'Idiopathic' crescentic glomerulonephritis. Circumferential crescent totally filling Bowman's space. The glomerular tuft is collapsed, making it difficult to recognize primary glomerulonephritis (Masson trichrome, ×250).

found two distinct morphological patterns. The first was characterized by typical pauci-immune necrotizing crescentic lesions, and, therefore, considered a renal-limited form of vasculitis. The second pattern was characterized by the absence of intracapillary necrosis, and by the presence of some mesangial proliferation, homogeneous circumferential crescents totally filling Bowman's space, and immune deposits more clearly demonstrable by immunofluorescence. The patients in the second group might still be called 'idiopathic', but probably have a non-definable primary chronic proliferative glomerulonephritis complicated by crescent formation. The difficulty in recognizing a clear pattern of primary glomerulonephritis is probably due to severe distortion of the glomerular tuft by massive crescent formation (Fig. 4.46).

References

Abe, T., Kida, H., Yoshimura, M., Yokoyama, H., Koshino, Y., Tomosugi, N. *et al.* (1986). Participation of extracapillary lesions (ECL) in progression of IgA nephropathy. *Clinical Nephrology*, **25**, 37–41.

Abreo, K., Abreo, F., Mitchell, B., and Schloemer, G. (1986). Idiopathic crescentic membranous glomerulonephritis. *American Journal of Kidney Diseases*, **8**, 257–61

Abuelo, J.G., Esparaza, A.R., Matarese, R.A., Endreny, R.G., Carvalho, J.S., and Allagra, S.R. (1984). Crescentic IgA nephropathy. *Medicine*, **63**, 396–406.

Adu, D., Howie, A.J., Scott, D.G.I., Bacon, P.A., McGonigle, R.J.S., and Michael, J. (1987). Polyarteritis and the kidney. *Quarterly Journal of Medicine*, **239**, 221–37.

Agodoa, L.C.Y., Striker, G.E., George, C.R.P., Glassock, R.G., and Quadracci, L.J. (1976). The appearance of non-linear deposits of immunoglobulins in Goodpasture's syndrome. *Clinical Nephrology*, **9**, 77–85.

Alwall, N., Erlanson, P., Tornberg, A., Fajers, C.M., and Moëll, H. (1958). Two cases of acute glomerular nephritis with severe oliguria for 75 days: Clinical course, roentgenological studies on kidney size, and postmortem findings. *Acta Medica Scandinavica*, **161**, 85–96.

Andres, G.A., Brentjens, J., Kohli, R., Anthone, R., Anthone, S., Baliah, T. *et al.* (1978). Histology of human tubulo-interstitial nephritis associated with antibodies to renal basement membrane. *Kidney International*, **13**, 480–91.

Appel, G.B., Silva, F.G., Pirani, C.L., Metzler, J.I., and Estes, D. (1978). Renal involvement in systemic lupus erythematosus. *Medicine*, **57**, 371–410.

Atkins, R.C. and Thomson, N.M. (1993). Rapidly progressive glomerulonephritis. In *Diseases of the kidney* (5th edn), (ed. R.W. Schrier and C.W. Gottschalk) pp. 1689–713. Little, Brown, Boston.

Atkins, R.C., Holdsworth, S.R., Glasgow, E.F., and Mathews, F.E. (1976). The macrophage in human rapidly progressive glomerulonephritis. *Lancet*, **i**, 830–2.

Bacani, R.A., Velasquez, F., Kanter, A., Pirani, C.L., and Pollak, V.E. (1968). Rapidly progressive (non-streptococcal) glomerulonephritis. *Annals of Internal Medicine*, **69**, 463–85.

Bailey, R.R., Simpson, I.J., Lynn, K.L., Neale, T.J., Doak, P.B., and McGiven, A.R (1981). Goodpasture's syndrome with normal renal function. *Clinical Nephrology*, **15**, 211–15.

Baldwin, D.S., Gluck, M-G., Lowenstein, J., and Gallo, G.R. (1977). Lupus nephritis: clinical causes as related to morphological forms and their transitions. *American Journal of Medicine*, **62**, 12–30.

Baldwin, D.S., Neugarten, J., Feiner, H.D., Gluck, M., and Spinowitz, B. (1987). The existence of a protracted course in crescentic glomerulonephritis. *Kidney International*, **31**, 790–4.

Balow, J.E. (1985). Renal vasculitis. *Kidney International*, **27**, 954–64.

Bathena, D.B., Migdal, S.D., Julian, B.A., McMorrow, R.G., and Baehler, R.W. (1987). Morphological and immunohistochemical observations in granulomatous glomerulonephritis. *American Journal of Pathology*, **126**, 581–91.

Beirne, G.J., Wagnild, J.P., Zimmerman, S.W., Mackem, P.D., and Burkholder, P.M. (1977). Idiopathic crescentic glomerulonephritis. *Medicine*, **56**, 349–81.

Bennett, W.M. and Kincaid-Smith, P. (1983). Macroscopic haematuria in mesangial IgA nephropathy: correlation with glomerular crescents and renal dysfunction. *Kidney International*, **23**, 393–400.

Berlyne, G. and Baker, J.S. (1964). Acute anuric glomerulonephritis. *Quarterly Journal of Medicine*, **33**, 105–15.

Bindi, P., Mougenot, B., Mentre, F., Noel, L.H., Peraldi, M.N., Vanhille, P. *et al.* (1993). Necrotizing crescentic glomerulonephritis without significant immune deposits: a clinical and serological study. *Quarterly Journal of Medicine*, **86**, 55–68.

Bohman, S.O., Olsen, S., and Petersen, V.P. (1974). Glomerular ultrastructure in extracapillary glomerulonephritis. *Acta Pathologica et Microbiologica Scandinavica*, **249**, 29–54.

Bolton, W.K., Innes, D.J., Jr., Sturgill, B.C., and Kaiser, D.L. (1987). T-cells and macrophages in rapidly progressive glomerulonephritis: clinicopathologic correlations. *Kidney International*, **32**, 869–76.

Bonsib, S.M. (1985). Glomerular basement membrane discontinuities. Scanning electron microscopy study of acellular glomeruli. *American Journal of Pathology*, 119, 357–60.

Bonsib, S.M. (1988). Glomerular basement membrane necrosis and crescent organization. *Kidney International*, 33, 966–74.

Border, W.A., Baehler, R.W., Bathena, D., and Glassock, R.J. (1979). IgA antibasement membrane nephritis with pulmonary hemorrhage. *Annals of Internal Medicine*, 91, 21–5.

Boucher, A., Droz, D., Adafer, E., and Noel, L.H. (1987). Relationship between the integrity of Bowman's capsule and the composition of cellular crescents in human crescentic glomerulonephritis. *Laboratory Investigation*, 56, 526–33.

Briggs, W.A., Johnson, J.P., Teichman, S., Yeager, H.C., and Wilson, C.B. (1979). Antiglomerular basement membrane antibody-mediated glomerulonephritis and Goodpasture's syndrome. *Medicine*, 58, 348–61.

Brun, C., Gormsen, H., Hilden, T., Iversen, P., and Raaschou, F. (1958). Kidney biopsy in acute glomerulonephritis. *Acta Medica Scandinavica*, 160, 155–64.

Burkholder, P.M. (1969). Ultrastructure demonstration of injury and perforation of the glomerular capillary basement membrane in acute proliferative glomerulonephritis. *American Journal of Pathology*, 56, 251–65.

Cameron, J.S. (1984). Henoch–Schönlein purpura: clinical presentation. *Contributions to Nephrology*, 40, 246–9.

Cameron, J.S. (1988). Renal disease and vasculitis. *Pediatric Nephrology*, 2, 490–7.

Cameron, J.S. (1991). New horizons in renal vasculitis. *Klinische Wochenschrift*, 69, 536–51.

Cameron, J.S., Turner, D.R., Ogg, C.S., Williams, D.G., Lessof, M.H., Chantler, C. *et al.* (1979). Systemic lupus with nephritis: a long-term study. *Quarterly Journal of Medicine*, 48, 1–24.

Cameron, J.S., Turner, D.R., Heaton, J., Williams, D.G., Ogg, C.S., Chantler, C. *et al.* (1983). Idiopathic mesangiocapillary glomerulonephritis. Comparison of Types I and II in children and adults and long-term prognosis. *American Journal of Medicine*, 74, 175–92.

Cattell, V. (1994). Macrophages in acute glomerular inflammation. *Kidney International*, 45, 945–52.

Cattell, V. and Jamieson, S.W. (1978). The origin of glomerular crescents in experimental nephrotoxic serum nephritis in the rabbit. *Laboratory Investigation*, 391, 589–90.

Chumbley, L.C., Harrison, E.G., and DeRemee, R.A. (1977). Allergic granulomatosis and angiitis (Churg–Strauss syndrome). Report and analysis of 30 cases. *Mayo Clinic Proceedings*, 52, 477–84.

Clarke, B.E., Ham, K.N., Tange, J.D., and Ryan, G.B. (1983). Origin of glomerular crescents in rabbit nephrotoxic nephritis. *Journal of Pathology*, 139, 247–58.

Clarkson, A.R. (1987). Henoch–Schönlein purpura and IgA nephropathy: to separate or unify? In *IgA nephropathy*, (ed. A.R. Clarkson) pp. 39–46. Martinus Nijhoff, Boston.

Clutterbuck, E.J., Evans, D.J., and Pusey, C.D. (1990). Renal involvement in Churg–Strauss syndrome. *Nephrology Dialysis Transplantation*, 5, 1–7.

Cohen, A.H., Border, W.A., Shankel, E., and Glassock, R.J. (1981). Crescentic glomerulonephritis: Immune versus non-immune mechanisms. *American Journal of Nephrology*, 1, 78–83.

Cohen Tervaert, J.W., Goldschmeding, R., Elema, J.D., van der Giessen, M., Huitema, M.G., van der Hem, G.K. *et al.* (1990). Autoantibodies against myeloid lysosomal enzymes in crescentic glomerulonephritis. *Kidney International*, 37, 799–806.

Couser, W.G. (1988). Rapidly progressive glomerulonephritis: Classification, pathogenetic mechanisms, and therapy. *American Journal of Kidney Diseases*, 11, 449–64.

Coward, R.A., Hamdy, N.A.T., Shortland, J.S., and Brown, C.B. (1986). Renal micropolyarteritis: a treatable condition. *Nephrology Dialysis Transplantation*, 1, 31–7.

Croker, B.P., Lee, T., and Gunnels, J.C. (1987). Clinical and pathological features of polyarteritis nodosa and its renal-limited variant: primary crescentic and necrotizing glomerulonephritis. *Human Pathology*, 18, 38–44.

D'Agati, V., Chander, P., Nash, M., and Mancilla-Jimanez, R. (1986). Idiopathic microscopic polyarteritis nodosa: ultrastructural observations on the renal vascular and glomerular lesions. *American Journal of Kidney Diseases*, 7, 95–110.

D'Amico, G., Ferrario, F., Colasanti, G., Ragni, A., and Bestetti-Bosisio, M. (1981). IgA-mesangial nephropathy (Berger's disease) with rapid decline in renal function. *Clinical Nephrology*, 16, 251–7.

D'Amico, G., Colasanti, G., Ferrario, F., and Sinico, R.A. (1989). Renal involvement in essential mixed cryoglobulinemia. *Kidney International*, 35, 1004–14.

Davson, J., Ball, J., and Platt, R. (1948). The kidney in periarteritis nodosa. *Quarterly Journal of Medicine*, 67, 175–202.

Dean, S.E., Saha, S.R., and Ramirez, G. (1991). Systemic vasculitis in Goodpasture's disease. *South Medical Journal* 84, 1387–90.

El Nahas, A.M., Muchaneta-Kubara, E.C., Zhang, G.Z., Adam, A., and Goumenos, D. (1996). Phenotypic modulation of renal cells during experimental and clinical renal scarring. *Kidney International*, 49, S23–7.

Ellis, A. (1942). Natural history of Brights' disease. Clinical, histological and experimental observations. *Lancet*, i, 34–6.

Fairley, C., Mathewson, D.C., and Becker, G.J. (1987). Rapid development of diffuse crescents in post-streptococcal glomerulonephritis. *Clinical Nephrology*, 28, 256–60.

Falk, R.J. and Jennette, J.C. (1988). Anti-neutrophil cytoplasmic autoantibodies with specificity for myeloperoxidase in patients with systemic vasculitis and idiopathic necrotizing and crescentic glomerulonephritis. *New England Journal of Medicine*, 318, 1651–7.

Fauci, A.S. (1978). The spectrum of vasculitis. *Annals of Internal Medicine*, 89, 660–76.

Ferrario, F., Castiglione, A., Colasanti, G., Barbiano di Belgioioso, G., Bertoli, S., and D'Amico, G. (1985). The detection of monocytes in human glomerulonephritis. *Kidney International*, 28, 513–19.

Ferrario, F., Colasanti, G., Barbiano di Belgioioso, G., Banfi, G., Campise, M.R., Confalonieri, R. *et al.* (1986). Histological and immunohistological features in essential mixed cryoglobulinemia glomerulonephritis. In *Antiglobulins, cryoglobulins and glomerulonephritis*, (ed. C. Ponticelli, L. Minetti, and G. D'Amico) pp. 193–202. Martinus Nijhoff, Dordrecht.

Ferrario, F., D'Amico, G., Napodano, P., Tadros, M., Rastaldi, M.P., and Sinico, R.A. (1993). Morphological basis for a new classification of rapidly progressive glomerulonephritis. In *Issues in nephrosciences*, (ed. G. D'Amico and G. Colasanti) pp. 3–11. Wichtig, Milan.

Ferrario, F., Tadros, M.T., Napodano, P., Sinico, R.A., Fellin, G., and D'Amico, G. (1994). Critical re-evaluation of 41 cases of 'idiopathic' crescentic glomerulonephritis. *Clinical Nephrology*, 41, 1–9.

Ferrario, F., Napodano, P., Rastaldi, M.P., and D'Amico, G. (1995). Capillaritis in IgA nephropathy. In *IgA nephropathy: pathogenesis and treatment. Contributions to nephrology*, (ed. A.R. Clarkson and A.J. Woodroffe). Vol. III, pp. 8–12. Karger, Basel.

Ferrario, F., Rastaldi, M.P., and D'Amico, G. (1996). The crucial role of renal biopsy in the management of ANCA-associated renal vasculitis. *Nephrology Dialysis Transplantation*, **11**, 726–8.

Fogazzi, G.B., Pasquali, S., Moriggi, M., Casanova, S., Damilano, I., Mihatsch, M.J. *et al.* (1989). Long-term outcome of Schönlein-Henoch nephritis in the adult. *Clinical Nephrology*, **31**, 60–6.

Fuiano, G., Cameron, J.S., Raftery, M., Hartley, B.H., Williams, D.G., and Ogg, C.S. (1988). Improved prognosis of renal microscopic polyarteritis in recent years. *Nephrology Dialysis Transplantation*, **3**, 383–91.

Furlong, T.J., Ibels, L.S., and Eckstein, R.P. (1987). The clinical spectrum of necrotizing glomerulonephritis. *Medicine*, **66**, 192–201.

Gans, R.O.B., Kuizinga, M.C., Goldschmeding, R., Assmann, K., Huysmans, F.T.M., Gerlag, P.G.G. *et al.* (1993). Clinical features and outcome in patients with glomerulonephritis and antineutrophil cytoplasmic autoantibodies. *Nephron*, **64**, 182–8.

Gill, D.G., Turner, D.R., Chantler, C., and Cameron, J.S. (1977). The progression of acute proliferative poststreptococcal glomerulonephritis to severe epithelial crescent formation. *Clinical Nephrology*, **8**, 449–52.

Glassock, R.G. (1978). A clinical and immunopathological dissection of rapidly progressive glomerulonephritis. *Nephron*, **22**, 253–65.

Glassock, R.G. (1985). Natural history and treatment of primary proliferative glomerulonephritis: a review. *Kidney International*, **17**, S136–142.

Glassock, R.G., Cohen, A.H., Adler, S.G., and Ward, H.J. (1991). Secondary glomerular diseases. In *The kidney* (4th edn.), (ed. B.M. Brenner and F.C. Rector, Jr.) pp. 1280–1368. Saunders, Philadelphia.

Gordon, M., Luqmani, R.A., Adu, D., Greaves, I., Richards, N., Michael, J. *et al.* (1993). Relapses in patients with a systemic vasculitis. *Quarterly Journal of Medicine*, **86**, 779–89.

Gorevic, P.D., Kassab, H.J., Levo, Y., Kohn, R., Meltzer, M., Prose, P. *et al.* (1980). Mixed cryoglobulinemia: clinical aspects and long-term follow-up of 40 patients. *American Journal of Medicine*, **69**, 287–308.

Gris, P., Pirson, Y., Hamels, J., Vaerman, J.P., Quiodbach, A., and Demol, H. (1991). Antiglomerular basement membrane nephritis induced by IgA1 antibodies. *Nephron*, **58**, 418–24.

Guettier, C., Nochy, D., Jacquot, C., Mandet, C., Camilleri, J.P., and Bariety, J. (1986). Immunohistochemical demonstration of parietal epithelial cells and macrophages in human proliferative extra-capillary lesions. *Virchows Archive (Pathology and Anatomy)*, **409**, 739–48.

Hamburger, J. (1956). Les glomerulo-nephrites malignes. In *Entretiens de Bichat*, Vol. 1. Expansion, Paris.

Hancock, W.W. and Atkins, R.C. (1984). Cellular composition of crescents in human rapidly progressive glomerulonephritis identified using monoclonal antibodies. *American Journal of Nephrology*, **3**, 177–81.

Harrison, C.V., Loughridge, L.W., and Milne, M.D. (1964). Acute oliguric renal failure in acute glomerulonephritis and polyarteritis. *Quarterly Journal of Medicine*, **129**, 39–55.

Harrison, D.J. and MacDonald, M.K. (1986). The origin of cells in the glomerular crescent investigated by the use of monoclonal antibodies. *Histopathology*, **10**, 945–52.

Heptinstall, R.H. (1992). Crescentic glomerulonephritis. In *Pathology of the kidney* (4th edn), (ed. R.H. Heptinstall) pp. 627–75. Little, Brown, Boston.

Hill, G.S. (1992). Systemic lupus erythematosus and mixed connective-tissue disease. In *Pathology of the kidney* (4th edn), (ed. R.H. Heptinstall) pp. 871–950. Little, Brown, Boston.

Hoffman, G.S., Leavitt, R.Y., Fleisher, T.A., Minor, J.R., and Fauci, A.S. (1990). Treatment of Wegener's granulomatosis with intermittent high-dose intravenous cyclophosphamide. *American Journal of Medicine*, **89**, 403–10.

Hoffman, G.S., Kerr, G.S., Leavitt, R.Y., Hallahan, C.W., Lebovics, R.S., Travis, W.D. *et al.* (1992). Wegener's granulomatosis: an analysis of 158 patients. *Annals of Internal Medicine*, **116**, 488–98.

Holdsworth, S.R., Allen, D., Thomson, N.M., Glasgow, E.F., and Atkins, R.C. (1980). Histochemistry of glomerular cells in animal models of crescentic glomerulonephritis. *Pathology*, **12**, 339–346.

Hooke, D.H., Gee, D.C., and Atkins, R.C. (1987). Leukocyte analysis using monoclonal antibodies in human glomerulonephritis. *Kidney International*, **31**, 964–72.

Jennette, J.C. (1991). Antineutrophil cytoplasmic autoantibody-associated diseases: a pathologist's perspective. *American Journal of Kidney Diseases*, **18**, 164–70.

Jennette, J.C. and Falk, R.J. (1994). The pathology of vasculitis involving the kidney. *American Journal of Kidney Diseases*, **24**, 130–41.

Jennette, J.C. and Hipp, C.G. (1985). The epithelial cell antigen phenotype of glomerular crescent cells. *American Journal of Clinical Pathology*, **86**, 274–80.

Jennette, J.C., Falk, R.J., Andrassy, K., Bacon, P.A., Churg, J., Gross, W.L. *et al.* (1994). Nomenclature of systemic vasculitides: Proposal of an international consensus conference. *Arthritis and Rheumatism*, **37**, 187–92.

Juncos, L.I., Alexander, R.W., and Marbury, T.C. (1979). Intravascular clotting preceding crescent formation in a patient with Wegener's granulomatosis and rapidly progressive glomerulonephritis. *Nephron*, **24**, 17–20.

Kaslowsky, S., McKay, D.G., Howes, E.L. Jr, Csavossy, I., and Wolfson, M. (1976). Multinucleated giant cells in antiglomerular basement membrane antibody-induced glomerulonephritis. *Nephron*, **16**, 415–26.

Katafuchi, R., Oh, Y., Hori, K., Komota, T., Yanase, T., Ikeda, K. *et al.* (1994). An important role of glomerular segmental lesions on progression of IgA nephropathy: a multivariate analysis. *Clinical Nephrology*, **41**, 191–8.

Kleinknecht, D., Kourilsky, O., Morel-Maroger, L., Adhemar, J.P., Droz, D., Masselot, J.P. *et al.* (1980). Dense deposit disease with rapidly progressive renal failure in a narcotic addict. *Clinical Nephrology*, **14**, 309–12.

Koethe, J.D., Gerig, J.S., Glickman, J.L., Sturgill, B.C., and Bolton, W.K. (1986). Progression of membranous nephropathy to acute crescentic rapidly progressive glomerulonephritis and response to pulse methylprednisolone. *American Journal of Nephrology*, **6**, 224–8.

Korzets, Z., Bernheim, J., and Bernheim, J. (1987). Rapidly progressive glomerulonephritis (crescentic glomerulonephritis) in the course of type I idiopathic membranoproliferative glomerulonephritis. *American Journal of Kidney Diseases*, **10**, 56–61.

Kurky, P., Helve, T., von Bonsdorff, M., Tornroth, T., Pettersson, E., Riska, H. *et al.* (1984). Transformation of membranous glomerulonephritis into crescentic glomerulonephritis with glomerular basement membrane antibodies: serial determinations of anti-GBM before the transformation. *Nephron*, **38**, 134–7.

Lan, H.Y., Paterson, D.J., and Atkins, R.C. (1991). Initiation and evolution of interstitial leukocytic infiltration in experimental glomerulonephritis. *Kidney International*, **40**, 425–433.

Langhans, T. (1885). Über die entzündlichen Veränderungen der Glomeruli und die acute Nephritis. *Virchows Archive (Pathology and Anatomy)*, **99**, 193–204.

Lanham, J.G., Elkon, K.B., Pusey, C.D., and Hughes, G.R. (1984). Systemic vasculitis with asthma and eosinophilia: a clinical approach to the Churg–Strauss syndrome. *Medicine*, **63**, 65–81.

Levy, M. and the French Cooperative Group of the Society of Nephrology. (1989). Familial cases of Berger's disease and anaphylactoid purpura: more frequent than previously thought. *American Journal of Medicine*, **87**, 246–8.

Levy, M., Broyer, M., Arsan, A., Levy-Bentolila, D., and Habib, R. (1976). Anaphylactoid purpura nephritis in childhood: natural history and immunopathology. *Advances in Nephrology*, **6**, 183–228.

Levy, M., Broyer, M., and Habib, R. (1979). Pathology and immunopathology of Schönlein–Henoch nephritis. In *Progress in glomerulonephritis*, (ed. P. Kincaid-Smith, A.J.F. D'Apice, and R.C. Atkins) pp. 261–81. Wiley, New York.

Levy, M., Gonzales-Burchard, G., Broyer, M., Dommergues, J.P., Foulard, M., Sorez, J.P. *et al.* (1985). Berger's disease in children: natural history and outcome. *Medicine*, **64**, 157–80.

Li, H.L., Hancock, W.W., Hooke, D.H., Dowling, J.P., and Atkins, R.C. (1990). Mononuclear cell activation and decreased renal function in IgA nephropathy with crescents. *Kidney International*, **37**, 1552–6.

Lölein, M. (1910). Über Nephritis nach dem heutigen Stande der pathologischanatomischen Forschung. *Ergeb. Inn. Med. Kinderheilkd.*, **5**, 411–23.

Magil, A.B. and Wadsworth, L.D. (1982). Monocyte involvement in glomerular crescents. *Laboratory Investigation*, **47**, 160–6.

McCluskey, R.T., Brentjens, J., and Andres, G.A. (1974). Tubular and interstitial renal diseases produced by immunologic mechanisms. *La Ricerca Clinica e di Laboratorio*, **4**, 795–821.

McCoy, R., Clapp, J., and Seigler, H.F. (1975). Membranoproliferative glomerulonephritis. Progression from the pure form to the crescentic form with recurrence after transplantation. *American Journal of Medicine*, **59**, 288–92.

McLeish, K.R., Yum, M.N., and Luft, F.C. (1978). Rapidly progressive glomerulonephritis in adults: clinical and histologic correlations. *Clinical Nephrology*, **10**, 43–50.

McPhaul, J.J., Jr. and Mullins, J.D. (1976). Glomerulonephritis mediated by antibody to glomerular basement membrane: immunological, clinical, and histopathological characteristics. *Journal of Clinical Investigation*, **57**, 351–61.

Meadow, S.R. and Scott, D.G. (1985). Berger disease: Henoch–Schönlein syndrome without the rash. *Journal of Pediatrics*, **106**, 27–32.

Meadow, S.R., Glasgow, E.F., White, R.H.R., Moncrieff, M.W., Cameron, J.S., and Ogg, C.S. (1972). Schönlein–Henoch nephritis. *Quarterly Journal of Medicine*, **41**, 241–258.

Min, K.W., Györkey, F., Györkey, P., Yium, J.J., and Eknoyan, G. (1974). The morphogenesis of glomerular crescents in rapidly progressive glomerulonephritis. *Kidney International*, **5**, 47–56.

Monga, G., Mazzucco, G., Coppo, R., Piccoli, G., and Coda, R. (1976). Glomerular findings in mixed IgG-IgM cryoglobulinemia. Light, electron microscopy, immunofluorescence and histochemical correlations. *Virchows Archive (Cell Pathology)*, **20**, 185–96.

Montoliou, J., Lens, X.M., Torras, A., and Revert, L. (1990). Henoch–Schönlein purpura and IgA nephropathy in father and son. *Nephron*, **54**, 77–9.

Moorthy, A.V., Zimmerman, S.W., Burkholder, P.M., and Harrington, A.R. (1975). Association of crescentic glomerulonephritis with membranous nephropathy: a report of three cases. *Clinical Nephrology*, **6**, 319–25.

Morita, T., Suzuki, Y., and Churg, J. (1973). Structure and development of the glomerular crescent. *American Journal of Pathology*, **72**, 349–59.

Morrin, P.A., Hinglais, N., Nabarra, B., and Kreis, H. (1978). Rapidly progressive glomerulonephritis. A clinical and pathologic study. *American Journal of Medicine*, **65**, 446–60.

Mota-Hernandez, F., Valbuena-Paz, R., and Gordillo-Paniagua, G. (1975). Long-term prognosis of anaphylactoid purpura nephropathy. *Pediatrician*, **4**, 52–9.

Müller, G.A., Müller, C.A., Markovic-Lipkovski, J., Kilper, R.B., and Risler, T. (1988). Renal major histocompatibility complex antigens and cellular components in rapidly progressive glomerulonephritis identified by monoclonal antibodies. *Nephron*, **49**, 132–9.

Nachman, P.H., Hogan, S.L., Jennette, J.C., and Falk, R. (1996). Treatment response and relapse in antineutrophil cytoplasmic autoantibody-associated microscopic polyangiitis and glomerulonephritis. *Journal of the American Society of Nephrology*, **7**, 33–9.

Neild, G.H., Cameron, J.S., Ogg, C.S., Turner, D.R., Williams, D.G., Brown, C.B. *et al.* (1983). Rapidly progressive glomerulonephritis with extensive glomerular crescent formation. *Quarterly Journal of Medicine*, **52**, 395–416.

Nicholson, G.D., Amin, U.F., and Alleyne, G.A. (1975). Membranous glomerulonephropathy with crescents. *Clinical Nephrology*, **4**, 198–201.

Nolasco, F.E.B., Cameron, J.S., Hartley, B., Coelho, A., Hildreth, G., and Reuben, R. (1987). Intraglomerular T cells and monocytes in nephritis: study with monoclonal antibodies. *Kidney International*, **31**, 1160–6.

Nölle, B., Specks, U., Lüdemann, J., Rohrbach, M.S., DeRemee, R.A., and Gross, W.L. (1989). Anticytoplasmic autoantibodies: their immunodiagnostic value in Wegener's granulomatosis. *Annals of Internal Medicine*, **111**, 28–40.

Pasternack, A., Tornroth, T., and Linder, E. (1978). Evidence of both anti-GBM and immune complex mediated pathogenesis in the initial phase of Goodpasture's syndrome. *Clinical Nephrology*, **9**, 77–85.

Pettersson, E. and Heigl, Z. (1992). Antineutrophil cytoplasmic antibody (cANCA and pANCA) titers in relation to disease activity in patients with necrotizing vasculitis: a longitudinal study. *Clinical Nephrology*, **37**, 219–28.

Pettersson, E., Tornroth, T., and Miettinen, A. (1984). Simultaneous antiglomerular basement membrane and membranous glomerulonephritis: case report and literature review. *Clinical Immunology and Immunopathology*, **31**, 171–80.

Pettersson, E., Sundelin, B., and Heigl, Z. (1995). Incidence and outcome of pauci-immune necrotizing and crescentic glomerulonephritis in adults. *Clinical Nephrology*, **43**, 141–9.

Pollak, V.E. and Pirani, C.L. (1969). Renal histologic findings in systemic lupus erythematosus. *Mayo Clinic Proceedings*, **44**, 630–44.

Poskitt, T.R. (1970). Immunologic and electron microscopy findings in Goodpasture's syndrome. *American Journal of Medicine*, **49**, 250–7.

Pusey, C.D., Rees, A.J., Evans, D.J., Peters, D.K., and Lockwood, C.M. (1991). Plasma exchange in focal necrotizing glomerulonephritis without anti-GBM antibodies. *Kidney International*, **40**, 757–63.

Rastaldi, M.P., Ferrario, F., Tunesi, S., Yang, L., and D'Amico, G. (1996). Intraglomerular and interstitial leukocyte infiltration, adhesion molecules, and interleukin-1α expression in 15 cases of antineutrophil cytoplasmic autoantibody-associated renal vasculitis. *American Journal of Kidney Diseases*, **27**, 48–57.

Rees, A.J. and Cameron, J.S. (1992). Crescentic glomerulonephritis. In *Oxford textbook of clinical nephrology*, (ed. J.S. Cameron, A.M. Davison, J.P. Grunfeld, D. Kerr, and E. Ritz) pp. 418–38. Oxford University Press.

Rees, A.J., Lockwood, C.M., and Peters, D.K. (1977). Enhanced allergic tissue damage in Goodpasture's syndrome by intercurrent bacterial infection. *British Medical Journal*, ii, 723–6.

Richman, A.V., Rifkin, S.T., and McAllister, C.J. (1981). Rapidly progressive glomerulonephritis: combined antiglomerular basement membrane antibody and immune complex pathogenesis. *Human Pathology*, **12**, 597–604.

Ronco, P., Verroust, P., Mignon, F., Kourilsky, O., Vanhille, P., Meyrier, A. *et al.* (1983). Immunopathological studies of polyarteritis nodosa and Wegener's granulomatosis: a report of 43 patients with 51 renal biopsies. *Quarterly Journal of Medicine*, **52**, 212–23.

Salant, D.J. (1987). Immunopathogenesis of crescentic glomerulonephritis and lung purpura. *Kidney International*, **32**, 408–25.

Saraf, P., Berger, H.W., and Thung, S.N. (1978). Goodpasture's syndrome with no overt renal disease. *Mount Sinai Journal of Medicine*, **45**, 451–4.

Savage, C.O.S., Winearls, C.G., Evans, D.J., Rees, A.J., and Lockwood, C.M. (1985). Microscopic polyarteritis: presentation, pathology and prognosis. *Quarterly Journal of Medicine*, **56**, 467–83.

Savage, C.O.S., Pusey, C.D., Bowman, C., Rees, A.J., and Lockwood, C.M. (1986). Antiglomerular basement membrane antibody mediated disease in the British Isles 1980–1984. *British Medical Journal*, **292**, 301–4.

Serra, A., Cameron, J.S., Turner, D.R., Hartley, B., Ogg, C.S., Neild, G.H. *et al.* (1984). Vasculitis affecting the kidney: Presentation, histopathology and long-term outcome. *Quarterly Journal of Medicine*, **210**, 181–207.

Shigematsu, H., Kobayashi, Y., Tateno, S., Hiki, Y., and Kuwao, S. (1982). Ultrastructural glomerular loop abnormalities in IgA nephropathy. *Nephron*, **30**, 1–7.

Silva, F.G., Hoyer, J.R., and Pirani, C.L. (1984). Sequential studies of glomerular crescent formation in rats with antiglomerular basement membrane-induced glomerulonephritis and the role of coagulation factors. *Laboratory Investigation*, **51**, 404–15.

Sinico, R.A., Radice, A., Pozzi, C., Ferrario, F., Arrigo, G., and the Italian Group of Renal Immunopathology (1994). Diagnostic significance and antigen specificity of antineutrophil cytoplasmic antibodies in renal diseases. A prospective multicentre study. *Nephrology Dialysis Transplantation*, **9**, 505–10.

Sinniah, R., Feng, P.H., and Chen, B.T.M. (1978). Henoch–Schönlein syndrome: a clinical and morphologic study of renal biopsies. *Clinical Nephrology*, **9**, 219–28.

Stachura, I., Si, L., and Whiteside, T.L. (1984). Mononuclear-cell subsets in human idiopathic crescentic glomerulonephritis (ICGN): analysis in tissue sections with monoclonal antibodies. *Journal of Clinical Immunology*, **4**, 202–8.

Stave, G.M. and Crocker, B.P. (1984). Thrombotic microangiopathy in antiglomerular basement membrane glomerulonephritis. *Archives of Pathology and Laboratory Medicine*, **108**, 747–51.

Stejskal, J., Pirani, C.L., Okada, M., Mandelenakis, N., and Pollak, V.E. (1973). Discontinuities (gaps) of the glomerular capillary wall and basement membrane in renal diseases. *Laboratory Investigation*, **28**, 149–69.

Stilmant, M.M., Bolton, W.K., Sturgill, B.C., Schmitt, G.W., and Couser, W.G. (1979). Crescentic glomerulonephritis without immune deposits: clinicopathologic features. *Kidney International*, **15**, 184–95.

Striker, L., Killen, P.D., Chi, E., and Striker, G.E. (1984). The composition of glomerulosclerosis: I. Studies in focal sclerosis, crescentic glomerulonephritis, and membranoproliferative glomerulonephritis. *Laboratory Investigation*, **51**, 181–92.

Teague, C., Doak, P., Simpson, I., Rainer, S., and Herdson, D. (1978). Goodpasture's syndrome: analysis of 29 cases. *Kidney International*, **13**, 492–503.

Velosa, J.A. (1987). Idiopathic crescentic glomerulonephritis or systemic vasculitis. *Mayo Clinic Proceedings*, **62**, 145–7.

Volhard, F. and Fahr, T. (1914). *Die Brightsche Nierenkrankheit*. Springer, Berlin.

Waldo, F.B. (1988). Is Henoch–Schönlein purpura the systemic form of IgA nephropathy? *American Journal of Kidney Diseases*, **12**, 373–7.

Wahls, T.L., Bonsib, S.M., and Schuster, V.L. (1987). Coexistent Wegener's granulomatosis and anti-glomerular basement membrane disease. *Human Pathology*, **18**, 202–5.

Welch, T.R., McAdams, A.J., and Berry, A. (1988). Rapidly progressive IgA nephropathy. *American Journal of Diseases of Childhood*, **142**, 789–93.

Wilkowsky, M.J., Velosa, J.A., Holley, K.E., Offord, K.P., Chu, C., Torres, V.E. *et al.* (1989). Risk factors in idiopathic renal vasculitis and glomerulonephritis. *Kidney International*, **36**, 1133–41.

Wilson, C.B. (1991). The renal response to immunological injury. In *The kidney*. (4th edn), (ed. B.M. Brenner and F.C. Rector, Jr.) pp. 1062–181. Saunders, Philadelphia.

Wilson, C.B. and Dixon F.J. (1986). The renal response to immunological injury. In *The kidney*, (3rd edn), (ed. B.M. Brenner and F.C. Rector) pp. 800–900. Saunders, Philadelphia.

Wilson, C.B. and Dixon, F.J. (1973). Antiglomerular basement membrane antibody-induced glomerulonephritis. *Kidney International*, **3**, 74–89.

Wilson, C.B. and Dixon, F.J. (1979). Renal injury from immune reactions involving antigens in or of the kidney. In *Immunologic mechanisms of renal disease*, (ed. C.B. Wilson, B.M. Brenner, and J.H. Stein) pp. 35–66. Churchill Livingstone, New York.

Whitworth, J.A., Morel-Maroger, L., Mignon, F., and Richet, G. (1976). The significance of extracapillary proliferation. Clinicopathological review of 60 patients. *Nephron*, **16**, 1–19.

Yoshioka, K., Takemura, T., Akano, N., Miyamoto, H., Iseki, T., and Maki, S. (1987). Cellular and non-cellular composition of crescents in human glomerulonephritis. *Kidney International*, **32**, 284–91.

Yoshioka, K., Takemura, T., Tohda, M., Akano, N., Miyamoto, H., Ooshima, A. *et al.* (1989). Glomerular localization of type III collagen in human kidney disease. *Kidney International*, **35**, 1203–10.

Zeek, P.M. (1953). Periarteritis nodosa and other forms of necrotizing angitis. *New England Journal of Medicine*, **248**, 764–72.

5

Anti-glomerular basement membrane disease

A. Neil Turner and Andrew J. Rees

Ernest Goodpasture reported a single patient with lung haemorrhage and rapidly progressive glomerulonephritis (RPGN) while on leave from his residency at the Massachusetts General Hospital as a pathologist at the Chelsea Naval Hospital (Goodpasture 1919). In retrospect, the patient probably had systemic vasculitis. Goodpasture went on to become a pioneer in developing culture techniques for pathogenic viruses, but his name has remained attached to anti-GBM disease since it was applied by Stanton and Tange (Stanton and Tange 1958). Subsequently, it has become apparent that systemic vasculitis is a more common cause of lung haemorrhage and RPGN than anti-GBM disease, and it has become necessary to distinguish that syndrome (Goodpasture's syndrome) from anti-GBM disease (Goodpasture's disease), as his name is now firmly associated with the rarer, but better understood, disorder.

Although uncommon, Goodpasture's disease has long served as a model of immune glomerular injury, and has been studied extensively in animal models as well as in man. Treatment originally developed for this disease has been adapted for use in other types of RPGN, and in some instances has been even more successful. In this chapter we discuss the features of spontaneous Goodpasture's disease, then consider two special examples: anti-GBM disease occurring in the setting of systemic vasculitis; and that occurring after renal transplantation in patients with Alport's syndrome.

Clinical features

A number of accounts have described the common features of Goodpasture's disease. Some recent series have contributed extra information on epidemiology and outcome (Beirne *et al.* 1977; Heptinstall 1983; Herody *et al.* 1993; Johnson *et al.* 1985; Kelly and Haponik 1994; Peters *et al.* 1982; Turner and Rees 1996; Wakui *et al.* 1992; Walker *et al.* 1985; Wilson and Dixon 1973; Wilson and Dixon 1981).

While most histological features are similar to those of other types of RPGN, the disease has certain characteristic features, which including the following:

- progression is often very rapid
- biopsy shows many crescents of the same age
- a history suggestive of lung haemorrhage for by months or years

- iron deficiency anaemia (another consequence of lung haemorrhage)
- lung haemorrhage is largely confined to smokers
- lung haemorrhage may occur in isolation, usually subacutely
- renal disease may occur in isolation, usually recognized as RPGN
- lack of other specific symptoms
- renal prognosis is worse than in vasculitis-associated RPGN

Commonly, the disease presents at a time of rapid upregulation of disease severity; lung haemorrhage (when present) becomes severe, and glomerulonephritis becomes crescentic. Either may be life-threatening, and the need for treatment is urgent.

Lungs

Lung haemorrhage occurs in 50–70% of patients, and is largely restricted to cigarette smokers (this is not the case in systemic vasculitis) (Donaghy and Rees 1983; Herody *et al.* 1993). Pulmonary haemorrhage causes breathlessness and cough, while haemoptysis is a late feature in many patients. Radiology shows alveolar shadowing, which may be patchy and asymmetrical, and closely resembles pulmonary oedema (Fig. 5.1). While sparing of peripheries and lung apices is typical, no features reliably distinguish it from other causes of alveolar shadowing. Changes may be brief and resolve within 48 hours after a minor episode of lung haemorrhage (Bowley *et al.* 1979). Infective changes and volume overload will precipitate or exacerbate lung haemorrhage, and may therefore coexist. Every year the literature contains one or two case reports of patients with the entirely typical presentation of lung haemorrhage in the absence of significant renal disease. Almost all of these have minor haematuria, and on renal biopsy linear fixation of anti-GBM antibody can be seen. In a proportion of patients there is a long history, sometimes years, of recurrent haemoptysis, breathlessness, and iron deficiency anaemia, suggestive of longstanding subacute lung haemorrhage. In the absence of overt renal disease, it resembles idiopathic pulmonary haemosiderosis (Rosenblum 1993). Fresh haemoptysis identifies recurrent lung haemorrhage, and a drop in haemoglobin may indicate quite a sizeable bleed. However these are both quite gross signs. In patients who are not critically ill, monitoring the ability of the lungs to exchange carbon monoxide, corrected for haemoglobin and lung volumes (the transfer factor, KCO) can identify the occurrence of lesser haemorrhage.

Kidneys

As in other causes of isolated RPGN, symptoms occur only late in the progression of disease, when renal impairment is advanced. As early treatment is essential for preservation of renal function, it is paradoxical that this is more likely to be achieved in patients who present with lung haemorrhage, because it leads them to seek medical attention earlier. Occasional patients with a very acute course will complain of loin pain or of macroscopic haematuria, progressing to

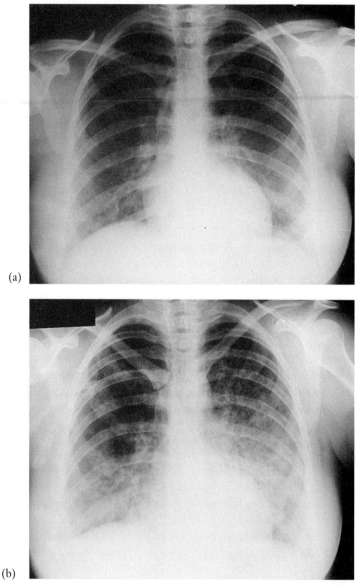

(a)

(b)

Fig. 5.1 Chest radiographs of a 23-year-old woman who presented with pulmonary haemorrhage (a) 1 week before admission and (b) on admission with a 2 week history of breathlessness and three minor episodes of haemoptysis over 3 months, the last 4 days previously. She had a haemoglobin of 5.4 g/dl with indicators of iron deficiency. By light microscopy her glomeruli appeared normal; she had microscopic haematuria but her serum creatinine was normal at 69 μmol/l. Circulating anti-GBM antibodies were detected by radio-immunoassay, and direct immunofluorescence of the renal biopsy showed linear fixation of IgG and C3 to the GBM. The radiological changes resolved on treatment with cyclophosphamide, prednisolone, and plasma exchange, but 2 weeks later she had a relapse with pulmonary haemorrhage 1 day after resuming smoking.

oliguria. As in other types of RPGN, severe hypertension is rarely a primary feature. There may be a long period of minor signs, but presentation either effectively at end-stage renal failure, or during a phase of accelerated disease tempo, are much the most common.

Diagnostic and pathological features

Even very low circulating levels of anti-GBM antibody are concentrated onto the GBM, where they can be identified by direct immunohistology. This is probably the most sensitive technique for identifying the antibodies, but the appearance is not specific, and has been reported in transplant biopsies, normal autopsy kidneys, diabetes, systemic lupus erythematosus, and fibrillary nephritis. Where the binding is accompanied by features of RPGN, or earlier inflammatory changes, there is little doubt about the nature of the disease. Otherwise, supporting evidence should be sought—most simply an immunoassay for circulating antibodies.

The pattern of antibody binding is usually strongly to the basement membrane of the glomerulus, sometimes weakly to Bowman's capsule, and sometimes also to some tubular basement membranes. IgG is usually the major component, often with C3, but other immunoglobulins may be found, and occasionally predominate. Circulating antibodies can be demonstrated by one of a variety of immunoassays based on published protocols or using commercial reagents. These may differ importantly in their sensitivity and specificity, and if there is any doubt then results should be checked at a reference centre by another assay and/or by Western blotting. Patients most likely to give false positive results in some assays include those with systemic inflammatory or infective disease, whereas false negative results are most likely in patients with subacute (sometimes lung only) disease. Patients with RPGN or severe lung haemorrhage are likely to have high titres of antibodies which few assays should miss.

Levels of other autoantibodies, total immunoglobulin levels, rheumatoid factor, complement components, and other tests are usually normal. There is usually no evidence of a marked acute phase response unless infective complications have developed.

Almost all patients with the disease, even when it appears to affect the lungs almost exclusively, have microscopic haematuria with the morphological features of glomerular bleeding. The histological features vary from mild focal and segmental proliferative changes to 100% involvement of glomeruli by crescents (Fig. 5.2). A similar degree of evolution of the lesions in different glomeruli is characteristic, dating the rapid progression of the disease to a short and severe episode. Fresh blood in the alveoli leads to an abrupt rise in KCO (which is usually depressed in renal failure), followed within days by a fall if there is no further haemorrhage (Bowley *et al.* 1979; Ewan *et al.* 1976). While bronchoscopic biopsy may show evidence of antibody fixation to the alveolar basement membrane, this is usually patchy, and absence of binding does not therefore exclude the diagnosis. The presence of haemosiderin-laden macrophages in biopsies or in bronchoalveolar lavage fluid supports the diagnosis of lung haemorrhage but gives no clue to the cause.

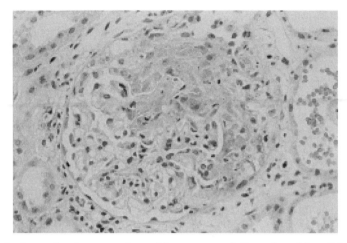

Fig. 5.2　A glomerulus from a patient with severe renal disese (requiring dialysis at presentation). There is segmental necrosis with extracapillary proliferation. Seventy per cent of the glomeruli showed crescent formation. However, there are still patent capillary loops in this and many other glomeruli, and the crescents were generally cellular. With intensive treatment, renal function improved to a creatinine of 255 μmol/l at 8 weeks and 168 μmol/l at 1 year. (By courtesy of Dr Mary Thompson.)

Treatment and outcome

The outcome of early series of patients with Goodpasture's disease was very poor, with mortalities approaching 100% through lung haemorrhage and renal failure. The advent of dialysis reduced the latter, but failure of treatments based on corticosteroids and azathioprine in varying combinations led to advocacy of bilateral nephrectomy as a way of arresting lung haemorrhage. Unfortunately even this drastic measure was not always successful. Effective treatment was developed in the early 1970s, based on the premise that if antibodies were damaging, removal and prevention of resynthesis was a rational objective. Similar regimens, based on cyclophosphamide, plasma exchange and corticosteroid therapy, have been widely found to be effective in arresting lung haemorrhage and preventing further renal damage. Where lung haemorrhage continues despite intensive treatment, attention to exacerbating factors, such as volume overload and infection, usually leads to eventual resolution.

We use a regimen comprising plasma exchange (4l daily for 14 days; replacing with human albumin solution, supplemented by fresh frozen plasma in the presence of active bleeding or recent invasive procedure); cyclophosphamide (2.5 mg/kg/day rounded down to the nearest 50 mg; reduced in patients over 55 years, and monitoring to ensure wbc > 3.5); and corticosteroids (prednisolone 60 mg daily, reducing at weekly intervals to 45, 30, 25, 20 mg and more slowly thereafter). All three elements are probably necessary for good results in severe disease. However avoidance of circumstances known to aggravate injury caused by anti-GBM antibodies is as crucial to effective management as attempts to control antibody levels and to suppress inflammation. These include prevention and prompt treatment of infection, and for lung haemorrhage, avoidance of fluid overload, oxygen toxicity (in ventilated patients try to keep inspired oxygen concentration as low as is compatible with adequate tissue oxygenation), and other potential pulmonary insults. Patients with less severe renal disease and without lung haemorrhage may do equally well with or without plasma exchange (Johnson *et al.* 1985). Immunoadsorption against protein A has been used as an alternative to plasma exchange (Bygren *et al.* 1985). It is certainly effective at removing antibodies, but its expense and technical difficulty have prevented its widespread application. There is little experience with additional or alternative agents to cyclophosphamide in this uncommon disease, although anecdotal accounts of good and bad results with cyclosporin have been reported.

While the use of pulses of methylprednisolone has been advocated, this may carry a substantially increased risk of infection and fluid retention, and either of these may have serious consequences for lung haemorrhage and for disease modulation in general. The rarity of the disease makes it difficult to compare treatments adequately, but failure of methylprednisolone pulses to arrest lung haemorrhage in two patients was reported by Williams *et al* (Williams *et al.* 1988).

Unfortunately most dialysis-dependent patients, and even most patients with serum creatinine greater than 600 μmol/l, do not recover renal function despite the best current treatment (Table 5.1). This is in marked contrast to the outcome of patients with idiopathic RPGN and a similar level of renal function or crescent score at presentation. It may be that these similarities mask a difference in the underlying structural damage to the glomeruli in the two types of disorder, but the difference in prognosis has important implications for treatment. It is not justifiable to expose patients with little chance of renal recovery to the risk of immunosuppression unless they have lung haemorrhage. However some patients have superimposed acute tubular necrosis on an underlying nephritis milder than the renal function suggests. Others have very cellular crescents of a similar age and obviously recent development; these may resolve with treatment. Renal biopsy is, therefore, an essential part of the assessment of patients with possible or definite anti-GBM disease. Finally, all patients who also have positive tests for ANCA should be given a trial of treatment unless the biopsy shows extensive scarring or there are other contraindications, as their renal prognosis may be much better. Where there is any doubt about the appropriateness of treatment, it should be commenced, as there is clear evidence that earlier treatment is more effective. It can always be stopped when all the evidence is assembled and found to favour non-treatment, and there is relatively little risk from a few days of therapy.

For patients with creatinine less than 600 μmol/l when treatment is begun, the best series show a survival rate with independent renal function at one year of 80–90%, whereas with creatinine greater than 600, the proportion with independent renal function is only 0–18%. Some series show much worse outcomes than this. The difference between the best and the worst results, and the poor overall outcome in large series across many centres, suggests that experience of managing severely affected patients is invaluable. Advice from centres with such experience may be helpful if the patient cannot be transferred. Lung recovery,

Table 5.1 Results of treatment in recent series using immunosuppression and plasma exchange*

Series	Percentage with independent renal function at 1 year according to initial creatinine level		Notes on treatment given
	<600 μmol/litre	>600 μmol/litre	
Briggs *et al.* (1979) (*n* = 15)	36 (11)	0 (4)	Only 4/15 received plasma exchange
Simpson *et al.* (1982) (*n* = 12)	70 (10)	0 (2)	8/12 received plasma exchange
Johnson *et al.* (1985) (*n* = 17)	69 (13)	0 (4)	Less cyclophosphamide than suggested in text. Half received plasma exchange, but only every third day and using frozen plasma
Walker *et al.* (1985) (*n* = 22)	82 (11)	18 (11)	Slightly less cyclophosphamide and plasma exchange than suggested in text
Hammersmith (1976–88) (*n* = 56)	90 (21)	11 (35)	As in text, except that some also received azathioprine 1 mg/kg/day
Herody *et al.* (1993) (*n* = 29)	93 (14)	0 (15)	Variable amounts of plasma exchange and different immunosuppressive regimens were used

* Untreated patients have been excluded. Treated patients are divided into two groups according to their creatinine at the time that treatment commenced or at presentation if this is not available (number in each group in parentheses). The percentage of patients who were alive and not requiring dialysis at 1 year is shown.

unlike that of the kidney, is generally clinically complete, although residual abnormalities on formal testing have been reported (Conlon *et al.* 1994).

Treatment usually needs to be continued for only 3 months, and recurrence of antibody production after this time is uncommon. We stop cyclophosphamide at that stage, and rapidly reduce and stop prednisolone. In the absence of treatment, antibody levels fall over 1–3 years. Recurrences of disease after renal transplantation have been described, but probably occurred when it was undertaken in the face of continuing antibody production. Renal transplantation appears to be safe once anti-GBM antibody levels have fallen to background levels, whether through treatment or time.

Epidemiology and pathogenesis

A bimodal incidence has been described in several different series, with peaks in the third and sixth-seventh decades. Men are slightly more commonly affected than women. The disease is very unusual in patients under 10 or over 70 years of age. It is uncommon, with an incidence of 0.5–1 cases per million population per year in various white populations (Andrassy *et al.* 1991; Segelmark *et al.*

1990; Turner and Rees 1996). Outside this racial group it is very rare. Cases of this rare disease occurring within families have been reported, and identical twins both concordant and discordant for the disease have been described. The strongest known risk factor is HLA type; HLA-DR15 confers the greatest risk, with a lesser association with DR4 and negative associations with DR1 and DR7 (Burns *et al.* 1995; Dunckley *et al.* 1991; Huey *et al.* 1993; Fisher *et al.* 1997). A very small proportion of patients have neither of the positively associated DR types, 3–10% in different series. However these DR types are common, and other factors, probably both genetic and environmental, must be involved. One other genetic influence, immunoglobulin allotypes, has been suggested (Rees *et al.* 1984). Some clues to possible environmental influences come from the associations of Goodpasture's disease, described below.

Associated diseases and environmental factors

Goodpasture's disease is uncommonly associated with other autoimmune disorders. Associations with two other renal diseases have been described, however. Membranous nephropathy with 'crescentic transformation' was first reported in 1974 (Klassen *et al.* 1974). Several cases with anti-GBM antibodies were described over the following years, although curiously we are aware of only one reported case in recent years. Much more common is an association of anti-GBM antibodies with systemic vasculitis, usually with anti-myeloperoxidase antibodies and a perinuclear ANCA pattern, and falling into the category of microscopic polyarteritis. There is evidence that in the majority of patients the anti-GBM antibody response is a secondary phenomenon (see below), and it is possible that both membranous nephropathy and vasculitis damage the GBM and lead to the development of an anti-GBM response. This interpretation is supported by two anecdotes describing patients developing Goodpasture's disease shortly after lithotripsy for intrarenal stones (Guerin *et al.* 1990; Umekawa *et al.* 1993).

Several attempts to look for associations with specific viral infections have been fruitless. There is a general epidemiological association of glomerulonephritis with exposure to organic solvents and hydrocarbon fumes, and Goodpasture's disease has been specifically implicated in some anecdotes. However it is difficult to come to firm conclusions on the scanty evidence in this rare disease, particularly as it is clear that such exposure may precipitate lung haemorrhage in those who have the disease subclinically already.

The Goodpasture antigen

While many glomerular diseases are believed to have an autoimmune etiology, the evidence is unequivocal for Goodpasture's disease. The absence of immunostaining for the Goodpasture antigen in Alport's syndrome strengthened the likelihood that the target of autoantibodies was a new, tissue-specific basement membrane component. By the late 1980s work from Kansas was suggesting that the antigen was carried on a tissue-specific basement membrane type IV collagen chain, $\alpha 3(IV)$. Type IV collagen is the major structural component of all basement membranes, and forms a 'chickenwire'-like network through associations end to end and side to side with adjacent type IV collagen molecules. cDNAs encoding the antigen-bearing NC1 domain of the α3-chain were isolated in the early 1990s, confirming the identity of the antigen (Morrison *et al.* 1991; Turner *et al.* 1992). Confusingly, the molecule most often implicated in Alport's syndrome is a homologous but distinct chain, α5(IV). It appears that three tissue-specific chains, α3, α4 and α5, form a specialized type IV collagen network in some basement membranes, including those of the glomerulus and the alveolus. Mutations in any of these three may cause Alport's syndrome, presumably by disrupting the stability of the whole network. The gene encoding the α5 chain is on the X chromosome, and is mutated in the commonest inheritance pattern. Genes encoding α3 and α4 chains have so far only been implicated in much rarer autosomal recessive pedigrees (Aumailley 1995; Tryggvason 1995).

The α3 and α4 chains are co-expressed wherever they are found. In addition to the GBM, they are found in distal tubular basement membrane in the kidney, and in smaller quantities in Bowman's capsule. They are also found in the basement membranes of the alveolus, choroid plexus, cochlea, some basement membranes in the eye, and at the neuromuscular junction. The α5 chain is expressed in a common network with the α3 and α4 chains in some locations, but in others (Bowman's capsule, epidermal basement membrane, oesophagus, and other locations) seems to form a network with the α6 chain (Cashman *et al.* 1988; Kleppel *et al.* 1989; Miner and Sanes 1994; Nakanishi *et al.* 1994; Ninomiya *et al.* 1995).

The Goodpasture antigen is therefore one of four tissue-specific type IV collagen chains, α3–α6, and is co-distributed with another of these, α4. The antigenic region of the molecule is the 230 amino acid NC1 domain at the carboxy terminus, a region which is structurally high conserved from invertebrates to mammals. There is 55–85% sequence homology between the NC1 domains of different chains in man. Why only the α3 chain is associated with spontaneous autoimmune disease is a fascinating and possibly revealing question.

Pulmonary haemorrhage

Pulmonary haemorrhage is an inconstant feature of both human disease and of animal models of anti-GBM disease, and shows a poor correlation with anti-GBM antibody titres, unlike nephritis. Although it was originally suspected that this was due to differences in antibodies between patients, and in the antigenic targets in different tissues, it is now clear that the antigen is the same molecule in lung and in kidney. However the accessibility of the basement membrane in the two locations is quite different. Antibody with specificity for any GBM component will bind directly to the GBM after intravenous injection, apparently because of the fenestrated nature of the endothelial covering in the glomerulus. This is not true for the alveolar basement membrane, where antibodies will only bind if some kind of insult is delivered to the lung so that endothelial cells are damaged or made more permeable. The insult may be inhaled, for example, oxygen toxicity, gasoline, or cigarette smoke (Downie *et al.* 1982; Jennings *et al.* 1981; Yamamoto and Wilson 1987); or it may be systemic, for example certain cytokines (Queluz and Andres 1990).

Anti-GBM antibodies in patients with systemic vasculitis

The occasional coincidence of anti-GBM antibodies and systemic vasculitis, usually with anti-myeloperoxidase antibodies and pANCA, was mentioned above (Short *et al.*, Niles *et al.*). The incidence of the association varies, but in some series was found in a substantial minority of patients with RPGN and a positive ANCA. As microscopic polyarteritis commonly presents as RPGN, with or without lung haemorrhage, it is difficult to establish which is the primary pathology in an individual patient. However it seems likely that the majority have primary vasculitic disease, and that the anti-GBM response is a secondary phenomenon, as it may be in membranous nephropathy. The age distribution of the phenomenon suggests this (patients are older), but firmer evidence comes from observations that: (1) many such patients have clinical or histological evidence of systemic vasculitis affecting extraglomerular blood vessels in the kidney or in other organs; (2) anti-GBM antibody titres tend to be lower and are relatively easily suppressed by treatment; and (3) the response to treatment is more typical of systemic vasculitis (or 'idiopathic' pauci-immune RPGN) than of Goodpasture's disease. In particular, these patients may recover renal function with treatment despite being oliguric or dialysis-dependent (Bosch *et al.* 1991; Jayne *et al.* 1990; Saxena *et al.* 1991). It should therefore be mandatory to measure ANCA in all patients in whom the diagnosis of anti-GBM disease is contemplated, and the possibility of successful treatment reviewed in the light of these observations.

It is likely that older series of patients with Goodpasture's disease have included patients who fall into this category, and it is not clear how this may have distorted the impression gained of Goodpasture's disease itself. How much the anti-GBM response contributes to the overall disease picture in systemic vasculitis is not clear, but it may vary from patient to patient.

Alloimmunity to GBM in patients with Alport's syndrome

Most patients with Alport's syndrome lack detectable $\alpha 3$, $\alpha 4$ and $\alpha 5$ chains from their GBM, so that renal transplantation introduces an array of glomerular antigens that may be new to their immune systems. Despite this, most transplants pass uneventfully, and the overall results of renal transplantation in Alport's syndrome are at least as good as those in patients with other diagnoses. However a high incidence of linear antibody fixation to the allograft GBM, without nephritis, has been noted in Alport's syndrome (Querin *et al.* 1986), and a small proportion of patients develop an anti-GBM nephritis in their allografts that is indistinguishable from spontaneous Goodpasture's disease (Savage *et al.* 1986). Characteristically this occurs some months after a first transplant, and weeks or less after a second or subsequent graft. In almost all reported cases the grafts affected by the disease have been lost, although the diagnosis has often been made too late for treatment to have a great impact on outcome. However two of 10 reported second grafts have survived.

It has only recently become possible to analyse the precise molecular targets of the alloantibodies that develop in this remarkable human 'model' of anti-GBM disease. The literature has suggested that most are directed towards the Goodpasture antigen, although some patients have clearly had different targets, and our own work suggests that the majority of alloantibodies are usually directed towards the α5 chain, the gene for which is the most commonly implicated in the causation of the disease (Briggs *et al* 1997). It is important to be aware of this possibility when transplanting patients with Alport's syndrome, for two reasons. First, it is clear that only very early treatment can hope to influence the course of this disease if it develops, and second, the antibodies may not be identified by immunoassays optimized to identify the typical anti-α3 chain antibodies of spontaneous Goodpasture's disease. Recognition must therefore be by allograft biopsy, followed up if necessary by immunoassays using either crude human GBM preparations (which may in other patients give a high false-positive rate) or Western blotting, backed up if possible by assays using recombinant antigens.

Treatment along the lines of conventional treatment for Goodpasture's disease may be effective if introduced in time. It is not clear how long it needs to be continued. This may be an area where the induction of specific tolerance could be of particular value in the future.

Insights from models of Goodpasture's disease

Anti-GBM disease was described in animals before it was recognized in man, initially being induced by passively injecting anti-glomerular antibodies raised in another species. This 'nephrotoxic nephritis' has been used to study mechanisms of antibody-induced injury, and how it may be modulated (considered below). Anti-GBM antibodies in man are predominantly 1gG1, and therefore complement-fixing. Damage may therefore be mediated by the membrane attack complex, or by neutrophil chemotaxis with or without the intervention of complement, or by macrophage recruitment. All of these mechanisms probably occur (Turner and Pusey 1991), perhaps to a different extent in various circumstances. The discovery of anti-GBM antibodies in man led to the obvious experiment of testing whether antibodies isolated from patients were equally nephrotoxic in animals. In monkeys they did indeed seem to induce acute renal disease, although not identical to the nephritis seen in the original host (Lerner *et al.* 1967).

Active models, in which autoimmunity to GBM is induced by immunization with GBM or GBM components, were slower to be developed. Until recently the best model was that developed in sheep by Steblay. In that model, repeated injection of human GBM in adjuvant led to a fatal crescentic nephritis. Later analysis of the target of autoantibodies that the sheep developed showed them to be against tissue-specific type IV collagen chains, probably α3 and/or α4 (Bygren *et al.* 1987; Jeraj *et al.* 1982; Steblay and Rudofsky 1968). In more recent years rats have been used, and not unexpectedly it has become clear that while antibodies may certainly be nephritogenic (Sado *et al.* 1992; Sado *et al.* 1989), cell-mediated immunity, specifically T lymphocytes, are critical to the development of the disease (Reynolds *et al.* 1991; Reynolds and Pusey 1994). Evidence from the human disease in this area is rudimentary but developing (Derry *et al.* 1995;

Fisher *et al.* 1995; Merkel *et al.* 1994). Very recently a model in mice has been described (Kalluri *et al.* 1997). The susceptibility of different strains of mice varies, as predicted from other models of autoimmunity in rodents, and is likely to be multifactorial. However it should now be possible to study the role of a great array of different mediators and components of the immune system, which are much better described in the mouse, aided by the range of mice with specific gene knockouts which is now becoming available (Danoff *et al.* 1995).

Modulating influences on disease severity

Because of the clearcut effects of renal injury on renal function, and the ability to measure autoantibody levels in Goodpasture's disease, it has been possible to make a unique range of clinical observations on the effect of non-specific modulators of the injury produced by given immune response in man. The original observations were that, in several patients, infection developing during the course of Goodpasture's disease could lead to a worsening of renal function and lung haemorrhage despite unchanged titres of pathogenic autoantibodies (Fig. 5.3) (Rees *et al.* 1977). Experiments using the model of nephrotoxic nephritis have subsequently shown that these effects can be reproduced by varying doses of lipopolysaccharide, or more specifically by tumour necrosis factor or interleukin-1 (Tomosugi *et al.* 1989). Surprisingly, this work has also shown that it is very difficult to achieve any renal injury at all using nephrotoxic globulin unless there is some lipopolysaccharide in the system; this may be a reason for differences in the experience of different investigators. More useful clinically is the development of ways in which inflammation and injury can be down-regulated. This can be achieved with antibodies or natural antagonists to pro-inflammatory cytokines (Karkar *et al.* 1992; Lan *et al.* 1995), or by the use of the anti-inflammatory cytokine IL-6 (Karkar *et al.* 1993), illustrating how observations in a rare disease may be used to unravel mechanisms of potentially much wider significance.

Conclusions

Anti-GBM, or Goodpasture's, disease remains the best understood variety of glomerulonephritis. Studies of both the human disease, and of experimental models, have revealed the role and importance of autoantibodies, and how these may damage glomeruli, but have only given clues as to how the disease may be initiated. It was one of the first glomerular diseases for which effective therapy was available. This success led to the successful development of similar treatment protocols for other types of RPGN. However the disease remains rare in all populations. It is important to recognise the diagnosis early because death from pulmonary haemorrhage can be prevented, and irreversible renal damage may be avoided.

Acknowledgements

NT was a NKRF Senior Research Fellow.

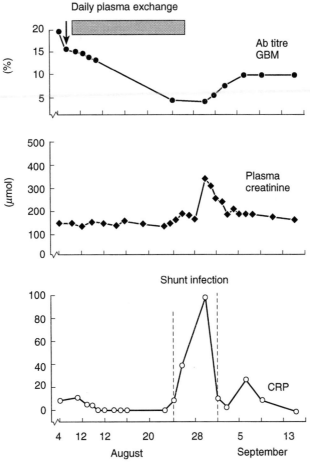

Fig. 5.3 The effect of intercurrent infection on tissue injury in Goodpasture's disease. Anti-GBM antibody titres (upper panel), creatinine (middle panel), and C-reactive protein (lower panel) in a patient with disease controlled by immunosuppressive agents and plasma exchange, who then developed an infection at the site of an arteriovenous shunt. (Reproduced with permission from Rees *et al.* 1997.)

References

Andrassy, K., Kuster, S., Waldherr, R., and Ritz, E. (1991). Rapidly progressive nephritis: analysis of prevalence and clinical course. *Nephron*, **59**, 206–12.

Aumailley, M. (1995). Structure and supramolecular organization of basement membranes. *Kidney International*, **47**, S4–S7.

Beirne, G.J., Wagnild, J.P., Zimmerman, S.W., Macken, P.D., and Burkholder, P.M. (1977). Idiopathic crescentic glomerulonephritis. *Medicine (Baltimore)*, **56**, 349–81.

Bosch, X., Mirapeix, E., Font, J., Borrrellas, X., Rodriguez, R., Lopez-Soto, A., Ingelmo, M., and Revert, L. (1991). Prognostic implication of anti-neutrophil cytoplasmic autoantibodies with myeloperoxidase specificity in anti-glomerular basement membrane disease. *Clinical Nephrology*, **36**, 107–13.

Bowley, N.B., Hughes, J.M., and Steiner, R.E. (1979). The chest X-ray in pulmonary capillary haemorrhage: correlation with carbon monoxide uptake. *Clinical Radiology*, **30**, 413–17.

Bowley, N.B., Steiner, R.E., and Chin, W.S. (1979). The chest X-ray in antiglomerular basement membrane antibody disease (Goodpasture's syndrome). *Clinical Radiology*, **30**, 419–29.

Briggs, W.A., Johnson, J.P., Teichman, S., Yeager, H.C., and Wilson, C.B. (1979). Antiglomerular basement membrane antibody-mediated glomerulonephritis and Goodpasture's syndrome. *Medicine (Baltimore)*, **58**, 348–61.

Burns, A.P., Fisher, M., Pusey, C.D., and Rees, A.J. (1995). Molecular analysis of HLA class II genes in Goodpasture's disease. *Quarterly Journal of Medicine*, **88**, 93–100.

Bygren, P., Freiburghaus, C., Lindholm, T., Simonsen, O., Thysell, H., and Wieslander, J. (1985). Goodpasture's syndrome treated with staphylococcal protein A immunoadsorption (letter). *Lancet*, **2**, 1295–6.

Bygren, P., Wieslander, J., and Heinegard, D. (1987). Glomerulonephritis induced in sheep by immunization with human glomerular basement membrane. *Kidney International*, **31**, 25–31.

Cashman, S.J., Pusey, C.D., and Evans, D.J. (1988). Extraglomerular distribution of immunoreactive Goodpasture antigen. *Journal of Pathology*, **155**, 61–70.

Conlon, P.J., Walshe, J.J., Daly, C., Carmody, M., Keogh, B., Donohoe, J., *et al.* (1994). Antiglomerular basement membrane disease: the long-term pulmonary outcome. *American Journal of Kidney Diseases*, **23**, 794–6.

Danoff, T.M., Cook, D.N., Neilson, E.G., and Kalluri, E. (1995). Murine anti-α3(IV) collagen disease is abrogated in MIP-1α deficient mice. *Journal of American Society Nephrology*, **6**, 827.

Derry, C.J., Ross, C.N., Lombardi, G., Mason, P.D., Rees, A.J., Lechler, R.I., *et al.* (1995). Analysis of T cell responses to the autoantigen in Goodpasture's disease. *Clinical and Experimental Immunology*, **100**, 262–8.

Donaghy, M., and Rees, A.J. (1983). Cigarette smoking and lung haemorrhage in glomerulonephritis caused by autoantibodies to glomerular basement membrane. *Lancet*, **2**, 1390–3.

Downie, G.H., Roholt, O.A., Jennings, L., Blau, M., Brentjens, J.R., and Andres, G.A. (1982). Experimental anti-alveolar basement membrane antibody-mediated pneumonitis. II. Role of endothelial damage and repair, induction of autologous phase, and kinetics of antibody deposition in Lewis rats. *Journal of Immunology*, **129**, 2647–52.

Dunckley, H., Chapman, J.R., Burke, J., Charlesworth, J., Hayes, J., Haywood, E., *et al.* (1991). HLA-DR and -DQ genotyping in anti-GBM disease. *Disease Markers*, **9**, 249–56.

Ewan, P.W., Jones, H.A., Rhodes, C.G., and Hughes, J.M. (1976). Detection of intrapulmonary hemorrhage with carbon monoxide uptake: application in Goodpasture's syndrome. *New England Journal of Medicine*, **295**, 1391–6.

Fisher, M., Pusey, C.D., and Rees, A.J. (1995). T cell receptors expressed by T cells proliferating to the Goodpasture antigen share common CDR3 sequences. *Journal of American Society Nephrology*, **6**, 828.

Fisher, M., Pusey, C.D., Vaughan, R.W., and Rees, A.J. (1997). Susceptibility to Goodpasture's disease is strongly associated with HLA-DRB1 genes. *Kidney International*, **51**, 222–9.

Goodpasture, E.W. (1919). The significance of certain pulmonary lesions in relation to the etiology of influenza. *American Journal of Medical Science*, **158**, 836–70.

Guerin, V., Rabin, C., Noel, L.H., Droz, D., Baron, C., Lallemand, F., and Jungers, P. (1990). Anti-glomerular basement membrane disease after lithotripsy. *Lancet*, **i**, 856–7.

Guerin, S., Noel, L.H., Grunfeld, J.P., Droz, D., Mahieu, P. and Berger J. (1986). Linear glomerular IgG fixation in renal allografts: incidence and significance in Alport's syndrome. *Clinical Nephrology*, **25**, 134–40.

Heptinstall, R.H. (1983). Schonlein–Henoch syndrome; lung hemorrhage and glomerulonephritis. In *Pathology of the Kidney*, (ed. R.H. Heptinstall) pp. 761–91. Little Brown, Boston.

Herody, M., Bobrie, G., Gouarin, C., Grunfeld, J.P., and Noel, L.H. (1993). Anti-GBM disease: Predictive value of clinical, histological and serological data. *Clinical Nephrology*, **40**, 249–55.

Huey, B., McCormick, K., Capper, J., Ratcliff, C., Colombe, B.W., Garoroy, M.R., *et al.* (1993). Associations of HLA-DR and HLA-DQ types with anti-GBM nephritis by sequence-specific oligonucleotide probe hybridization. *Kidney International*, **44**, 307–12.

Jayne, D.R.W., Marshall, P.D., Jones, S.J., and Lockwood, C.M. (1990). Autoantibodies to glomerular basement membrane and neutrophil cytoplasm in rapidly progressive glomerulonephritis. *Kidney International*, **37**, 965–70.

Jennings, L., Roholt, O.A., Pressman, D., Blau, M., Andres, G.A., and Brentjens, J.R. (1981). Experimental anti-alveolar basement membrane antibody-mediated pneumonitis. 1. The role of increased permeability of the alveolar capillary wall induced by oxygen. *Journal of Immunology*, **127**, 129–34.

Jeraj, K., Michael, A.F., and Fish, A.J. (1982). Immunologic similarities between Goodpasture's and Steblay's antibodies. *Clinical Immunology and Immunopathology*, **23**, 408–13.

Johnson, J.P., Moore, J.J., Austin, H.A., Balow, J.E., Antonovych, T.T., and Wilson, C.V. (1985). Therapy of anti-glomerular basement membrane antibody disease: analysis of prognostic significance of clinical, pathologic and treatment factors. *Medicine (Baltimore)*, **64**, 219–27 (abstract).

Kalluri, R., Damoff, T.M., and Neilson, E.G. (1997). Murine anti-α3(IV) collagen disease: a model of human Goodpasture syndrome and anti-GBM nephritis. *Journal of American Society Nephrology*, **6**, 833.

Karkar, A.M., Koshino, Y., Cashman, S.J., Bonnefoy, J., and Meager, A. (1992). Passive immunization against tumour necrosis factor-alpha (TNF-alpha) and IL-1 beta protects from LPS enhancing glomerular injury in nephrotoxic nephrits in rats. *Clinical and Experimental Immunology*, **90**, 312–18.

Karkar, A.M., Tam, F.W.K., Proudfoot, A., Meager, A., and Rees, A.J. (1993). Modulation of antibody-mediated glomerular injury *in vivo* by interleukin-6. *Kidney International*, **44**, 967–73.

Kelly, P.T., and Haponik, E.F. (1994). Goodpasture syndrome: molecular and clinical advances. *Medicine (Baltimore)*, **73**, 171–85.

Klassen, J., Elwood, C., Grossberg, A.L., Milgrom, F., Montes, M., Sepulveda, M., *et al.* (1974). Evolution of membranous nephropathy into anti-glomerular basement membrane glomerulonephritis. *New England Journal of Medicine*, **290**, 1340–4.

Kleppel, M.M., Santi, P.A., Cameron, J.D., Wieslander, J., and Michael, A.F. (1989). Human tissue distribution of novel basement membrane collagen. *American Journal of Pathology*, **134**, 813–25.

Lan, H.Y., Nikolic-Paterson, D.J., Mu, W., Vannice, J.L., and Atkins, R.C. (1995). Interleukin-1 receptor antagonist halts the progression of established crescentic glomerulonephritis in the rat. *Kidney International*, **47**, 1303–9.

Lerner, R.A., Glassock, R.J., and Dixon, F.J. (1967). The role of anti-glomerular basement membrane antibody in the pathogenesis of human glomerulonephritis. *Journal of Experimental Medicine*, **126**, 989–1004.

Merkel, F., Kalluri, R., Marx, M. (1996). Autoreactive T-cells in Goodpasture's syndrome recognise the N-terminal NCl domain α3 type IV collagen. *Kidney International*, **49**, 1127–33.

Miner, J.H., and Sanes, J.R. (1994). Collagen IV α3, α4, and α5 chains in rodent basal laminae: sequence, distribution, association with laminins, and developmental switches. *Journal of Cell Biology*, **127**, 879–91.

Morrison, K.E., Mariyama, M., Yang-Feng, T.L., and Reeders, S.T. (1991). Sequence and localization of a partial cDNA encoding the human α3 chain of type IV collagen. *American Journal of Human Genetics*, **49**, 545–54.

Nakanishi, K., Yoshikawa, N., Iijima, K., Kitagawa, K., Nakamura, H., Ito, H., *et al.* (1994). Immunohistochemical study of α1-5 chains of type IV collagen in hereditary nephritis. *Kidney International*, **46**, 1413–21.

Ninomiya, Y., Kagawa, M., Iyama, K., Naito, I., Kishiro, Y., Seyer, J.M., *et al.* (1995). Differential expression of two basement membrane collagen genes, COL4A6 and COL4A5, demonstrated by immunofluorescence staining using peptide-specific monoclonal antibodies. *Journal of Cell Biology*, **130**, 1219–29.

Peters, D.K., Rees, A.J., Lockwood, C.M., and Pusey, C.D. (1982). Treatment and prognosis in antibasement membrane antibody-mediated nephritis. *Transplantation Proceedings*, **14**, 513–21.

Queluz, T.T., and Andres, G. (1990). Pathogenesis of an experimental model of Goodpasture's haemorrhagic pneumonitis. *Nephrology Dialysis Transplantation*, 5, **S1**, 3–5.

Rees, A.J., Demaine, A.G., and Welsh, K.I. (1984). Association of immunoglobulin Gm allotypes with antiglomerular basement membrane antibodies and their titer. *Human Immunology*, **10**, 213–20.

Rees, A.J., Lockwood, C.M., and Peters, D.K. (1977). Enhanced allergic tissue injury in Goodpasture's syndrome by intercurrent bacterial infection. *British Medical Journal*, **2**, 723–6.

Reynolds, J., Cashman, S.J., Evans, D.J., and Pusey, C.D. (1991). Cyclosporin A in the prevention and treatment of experimental autoimmune glomerulonephritis in the brown Norway rat. *Clinical and Experimental Immunology*, **85**, 28–32.

Reynolds, J., and Pusey, C.D. (1994). *In vivo* treatment with a monoclonal antibody to T helper cells in experimental autoimmune glomerulonephritis. *Clinical and Experimental Immunology*, **95**, 122–7.

Rosenblum, N.D. (1993). Case records of the Massachusetts General Hospital. *New England Journal of Medicine*, **328**, 1183–90.

Sado, Y., Kagawa, M., Rauf, S., Naito, I., Moritoh, C., and Okigaki, T. (1992). Isologous monoclonal antibodies can induce anti-GBM glomerulonephritis in rats. *Journal of Pathology*, **168**, 221–7.

Sado, Y., Naito, I., and Okigaki, T. (1989). Transfer of anti-glomerular basement membrane antibody-induced glomerulonephritis in inbred rats with isologous antibodies from the urine of nephritic rats. *Journal of Pathology*, **158**, 325–32.

Savage, C.O., Pusey, C.D., Kershaw, M.J., Cashman, S.J., Harrison, P., Hartley, B., *et al.* (1986). The Goodpasture antigen in Alport's syndrome: studies with a monoclonal antibody. *Kidney International*, **30**, 107–12.

Saxena, R., Bygren, P., Rasmussen, N., and Wieslander, J. (1991). Circulating autoantibodies in patients with extracapillary glomerulonephritis. *Nephrology Dialysis Transplantation*, **6**, 389–97.

Segelmark, M., Butkowski, R., and Wieslander, J. (1990). Antigen restriction and IgG subclasses among anti-GBM autoantibodies. *Nephrology Dialysis Transplantation*, 5, 991–6.

Simpson, I.J., Doak, P.B., Williams, L.C., Blacklock, H.A., Hill, R.S., Herdson, P.B., *et al.* (1982). Plasma exchange in Goodpasture's syndrome. *American Journal of Nephrology*, 2, 301–11.

Stanton, M.C., and Tange, J.D. (1958). Goodpasture's syndrome (pulmonary haemorrhage associated with glomerulonephritis). *Australian New Zealand Journal of Medicine*, 7, 132–44.

Steblay, R.W., and Rudofsky, U. (1968). *In vitro* and *in vivo* properties of autoantibodies eluted from kidneys of sheep with autoimmune glomerulonephritis. *Nature*, 218, 1269–71.

Tomosugi, N.I., Cashman, S.J., Hay, H., Pusey, C.D., Evans, D.J., Shaw, A., *et al.* (1989). Modulation of antibody-mediated glomerular injury *in vivo* by bacterial lipopolysaccharide, tumor necrosis factor, and IL-1. *Journal of Immunology*, 142, 3083–90.

Tryggvason, K. (1995). Molecular properties and diseases of collagens. *Kidney International*, 47, S-24–28.

Turner, A.N., Brainwood, D., Gubler, M.C., Kashtan, C.E. (1996). Alloantibodies to $\alpha(IV)NCT$ in Alport post-transplant anti-GBM disease. *Journal of the American Society of Nephrology*, 7, 1724 (abstract).

Turner, A.N., and Rees, A.J. (1992). Antiglomerular basement membrane disease. In *Oxford textbook of nephrology*, (eds. J.S. Cameron, A.M. Davison, J.-P. Grunfeld, D.N.S. Kerr and E. Ritz) pp. 438–56. Oxford University Press, Oxford.

Turner, N., Mason, P.J., Brown, R., Fox, M., Povey, S., Rees, A.J., Pusey, C.D. (1992). Molecular cloning of the human Goodpasture antigen demonstrates it to be the $\alpha 3$ chain of type IV collagen. *Journal of Clinical Investigation*, 89, 592–601.

Turner, N., and Pusey, C.D. (1991). Anti-glomerular basement membrane disease. In *Immunology of renal disease*, (ed. C.D. Pusey) pp. 229–54. Kluwer Academic Publishers, Lancaster.

Umekawa, T., Kohri, K., Iguchi, M., Yoshioka, K., and Kurita, T. (1993). Glomerular-basement-membrane antibody and extracorporeal shock wave lithotripsy. *Lancet*, 341, 556.

Wakui, H., Chubachi, A., Asakura, K., Nishimura, S., Nakamoto, Y., and Miura, A.B. (1992). Goodpasture's syndrome: a report of an autopsy case and a review of Japanese cases. *Internal Medicine*, 31, 102–7.

Walker, R.G., Scheinkestel, C., Becker, G.J., Owen, J.E., Dowling, J.P., and Kincaid Smith, P. (1985). Clinical and morphological aspects of the management of crescentic anti-glomerular basement membrane antibody (anti-GBM) nephritis/Goodpasture's syndrome. *Quarterly Journal of Medicine*, 54, 75–89.

Williams, P.S., Davenport, A., McDicken, I., Ashby, D., and Bone, J.M. (1988). Increased incidence of anti-glomerular basement membrane antibody (anti-GBM) nephritis in the Mersey region, September 1984–October 1985. *Quarterly Journal of Medicine*, 68, 727–33.

Wilson, C.B., and Dixon, F.J. (1973). Anti-glomerular basement membrane antibody-induced glomerulonephritis. *Kidney International*, 3, 74–89.

Wilson, C.B., and Dixon, F.J. (1981). The renal response to immunological injury. In *The kidney*, (ed. B.M. Brenner and F.C. Rector) pp. 1237–350. W.B. Saunders, Philadephia, PA.

Yamamoto, T., and Wilson, C.B. (1987). Binding of anti-basement membrane antibody to alveolar basement membrane after intratracheal gasoline instillation in rabbits. *American Journal of Pathology*, 126, 497–505.

6

Pathogenesis of systemic vasculitis

Patrick Nachman, J. Charles Jennette, and Ronald J. Falk

Systemic vasculitides have a wide range of aetiologies and pathogenic mechanisms, and can be broadly divided into primary and secondary forms. Over the years, systemic vasculitides have been categorized according to a number of different classifications. In an effort to standardize the terminology of primary systemic vasculitides, an international consensus conference at Chapel Hill, North Carolina recently proposed a modified nomenclature. The Chapel Hill terminology is shown in Table 6.1, and the terms described therein will be used in this chapter (Jeanette *et al.* 1994). This nomenclature is based on histological characteristics of the inflammatory process and the size of the affected vessels. Each histological pattern of inflammation may result from a number of different pathogenic mechanisms. Other forms of vasculitides may be secondary to systemic autoimmune diseases, infectious agents, environmental toxins, or therapeutic agents (see also Fig. 6.1).

Vessel wall destruction can be mediated either by direct invasion and proliferation of bacterial pathogens (e.g. meningococcaemia), by immune complex deposition in the vessel wall (e.g. in cryoglobulinaemic vasculitis), by direct antibody-mediated destruction of the vessel wall (Goodpasture's disease), or may lack clear evidence of immune deposits or complexes—such as in pauci-immune vasculitides associated with antineutrophil cytoplasmic autoantibodies (ANCA). All of these different initiating mechanisms ultimately lead to a final common pathway of necrotizing vascular inflammation, which involves leucocyte and endothelial activation, leucocyte adhesion to endothelial cells, and injury to the vessel wall.

In this chapter, we review the pathogenesis of vasculitides grouped according to the putative mechanism of vascular injury.

Immune complex-mediated vasculitides

These vasculitides occur when immune complexes are deposited in vessel walls or form *in situ* within vessel walls. Regardless of their origin, immune complexes initiate acute inflammation via activation of the complement cascade, by attracting and activating leucocytes, and by stimulating various other phlogistic mediators.

Recently, Mozes *et al.* (1993) showed that major histocompatibility complex (MHC) class I-deficient mice were resistant to the development of experimental SLE after immunization with the human monoclonal anti-DNA antibody 16/6Id or anti-16/6Id. These mice were capable of producing antibodies to 16/6Id, but unlike normal mice did not develop any antibodies to DNA or nuclear extract. They also failed to respond at all to anti-16/6Id. These data demonstrate a key role of MHC class I in the induction of experimental autoimmune SLE. The authors proposed a model in which experimental SLE depends on the induction of an idiotype–anti-idiotype network, itself dependent on MHC class I peptide presentation. Once antigen and antibody tissue deposition have occurred, a variety of effector pathways result in tissue inflammation.

Humoral mediators

Activation of the complement system is an important pathogenetic mechanism that contributes to many forms of immune-mediated injury, including immune complex vasculitis. Complement activation causes tissue injury by generating: (1) anaphylotoxins, such as C4a, C3a, and C5a, and the kinin-like peptide C2b, which increase vascular permeability; (2) chemotaxins, such as C5a and C567, which induce leucocyte infiltration; (3) promoters of immune adherence, such as C3b and C4b, which cause leucocytes to localize at sites of immune deposition; and (4) the membrane attack complex (MAC), composed of C5b-9, which can cause cell lysis or non-lethal membrane perturbation leading to the release of inflammatory mediators. Thus, complement activation at sites of immune complex localization, such as glomeruli in immune complex vasculitis, causes inflammatory injury.

The complement system can also play a protective role in patients with circulating immune complexes, because it is important in opsonizing immune complexes so that they will be more efficiently removed from the circulation by erythrocyte adherence and phagocytosis by neutrophils and the mononuclear phagocyte system. A less well-defined, potentially protective role of the complement system in immune complex disease is its ability to solubilize immune complexes.

Coagulation system activation by the intrinsic and extrinsic pathways, platelet activation, and endothelial injury are involved in vascular inflammation, including that in immune complex vasculitis, such as seen sometimes in SLE. Many of the activated mediator systems and injurious events occurring in the vasculature of lupus patients promote activation of the coagulation system, both within the vasculature, and within tissues at sites of fibrinoid necrosis. This latter process results when plasma exudes from inflamed vessels or flows from ruptured vessels into adjacent issues, where it contacts thrombogenic substances, such as collagen and tissue thromboplastin, leading to fibrin formation. Fibrin formation in extravascular sites is followed by mesenchymal cell responses, for example, fibroplasia leading to glomerular scarring, and epithelial hyperplasia leading to glomerular crescent formation.

Intravascular activation of the coagulation system can lead to thrombosis. This is initiated by a variety of mechanisms, including activation of humoral mediator systems via Hageman factor, platelet activation, and endothelial damage. This latter event, in addition to exposing thrombogenic basement membrane constituents, disturbs the balance between endothelial cell-derived antithrombogenic prostacyclin and platelet-derived thrombogenic thromboxane.

In lupus patients, especially those with nephritis, there are prothrombotic abnormalities in the coagulation and plasmin systems, such as increased factor VIII complex activity and decreased plasminogen activator activity (Kant *et al.* 1981; Colasanti *et al.* 1987; Takemura *et al.* 1987). However, these humoral changes may be secondary to direct effects of immune pathogenetic mechanisms on endothelial cells and platelets. Lethal injury to endothelial cells in vessels, including glomerular capillaries, exposes the thrombogenic surfaces of vascular basement membranes that activate fibrin formation via the intrinsic coagulation system and initiate platelet activation via contact with matrix molecules such as fibronectin and vitronectin. Vascular necrosis leads to intravascular coagulation (thrombosis) and extravascular coagulation (fibrinoid necrosis) by bringing procoagulants into contact with fragmented collagenous matrix molecules and tissue thromboplastin, which initiates extrinsic system coagulation.

Sublethal endothelial cell injury is also prothrombotic and pro-inflammatory. Since endothelial cells synthesize factor VII complex, plasminogen activator, and prostacyclin, endothelial injury can cause abnormalities in these factors that will disturb haemostatic control. Injured endothelial cells are a source of platelet-activating factor (PAF), which not only causes platelet aggregation and secretion, but also causes chemotaxis and activation of mononuclear phagocytes and neutrophils. PAF also causes increased vascular permeability by inducing retraction and separation of endothelial cells, which may promote capillary wall immune complex deposition. Injured endothelium releases cytokine growth factors that could contribute to glomerular hypercellularity by stimulating proliferation of endothelial and mesangial cells. Injury-induced up-regulation of endothelial leucocyte adhesion molecules promotes infiltration of leucocytes, which could contribute to the glomerular leucocyte infiltration observed in proliferative immune complex vasculitis.

A mechanism of endothelial injury that may be important in lupus patients is endothelial injury caused by specific anti-endothelial antibodies and polyspecific antiphospholipid antibodies that bind to endothelial cell membranes. The polyspecificity of autoantibodies in SLE for a vary of polynucleotides and phospholipids can be explained by the presence of appropriately spaced phosphodiester groups in both polynucleotides and phospholipids (Shoenfeld *et al.* 1983). Lupus anticoagulant and anticardiolipin are examples of antiphospholipid antibodies that might have pathogenetic capabilities. For examples, lupus antiphospholipid antibodies can inhibit prostacyclin and plasminogen activator release by endothelial cells (Carreras *et al.* 1982; Le Roux *et al.* 1986), thus promoting thrombosis. Cines *et al.* (1984) have identified complement-fixing anti-endothelial antibodies in lupus patients that are capable of causing endothelial prostaglandin release, adherence of platelets to endothelial cells, and disruption of endothelial monolayers. They also demonstrated that heat-aggregated IgG, a model of immune complexes, had similar effects on endothelial cells. This suggests that binding of circulating immune complexes, such as those in lupus patients, to endothelial cells by mechanisms independent of specific antigen recognition can also effect endothelial cell function.

Leucocytes

As in all forms of necrotizing vasculitis, leucocytes are major pathogenetic effectors in immune complex vasculitis. Leucocyte chemo-attractants and activators are generated by all of the pathophysiological events of immune complex vasculitis that have been discussed thus far.

Mononuclear phagocytes are inflammatory effector cells, and have an extensive armamentarium of mediators capable of contributing to the tissue injury observed in immune complex vasculitis. Activated mononuclear phagocytes secrete a variety of hydrolytic enzymes, such as collagenase, elastase, plasminogen activator, and neutral proteases. In addition to lytic injury mediated by these enzymes, mononuclear phagocytes cause cell injury by generating toxic oxygen species, such as superoxide anion, hydrogen peroxide, and hydroxyl radical. They also release complement components (C2, C3, C4, C5, and factor B), lipid metabolites (prostaglandins), PAF, and cytokines, all of which are involved in mediating inflammation. Three important cytokines released by activated mononuclear phagocytes are interleukin-1 (IL-1), tumour necrosis factor (TNF), and interferon-γ. The chemotactic and activating properties of such cytokines could contribute to glomerular and tubulo-interstitial leucocyte influx, and their growth factor activities could lead to glomerular endothelial, mesangial, and epithelial (i.e. crescent) proliferation. Endothelial tubulo-reticular inclusions, which are another vascular structural change that is characteristic of lupus vasculitis, may be the result of cytokine (e.g. interferon-α) effects on endothelial cells (Feldman *et al.* 1988).

Activation of mononuclear phagocytes in lupus vasculitis has been demonstrated by measuring increased procoagulant activity in circulating monocytes. Activated mononuclear phagocytes secrete at least three procoagulant monokines: thromboplastin, factor X-activating factors, and a prothrombinase. Cole *et al.* (1985) demonstrated a 100-fold increase in the prothrombinase activity of circulating monocytes in 8/8 lupus patients with focal or proliferative glomerulonephritis, as compared with patients with non-lupus glomerulonephritis, or lupus patients without nephritis.

Cryoglobulinaemic vasculitis

Another form of immune complex vasculitis is caused by cryoglobulinaemia. Cryoglobulins are composed of different types of immunoglobulins which allow for their separation into three types. Type I is characterized by the presence of monoclonal immunoglobulin, usually IgM. Type II and type III are mixtures of monoclonal with polyclonal, or polyclonal with polyclonal immunoglobulins, respectively. In these types, the monoclonal component (type II) or one of the polyclonal components (type III) has rheumatoid factor activity. Type I cryo-globulins may occlude the microvasculature, but do not generally induce inflammation. Type II and type III cryoglobulins are immune complexes and therefore do incite vascular inflammation. Type I cryoglobulins are most often found in patients with lymphoproliferative disorders, such as multiple myeloma and Waldenstrom's macroglobulinaemia. Type II may be associated with viral infections, or with lymphoproliferative disorders (see below). Type III are most often found in patients with autoimmune disorders, chronic infections, or inflammatory disorders. Cryoglobulinaemic vasculitis is often characterized clinically by purpura, arthritis, systemic vasculitis, and nephritis. The most common renal lesion in patients with cryoglobulinaemia is type I membranoproliferative glomerulonephritis. Vasculitis of small arteries, arterioles and post-capillary venules is present in at lease one-third of the patients, especially in those with more severe disease. It is characterized by fibrinoid necrosis of the vessel wall with infiltrates of leucocytes. Electron microscopy reveals vascular electron-dense deposits. Immunohistology reveals granular staining of the vessel walls for immunoglobulin and complement (D'Amico *et al.* 1989).

Because of the monoclonal nature of the IgM rheumatoid factor, type II cryo-globulinaemia has been linked to lymphoproliferative disorders. Perl *et al.* (1989) reported the presence of clonal rearrangements of immunoglobulin genes in 4 out of 12 patients. However, the contention that type II cryoglobulinaemia is caused by a lymphoproliferative disorder is not supported by the low clinical incidence of lymphoproliferative disorders in all but one (Frankel *et al.* 1992) series of patients (Brouet *et al.* 1974; Invernizzi *et al.* 1983; D'Amico *et al.* 1989).

Type II cryoglobulinaemia has been associated with certain viral infections, including hepatitis B (Levo *et al.* 1977) and Epstein–Barr virus (Fiorini *et al.* 1986, 1988). A growing number of reports have linked hepatitis C virus (HCV) infection and type II cryoglobulinaemia (Pascuar *et al.* 1990; Ourand *et al.* 1991; Burstein and Rodby 1993). Misiani *et al.* (1992) studied the association between HCV infection and cryoglobulinaemia in 51 patients, using as controls 45 patients with non-cryoglobulinaemic glomerulonephritis. The authors looked for the presence of HCV by a number of different techniques, including two ELISAs (c100 ELISA and c22/c200 ELISA), a recombinant immunoblot assay (4-RIBA), and serum-HCV RNA by PCR. Anti-HCV antibodies were found in the cryoglobulins precipitated from patients with cryoglobulinaemia before and after the use of dithiothreitol, a substance which destroys the IgM antibodies with rheumatoid factor activity. Depending on the assay used, up to 98% of the patients with type II cryoglobulinaemia had evidence of HCV infection, whereas the rate of reactivity was only 2% in the control group. The study of cryoglobulin precipitates with the c100 ELISA revealed detectable anti-HCV activity in 94% of patients, with the use of dithiothreitol. These results are confirmed by the study of Agnello *et al.* (1992), who also demonstrated a lack of association between HCV and type I cryoglobulinaemia. In addition, the concentrations of HCV-RNA and anti-HCV antibody, but not antibodies to Epstein–Barr Virus (EBV) or rubella, were found to be much higher in the cryoglobulin precipitate than in the corresponding serum. The high prevalence of HCV infection in type II cryoglobulinaemia patients, as well as the demonstration of anti-HCV antibodies and HCV RNA in the cryoglobulin precipitate, provides compelling evidence for an association between HCV infection and the development of type II cryoglobulinaemia. The definitive role for these immune complexes in the generation of the pathological abnormalities of disease would require the demonstration of HCV antigens in the vascular or renal lesions. These data lend support to the concept that the development of the monoclonal rheumatoid factor is in response to the production of polyclonal IgGs, such as those related to viral infections, rather than the concept that the monoclonal rheumatoid factor is related to a primary lymphoproliferative disorder.

Henoch–Schönlein purpura

This disorder is usually attributed to the deposition of IgA-immune complexes and the subsequent activation of the complement system. However, despite numerous recent studies, the aetiology and pathogenesis of Henoch–Schönlein purpura (HSP) remains poorly understood. In addition, the common practice of grouping HSP with IgA nephropathy renders many of the study results difficult to interpret.

Since the report by Tanaka *et al.* (1969), linking HSP with an increase in serum IgA, substantial work has been done to define the role of circulating IgA or IgA-immune complexes in the pathogenesis of HSP. Despite reports of clustering of cases, and the recognition that HSP seems to follow upper respiratory tract infections, no specific exogenous antigenic or infectious precipitant has been consistently identified.

The existence and pathogenetic role of circulating IgA-immune complexes in patients with HSP remains unproven, mostly because earlier studies relied on the assessment of size or the activation of complement for the detection of immune complexes. Because of the presence of dimeric, trimeric, or tetrameric IgA in the circulation, 'molecular' size alone cannot be a reliable indicator of the presence of true IgA immune complexes that contain IgA bound to target antigen. In addition, IgA is a poor activator of the complement system, making assays based on complement activation unreliable. Despite these problems, there is evidence (Knight 1990) for :

(1) increased numbers of circulating IgA-producing B cells;

(2) the existence of IgA rheumatoid factor (binding to IgG) in the sera of patients with acute HSP, which disappears as the disease resolves. The IgG in these 'complexes' may be capable of complement binding and activation;

(3) the presence of IgA- and IgG-containing macromolecular aggregates in the serum of patients with HSP. The high molecular weight aggregates and the IgG-containing complexes seem to be features distinguishing HSP from IgA nephropathy; and

(4) the activation of the alternative pathway of complement, as suggested by the findings of low levels of properdin and elevated C3d (breakdown product of

C3) in the serum of patients with acute HSP, and the finding of C3 and properdin on glomerular immunohistology. The serum abnormalities also appear to return to normal with resolution of the disease.

There are now several reports of the presence of IgA ANCA in HSP, although this has not been confirmed in other series.

Hepatitis B-associated vasculitis

Hepatitis B virus (HBV) has been associated with the development of necrotizing vasculitis, as initially reported by Gocke *et al.* (1970). However, necrotizing vasculitis seems to be a rare complication of HBV infection. The annual incidence is estimated at 7.7 per 100 000 Alaskan Eskimos, a population in which HBV infection is hyperendemic (McMahon *et al.* 1989). In a prospective study of 1400 hepatitis B surface antigen-positive (HBsAg) native carriers, no cases of either cryoglobulinaemia or necrotizing vasculitis occurred over a period of 7815 carrier years (McMahon *et al.* 1990). Conversely, HBV infection has been reported to occur in about 30% of patients with polyarteritis (Sergent *et al.* 1976; Mayder and Keystone 1992). Marcellin *et al.* (1991) have reported a much higher prevalence (68%) of HBV infection in 28 patients with polyarteritis nodosa (versus only about 10% of 10 control patients with other systemic vasculitides) using very sensitive monoclonal RIA and DNA hybridization techniques.

The incidence of renal involvement in HBV-associated necrotizing vasculitis is unclear. In most series (Duffy *et al.* 1976; Sergent *et al.* 1976; McMahon *et al.* 1989, 1990), the incidence of renal involvement, as determined by proteinuria, haematuria, decreased creatinine clearance, or biopsy, seems to be about 38–44%. On the other hand, in Michalak's report of seven necropsy cases, six had glomerular HBsAg-immune complex deposits in addition to classical periarteritis nodosa (PAN) with documented HBsAg-immune complex deposition in the vessel wall (Michalak 1978).

The evidence for the association of HBV with necrotizing vasculitis extends beyond epidemiological data. In their initial report, Gocke *et al.* (1970) were able to demonstrate the presence of Australia-antigen-containing immune complexes in the serum, as well as Australia antigen positive IgM and B1C in the arterial wall from one patient. These findings are confirmed in the seven necropsy cases presented by Michalak (1978), in which he demonstrated HBsAg, IgG, IgM, B1C, and C1q in the walls of vessels. Michalak also documented fixation of heterologous complement, as well as the ability to elute the immune complexes from the tissue using buffers known to dissociate immune complexes (Glycine HC1; NaSCN; and KSCN) but not phosphate buffered saline.

Direct antibody attack-mediated vasculitis

Another pathogenetic mechanism of vascular inflammation is direct antibody binding to constituents of the vessel wall. This is, in essence, a form of *in situ*

immune complex formation, and would initiate the same inflammatory pathogenetic mechanisms as discussed previously. Two models of this pathogenetic
mechanism include Kawasaki's disease and anti-glomerular basement membrane
(anti-GBM) or Goodpasture's disease.

Anti-endothelial cell antibodies, sometimes referred to as AECA, are directed
against both constitutive and inducible endothelial antigens. Cytokine stimulation
with IL-1 or TNF induces the expression of a variety of endothelial antigens.
For instance, in Kawasaki's disease, AECA are directed against cytokine-induced
endothelial antigens (Leung *et al.* 1986, 1989). Whether this antibody-antigen
interaction is responsible for Kawasaki's disease is not certain.

In anti-GBM disease, the antibodies are directed against constituents of the
vascular basement membrane. These antibodies react with a 28 kDa monomeric
peptide, which is one of the three non-collagenous peptides in the globular
domain at the carboxy terminal of type IV collagen in the GBM (Weislander
et al. 1984*a,b*, 1985). The autoantigen has now been localized to the NCI domain
of the α3 chain of type IV collagen (see Chapter 5).

Certain factors have been implicated in the development and 'expression' of
anti-GBM disease, such as genetic predisposition, and exposure to environmental
toxins or pathogens. Rees *et al.* (1978, 1984) reported a strong association
between Goodpasture's disease and the HLA-DRw2 antigen, conferring a relative risk of 15.9. These authors also reported an increased incidence of HLA-B7,
which was associated with increased severity of disease.

Toxins (e.g. hydrocarbon solvents, tobacco smoking) or viral infections (e.g.
influenza A infection) may play a permissive role in the development of pulmonary haemorrhage (Churchill *et al.* 1983; Ravnskow *et al.* 1983; Daniell *et al.*
1988), possibly by the unmasking of the antigenic epitopes (Yoshioka *et al.* 1985),
thereby providing access for pulmonary localization of circulating anti-GBM
antibodies.

Vasculitis associated with antineutrophil cytoplasmic autoantibodies (ANCA)

Vasculitides associated with ANCA are characterized by the absence or paucity
of demonstrable vascular immune complexes or antibody deposition. ANCA are
found in the circulation of patients with Wegener's granulomatosis, microscopic
polyangiitis, Churg–Strauss syndrome, and idiopathic necrotizing glomerulonephritis. This association, along with the absence of evidence for immune
complex deposition or direct antibody binding to vessel walls, has led to the
hypothesis that ANCA are somehow pathogenic.

ANCA have multiple antigen specificities. There are, however, two major
specificities, which are for proteinase-3 (PR3) and myeloperoxidase (MPO). Both
proteins are found in the primary granules of neutrophils and the lysosomes of
monocytes. By indirect immunofluorescence (IIF), when alcohol-fixed neutrophils
are used as a substrate to detect ANCA, two different patterns of fluorescence

can be differentiated: a perinuclear staining (p-ANCA), or a cytoplasmic staining (c-ANCA). The c-ANCA pattern is caused by antibodies against PR3, whereas the p-ANCA pattern is most frequently caused by antibodies to MPO. There are other antigen specificities for ANCA, such as cathepsin G, elastase, lactoferrin, and bacteriocidal/permeability-inducing protein. Although there is substantial overlap, certain forms of ANCA-associated systemic vasculitis have a higher frequency of p-ANCA or c-ANCA. For example, c-ANCA is the most common form in Wegener's granulomatosis, whereas p-ANCA is usually associated with microscopic polyangiitis or renal-limited disease.

Because the ANCA antigens are inside neutrophils and monocytes, ANCA must either penetrate inside the cell or the antigens must translocate to the cell surface in order for ANCA to have an *in vivo* effect. Small amounts of cytokine (e.g. tumour necrosis factor or interleukin-1) or bacterial formyl peptides, at concentrations too low to cause neutrophil activation, are capable of inducing the externalization of small amounts of ANCA antigens to the cell surface. This can be detected by immuno-electron microscopy or flow cytometry (Falk *et al.* 1990*a*). Moreover, Csernok *et al.* (1991) demonstrated the increased presence of PR3 on the plasma membrane of neutrophils from patients with Wegener's granulomatosis, compared with patients with other autoimmune diseases or healthy donors, and found a correlation between the level of expression and clinical disease activity. Similarly, Guckian *et al.* (1993) demonstrated the expression of PR3 and MPO on the surface of neutrophils in patients with sepsis.

In the normal inflammatory response, priming of the neutrophils and monocytes facilitates their margination and diapedesis; however, full activation of the neutrophils with degranulation and respiratory burst does not occur until the leucocytes have exited the vasculature. If ANCA are able to induce activation and degranulation of the neutrophils and monocytes while they are traversing the vessel wall, the release of lytic enzymes and toxic oxygen metabolites could produce necrotizing inflammatory injury such as that observed in patients with ANCA-associated vasculitides.

There are several putative mechanisms of ANCA-mediated pathogenesis. These are not mutually exclusive and may, in fact, participate simultaneously in the destruction of vessel walls (Fig. 6.2):

1. *ANCA activate neutrophils and monocytes, which results in endothelial damage.* Falk and coworkers have demonstrated that MPO-ANCA can activate cytokine-primed neutrophils *in vitro* resulting in the release of their granule proteins and the production of oxygen radicals (Falk *et al.* 1990*a*; Charles *et al.* 1991). If such activation occurs *in vivo* prior to complete diapedesis, vessel wall damage would occur.

ANCA stimulation of neutrophils may be mediated by both F(ab')$_2$- and Fc-dependent mechanisms. Falk *et al.* (1990*a*) have concluded that F(ab')$_2$ of MPO-ANCA can induce *in vitro* activation of neutrophils but requires priming with tumour necrosis factor (TNF). However, in Mulder's research, F(ab')$_2$ ANCA could bind but not activate neutrophils (Mulder *et al.* 1993). A role for

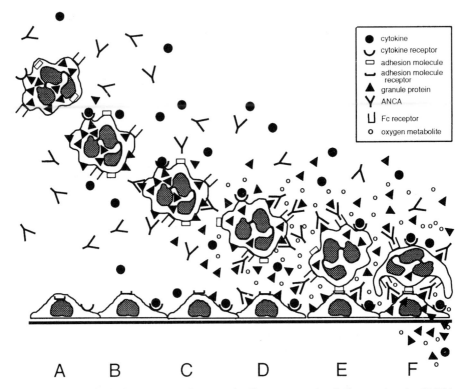

●	cytokine
◡	cytokine receptor
▫	adhesion molecule
‿	adhesion molecule receptor
▲	granule protein
Y	ANCA
⊔	Fc receptor
○	oxygen metabolite

A   B   C   D   E   F

Fig. 6.2 Hypothetical sequence of events leading to vascular inflammation in ANCA-associated vasculitis, based on *in vitro* data. (A) Circulating quiescent neutrophils containing cytoplasmic granule protein ANCA target antigens (e.g. MPO and PR3). (B) Priming of neutrophils by cytokines (e.g. IL-1 or TNF) results in translocation of the ANCA target antigens to the cell surface. (C) ANCA bind to target antigens at the cell surface. (D) Neutrophils are activated via Fc-independent and/or Fc-dependent events, resulting in degranulation and the release of toxic oxygen metabolites. (E) Adhesion of neutrophils to endothelial cells mediated by adhesion molecules and their ligands. (F) Additional activation occurs via interaction of ANCA with target antigens bound to or expressed on the endothelial cell surface. Endothelial cell and vascular tissue injury results. (Reprinted with permission from Jennette, J.C. *Laboratory Investigation*, 1994, **70**, 135–7.)

Fc receptor engagement in ANCA-induced leucocyte activation is supported by the observation that activation and the respiratory burst are diminished or inhibited by blockade of the Fc gamma IIA receptor on neutrophils (Mulder *et al.* 1993; Porges *et al* 1993). In addition, IgG3 ANCA, which bind well to the Fc gamma IIA receptor, have been associated with active disease (Mulder *et al.* 1995). Whether ANCA induce neutrophil activation via the $F(ab')_2$ or Fc portion of the immunoglobulin molecule, or both, remains a matter of active investigation.

Ewert *et al.* (1992*a*) have demonstrated that neutrophils activated by ANCA damage lipopolysaccharide-stimulated endothelial cells *in vitro*, as measured by the release of ^{51}Cr and and LDH. Control immunoglobulin from patients with ANCA-negative necrotizing glomerulonephritis failed to induce similar damage. Priming of the neutrophils was essential for endothelial damage to occur, and the amount of damage was dependent on the dose of anti-MPO antibody present. In a similar set of experiments, Savage *et al.* (1992) also demonstrated that anti-MPO and anti-PR3 antibodies, as well as p-ANCA and c-ANCA F(ab')$_2$, could stimulate PMA and ionomycin primed neutrophils to mediate injury to BCNU or TNF treated human umbilical vein endothelial cells (HUVEC) *in vitro*.

In an *in vivo* model of vascular permeability in the dermis of spontaneously hypertensive (SHR) rats, Kiser *et al.* (1992) demonstrated that anti-MPO antibodies and F(ab')$_2$ increased the permeability to [^{125}I]-aluminium, and [^{51}Cr]-labelled neutrophil accumulation at the site of injection. Thus, ANCA-induced neutrophil activation not only activates neutrophils *in vitro*, but also damages endothelial cell monolayers and increases vascular permeability *in vivo*.

2. *ANCA interact with target antigens on endothelial cells.* ANCA antigens may be liberated from neutrophils and monocytes at the time of degranulation and adhere to the endothelial cell surface, where they would act as ligands for ANCA. Vargunam *et al.* (1992) demonstrated that MPO could bind to cultured endothelial cells. This binding was inhibited by prior incubation of the cells in poly-D-lysine (poly-cation) suggesting that it is charge-mediated, MPO being a cationic protein. Similarly, Ballieux *et al.* (1993) have demonstrated that MPO, but not PR3, can bind to endothelial cells *in vitro*.

Another possible source of ANCA antigen on the endothelial cell surface is synthesis and expression of ANCA antigen by the endothelial cells themselves. This mechanism is suggested by work from Mayet *et al.* (1993), which demonstrated the capability of endothelial cells to express PR3 on their cell surface when stimulated by TNF-α, IL-1, and interferon-γ. However, others have not been able to reproduce these findings (King *et al.* 1995).

Whether the ANCA antigens on the endothelial cell membrane are derived from leucocytes or endothelial cells, the *in situ* formation of antibody-antigen complexes on endothelial cells would lead to inflammation via complement activation, or perhaps by direct antibody dependent cell-mediated cytotoxicity. There is little evidence for such immune complexes on endothelial cells in affected tissues from patients with ANCA-associated vasculitis. However, such complexes might be extremely short-lived *in vivo*, preventing their detection in biopsy material.

Anti-endothelial cell antibodies have been detected in some patients with microscopic polyangiitis and Wegener's granulomatosis (Savage *et al.* 1991; Varagunam *et al.* 1993). These antibodies may be directed against a heterogeneous group of as yet poorly characterized endothelial antigens unrelated to ANCA antigens (Del Papa *et al.* 1994), some of which may be exposed by the vascular damage itself (Direskeneli *et al.* 1994). Whether these antibodies participate in the pathogenesis of ANCA-associated diseases is uncertain (Varagunam *et al.* 1993).

Either mechanism mentioned above would induce adhesion of neutrophils and monocytes to endothelial cells. The neutrophil–endothelial cell interaction can occur at two levels: (1) low affinity apposition mediated by selectins; and (2) high affinity adhesion mediated by neutrophil integrins. The effect of ANCA on endothelial damage by neutrophils may be mediated in part by increasing neutrophil apposition and adhesion to endothelial cells. Ewert *et al.* (1992*b*) demonstrated that anti-MPO antibodies increased the adherence of neutrophils to endothelial cells *in vitro*. This effect involved the neutrophil adhesion molecule CDlla/18 and was blocked by an antibody to the common beta chain of β2-integrin. The ability of anti-MPO antibodies to induce expression of CDlla/18 on neutrophils was also confirmed by flow cytometry analysis. Similarly, Mayet and Mayer Zum Buschenfelde (1993) have demonstrated increased adherence of neutrophils to endothelial cells by prior incubation of the endothelial cells with anti-PR3 antibodies or TNFα, but not with antibodies to Ro (SS-A), La (SS-B), or RNP. This effect could be partially inhibited by pre-incubation of the endothelial cells with an antibody to E-selectin. Both TNFα and anti-PR3 antibodies increased the expression of E-selectin on the endothelial cell membrane with similar kinetics.

3. *ANCA inactivate the proteinases that control the enzymatic activity of ANCA antigens.* A third putative mechanism for ANCA pathogenesis involves inactivation of proteinases by ANCA. Van De Wiel *et al.* (1992) demonstrated an inhibitory effect of c-ANCA on the proteolytic activity of PR3. In addition, c-ANCA inhibit the complexing of PR3 to α1-proteinase, thereby impeding antigen inactivation and clearance. The authors suggested that 'persistence of antibody-protease complexes may lead to damage either through residual antibody-bound PR3 activity or through dissociation of active PR3 from the complex'. This mechanism is indirectly supported by work from Esnault *et al.* (1993), in which a high incidence of severe α-1-proteinase deficiency was found in a group of eight patients with Wegener's granulomatosis. More recent studies confirm this association (Elzouki *et al.* 1994).

Role of T cells in systemic vasculitis

It seems highly likely that T cells are involved in providing help for ANCA production, and they could also contribute directly to tissue injury. Cell-mediated immunity is suggested by the granuloma formation characteristic of Wegener's granulomatosis, and by reports that T cells form part of the glomerular infiltrate in crescentic nephritis. Peripheral blood T cells from patients with ANCA-positive vasculitis have been shown to proliferate *in vitro* to the appropriate auto-antigen, PR3 or MPO (Brouwer *et al.* 1994; Ballieux *et al.* 1995). There are also suggestions that peripheral blood T cells in vasculitis patients express receptors with limited Vβ families (Simpson *et al.* 1995), although this finding needs to be confirmed.

Animal models of ANCA-associated disease

Despite the *in vitro* evidence that ANCA may play a pathogenic role in the development of small vessel vasculitis, definite proof of such a role awaits an *in vivo* model of ANCA-associated disease. Brouwer *et al.* (1993) have reported that pauci-immune glomerulonephritis and vasculitis could be precipitated by infusing MPO, plus hydrogen peroxide, or a crude preparation of neutrophil granule enzymes, into the kidney of rats previously immunized with human MPO. However, Yang *et al.* (1994) demonstrated that this model led to the development of an immune complex-mediated glomerulonephritis, with the deposition of IgG and C3 as demonstrated by immunofluorescence microscopy. Whether subtle differences in methodology are responsible for these differences in results has yet to be determined.

Kobayashi *et al.* (1993) injected rabbit antibody specific to rat MPO into rats that subsequently received either rabbit serum containing high titers of anti-rat GBM antibodies (Masugi serum) or normal rabbit serum. Control animals were first injected with normal rabbit serum or the Masugi serum. In this model, the authors demonstrated an increase in neutrophil and fibrin accumulation in the glomeruli of rats first treated with anti-MPO antibodies, suggesting that anti-MPO antibodies aggravated rat Masugi nephritis.

In Brown–Norway rats, mercuric chloride induces a T cell-dependent polyclonal B cell activation, leading to the development of numerous autoantibodies to the GBM, ds-DNA, thyroid antigens, and MPO. Mathieson *et al.* (1992) and Esnault *et al.* (1992) reported the development of widespread inflammation, including necrotizing vasculitis, in BN rats treated with mercuric chloride, in the presence of anti-MPO antibodies and anti-GBM antibodies. The areas of vasculitis were mostly confined to the skin and gastrointestinal tract, and despite the presence of pneumonitis and interstitial nephritis, no vasculitis could be demonstrated in either organ. No immunofluorescence studies of the areas of necrotizing vasculitis in the skin and gastrointestinal tract were described, but immunofluorescence microscopy of the kidneys revealed linear IgG deposits along the capillary walls. This model does not appear to be that of a pauci-immune vasculitis and the role of anti-MPO antibodies in this setting is unclear.

Harper *et al.* (1993) report finding ANCA in 20% of female MRL lpr/lpr mice; however, the monoclonal IgG ANCA isolated from these mice bound non-specifically to MPO, lactoferrin, and DNA with equal affinity. Recently, Kinjoh *et al.* (1993) described an inbred strain of mice derived from the MRL and BXSB strains. These mice, named 'spontaneous crescentic glomerulonephritis-forming/Kinjoh' (or SCG/Kj), develop a severe crescentic glomerulonephritis with only small amounts of granular IgG and C3 deposits, and a systemic necrotizing vasculitis involving chiefly small arteries and arterioles. The evaluation of this strain as a model of ANCA-associated disease is currently under way.

Finally, Blanck *et al.* (1995) have described a murine model induced by immunization of mice with ANCA. They proposed that this led to the production of anti-ANCA antibodies (Ab2) and subsequently anti-anti-ANCA antibodies

(Ab3) via the idiotypic network. The Ab3 could then act as ANCA in initiating disease. However, the pathological findings were not typical of vasculitis found in man.

Drug-associated vasculitis

D-Penicillamine

There are several reports of pulmonary-renal vasculitis syndrome associated with treatment with D-penicillamine (Devogelaer *et al.* 1987; Macarron *et al.* 1992). This is characterized by haematuria, proteinuria, renal failure, and pulmonary haemorrhage. Cases of Goodpasture's disease with documented anti-GBM antibodies and/or linear antibody staining on immunofluorescence microscopy associated with D-penicillamine are rare (Peces *et al.* 1987). In most cases, however, ANCA tests were either not performed or performed late in the course of the disease. There are, nevertheless, two case reports of D-penicillamine-induced pulmonary-renal vasculitis syndrome with documented presence of p-ANCA and absence of anti-GBM antibodies (Lauque *et al.* 1990; Jones and Major 1992).

Propylthiouracil

Propylthiouracil (PTU) is a thionamide used in the treatment of hyperthyroidism. It has been associated with a number of complications or side-effects such as leucopenia, rash, fever, and, rarely, sicca-like syndrome and vasculitis. Two articles report the association of PTU therapy with ANCA-positive vasculitis and necrotizing glomerulonephritis. In Dolman *et al.*'s (1993) report, six patients treated with PTU developed a vasculitis-like disorder, although not all patients had biopsy-proven evidence of renal involvement. All six patients had evidence of presence of ANCA with specificity for human neutrophil elastase, sometimes simultaneously with anti-PR3 or anti-MPO antibodies. Vogt *et al.* (1994) report two adolescent patients who developed MPO-ANCA positive crescentic glomerulonephritis requiring immunosuppression. A previous report by Griswold *et al.* (1978) suggested that circulating immune complexes might play a part in the pathogenesis of PTU-associated vasculitis.

Hydralazine

The most common, and best-documented complication of hydralazine treatment is a lupus-like syndrome. This syndrome has been described since the mid 1950s, and was later recognized to be associated with higher doses, and to occur more commonly in slow acetylators. Hydralazine has also been associated with necrotizing vasculitis involving the skin, with or without associated focal necrotizing glomerulonephritis (Björck *et al.* 1983, 1985). In addition to antinuclear antibodies, patients with hydralazine-induced lupus-like syndrome also develop p-ANCA, usually with specificity for MPO (Nassberger *et al.* 1990). Whether hydralazine induces a focal necrotizing glomerulonephritis as the consequence of a lupus-like syndrome (Ihle *et al.* 1984), or in association with anti-MPO antibodies, is a matter for discussion.

Summary

The pathogenesis of systemic vasculitis is incompletely understood. It is clear, however, that multiple different mechanisms, many involving immunological events, cause vascular inflammation. There is substantial evidence that vasculitis can be mediated by immune complex deposition, direct binding of antibodies, or attack on vessel walls by ANCA-activated leucocytes. It is also likely that more than one mechanism may be at play simultaneously in any given setting. At this point, the elucidation of the aetiology and primary mechanisms of tissue injury awaits animal models of disease which more precisely mimic the human condition. Such models are, unfortunately, still lacking today.

References

Agnello, V., Chung, R.T., and Kaplan, L.M. (1992). A role for hepatitis C virus infection in type II cryoglobulinemia. *New England Journal of Medicine*, **327**, 1490–5.

Ballieux, B.E., van der Burg, S.H., Hagen, E.C., van der Woude, F.J., Melief, C.J., and Daha, M.R. (1995). Cell-mediated autoimmunity in patients with Wegener's granulomatosis (WG). *Clinical and Experimental Immunology*, **100**, 186–93.

Ballieux, B.E.P.B., Zondervan, K., Hagen, E.C., van der Woude, F.J., van Es, L.A., and Daha, M.R. (1993). Differential binding of MPO and PR3 to monolayers of endothelial cells. *Clinical and Experimental Immunology*, **93**, 17 (abstract).

Björck, S., Westberg, G., Svalander, C., and Mulec, H. (1983). Rapidly progressive glomerulonephritis after hydralazine. *Lancet*, **ii**, 42.

Björck, S., Svalander, C., and Westberg, G. (1985). Hydralazine associated glomerulonephritis. *Acta Medica Scandinavica*, **218**, 261–9.

Blanck, M., Tomer, Y., Stein, M., Kopolovic, J., Wiik, A., Meroni, P.L. *et al.* (1995). Immunization with anti-neutrophil cytoplasmic antibody (ANCA) induces the production of mouse ANCA and perivascular lymphocyte infiltration. *Clinical and Experimental Immunology*, **101**, 120–30.

Brouet, J-C., Clauvel, J-P., Danon, F., Klein, M., and Seligman, M. (1974). Biologic and clinical significance of cryoglobulins. *American Journal of Medicine*, **57**, 775–8.

Brouwer, E., Huitema, M.G., Klok, P.A. *et al.* (1993). Antimyeloperoxidase-associated proliferative glomerulonephritis: an animal model. *Journal of Experimental Medicine*, **177**, 905–14.

Brouwer, E., Stegeman, C.A., Huitema, M.G., Limburg, P.C., and Kallenberg, C.G. (1994). T cell reactivity to proteinase 3 and myeloperoxidase in patients with Wegener's granulomatosis (WG). *Clinical and Experimental Immunology*, **98**, 448–53.

Burstein, D.M., and Rodby, R.A. (1993). Membranoproliferative glomerulonephritis associated with Hepatitis C virus infection. *Journal of the American Society of Nephrology*, **4**, 1288–93.

Carreras, L.O., and Vermylen, J.G. (1982). Lupus anticoagulant and thrombosis—possible role of inhibition of prostacyclin formation. *Thrombosis and Haemostasis*, **48**, 38–40.

Charles, L.A., Caldas, M.L., Falk, R.J., Terrell, R.S., and Jennette, J.C. (1991). Antibodies against granule proteins activate neutrophils *in vitro*. *Journal of Leukocyte Biology*, **50**, 539–46.

Churchill, D.N., Fine, A., and Gault, M.H. (1983). Association between hydrocarbon exposure and glomerulonephritis: an appraisal of the evidence. *Nephron*, **33**, 169–72.

Cines, D.B., Lyss, A.P., Reeber, M., Bina, M., and Dehoratius, R.I. (1984). Presence of complement fixing anti-endothelial cell antibodies in systemic lupus erythematosus. *Journal of Clinical Investigation*, **73**, 611–25.

Colasanti, G., Morel Maroger, L., and D'Amico, G. (1987). Deposition of fibrin-stabilizing factor (F XIIIA and S), fibrinogen-related antigens, fibrinogen degradation products (FDPd and FDPe) and antihemolytic factor (F VIII) in renal disease: analysis of 161 cases by immunofluorescence microscopy. *Clinical Nephrology*, **28**, 28–34.

Cole, E.H., Schulman, J., Urowitz, M., Keystone, E., Williams, C., and Levy, G.A. (1985). Monocyte procoagulant activity in glomerulonephritis associated with systemic lupus erythematosus. *Journal of Clinical Investigation*, **75**, 861–8.

Csernok, E.M., Schmitt, E.W.H., Bainton, D., and Gross, W.L. (1991). Translocation of proteinase 3 on the cell surface of neutrophils: association with disease activity in Wegener's granulomatosis. *Arthritis and Rheumatism*, **31** (suppl.1), 71.

D'Amico, G., Colasanti, G., Ferrario, F., and Sinico, R.A. (1989). Renal involvement in essential mixed cryoglobulinemia. *Kidney International*, **35**, 1004–14.

Daniell, W.E., Couser, W.G., and Rosenstock, L. (1988). Occupational solvent exposure and glomerulonephritis. A case report and review of the literature. *Journal of the American Medical Association*, **259**, 2280–3.

Davies, K.A., Hird. V., Stewart, S. *et al.* (1990). A study of *in vivo* immune complex formation and clearance in man. *Journal of Immunology*, **144**, 4613–20.

Del Papa, N., Conforti, G., Gambini, D. *et al.* (1994). Characterization of the endothelial surface proteins recognized by anti-endothelial antibodies in primary and secondary autoimmune vasculitis. *Clinical Immunology and Immunopathology*, **70**, 211–16.

Devogelaer, J.P., Pirson, Y., Vandenbroucke, J.M., Cosyns, J.P., Brichard, S., and Nagant de Deuxchaisnes, C. (1987). D-penicillamine induced crescentic glomerulonephritis: report and review of the literature. *Journal of Rheumatology*, **14**, 1036–41.

Direskeneli, H., De Cruz, D, Khamashta, M.A., and Hughes, G.R. (1994). Auto-antibodies against endothelial cells, extracellular matrix, and human collagen type IV in patients with systemic vasculitis. *Clinical Immunology and Immunopathology*, **70**, 206–10.

Dolman, K.M., Gans, R.O., Vervaat, T.J. *et al.* (1993). Vasculitis and antineutrophil cytoplasmic autoantibodies associated with propylthiouracil therapy. *Lancet*, **342**, 651–2.

Duffy, J., Lidsky, M.D., Dharp, J.T., Davis, J.S. Person, D.A., Hollinger, F.B. *et al.* (1976). Polyarthritis, polyarteritis and hepatitis B. *Medicine*, **55**, 19–37.

Durand, J.M., Lefevre, P., Harle, J.R., Boucrat, J., Vitviski, L., and Soubeyrand, J. (1991). Cutaneous vasculitis and cryoglobulinaemia type II associated with hepatitis C virus infection. *Lancet*, **337**, 499–500 (letter).

Elzouki, A.N., Segelmark, M., Wieslander, J., and Eriksson, S. (1994). Strong link between the alpha 1-antitrypsin PiZ allele and Wegener's granulomasosis. *Journal of Internal Medicine*, **236**, 543–8.

Esnault, V.L., Mathieson, P.W., Thiru, S., Oliveira, D.B., and Lockwood, M.C. (1992). Autoantibodies to myeloperoxidase in brown Norway rats treated with mercuric chloride. *Laboratory Investigation*, **67**, 114–20.

Esnault, V.L., Testa, A., Audrain, M. *et al.* (1993). Alpha 1-antitrypsin genetic polymorphism in ANCA-positive systemic vasculitis. *Kidney International*, **43**, 1329–32.

Ewert, B.H., Jennette, J.C., and Falk R.J. (1992*a*). Anti-myeloperoxidase antibodies stimulate neutrophils to damage human endothelial cells. *Kidney International*, **41**, 375–83.

Ewert, B.H., Becker, M., Jennette, J.C., and Falk, R.J. (1992*b*). Anti-myeloperoxidase antibodies (aMPO) stimulate neutrophils to adhere to cultured human endothelial cells utilizing the beta-2-integrin CD11/18. *Journal of the American Society of Nephrology*, **3**, 585.

Falk, R.J., Terrell, R.S., Charles, L.A., and Jennette, J.C. (1990*a*). Anti-neutrophil cytoplasmic autoantibodies induce neutrophils to degranulate and produce oxygen radicals *in vitro*. *Proceedings of the National Academy of Science USA*, **87**, 4115–19.

Feldman, D., Goldstein, A.L., Cox, D.C., and Grimley, P.M. (1988). Cultured human endothelial cells treated with recombinant leukocyte A interferon. Tubuloreticular inclusion formation, antiproliferative effect, and $2'-5'$ oligoadenylate synthetase induction. *Laboratory Investigation*, **58**, 584–9.

Fiorini, G., Bernasconi, P., Sinico, R.A., Chianese, R., Pozzi, F., and D'Amico, G. (1986). Increased frequency of antibodies to ubiquitous viruses in essential mixed cryoglobulinemia. *Clinical and Experimental Immunology*, **64**, 65–70.

Fiorini, G.F., Sinico, R.A., Winearls, C., Custode, P., DeGiuli-Morghen, C., and D'Amico, G. (1988). Persistent Epstein–Barr virus in patients with type II essential mixed cryoglobulinemia. *Clinical Immunology and Immunopathology*, **47**, 262–9.

Frankel, A.H., Singer, D.R., Winearls, C.G., Evans, D.J. Rees, A.J., and Pusey, C.D. (1992). Type II essential mixed cryoglobulinaemia: presentation, treatment and outcome in 13 patients. *Quarterly Journal of Medicine*, **82**, 101–24.

Gocke, D.J., Hsu, K., Morgan, C., Bombardieri, S., Lockshin, M., and Christian, C.L. (1970). Association between polyarteritis and Australia antigen. *Lancet*, **ii**, 1149–53.

Griswold, W.R., Mendoza, S.A., Johnston, W., and Steven Nichols, L.C.D.R. (1978). Vasculitis associated with propylthiouracil–Evidence for immune complex pathogenesis and response to therapy. *Western Journal of Medicine*, **128**, 543–6.

Guckian, M., and O'Donoghue, D.J. (1993). Membrane surface ANCA antigen expression on human neutrophils *in vivo*. *Clinical and Experimental Immunology*, **93** (suppl.1), 25 (abstract).

Harper, J.M., Lockwood, C.M., and Cooke, A. (1993). Anti-neutrophil cytoplasm antibodies in MRL- lpr/lpr mice *Clinical and Expermental Immunology*, **93**(suppl.1), 22 (abstract).

Ihle, B.U., Whitworth, J.A., Dowling, J.P., and Kincaid-Smith, P. (1984). Hydralazine and lupus nephritis. *Clinical Nephrology*, **22**, 230–8.

Invernizzi, F., Galli, M., Serino, G., Monti, G., Meroni, P.L., Granatieri, C. *et al.* (1983). Secondary and essential cryoglobulinemias. Frequency, nosological classification and long-term follow-up. *Acta Haematologica*, **70**, 73–82.

Jennette, J.C., Falk, R.J., Andrassy, K., Bacon, P.A., Churg, J., Gross, W.L. *et al.* (1994). Nomenclature of systemic vasculitides: The proposal of an international consensus conference. *Arthritis and Rheumatism*, **37**, 187–92.

Jones, B.F., and Major, G.A.C. (1992). Crescentic glomerulonephritis in a patient taking penicillamine associated with antineutrophil cytoplasmic antibody. *Clinical Nephrology*, **38**, 293.

Kant, K.S., Pollak, V.E., Weiss, M., Glueck, H.I., Miller, M.A., and Hess, E.V. (1981). Glomerular thrombosis in systemic lupus erythematosus: Prevalence and significance. *Medicine*, **60**, 71–86.

King, W.J., Adu, D., Daha, M.R., Brooks, C.J., Radford, D.J., Pall, A.A. *et al.* (1995). Endothelial cells and renal epithelial cells do not express the Wegener's autoantigen, proteinase 3. *Clinical and Experimental Immunology*, **102**, 98–105.

Kinjoh, K., Kyogoku, M., and Good, R.A. (1993). Genetic selection for crescent formation yields mouse strain with rapidly progressive glomerulonephritis and small vessel vasculitis. *Proceedings of the National Academy of Science USA*, **90**, 3413–17.

Kiser, M.A., Jennette, J.C., and Falk, R.J. (1992). Effects of antibodies to myeloperoxidase (aMPO) on vascular permeability and neutrophil accumulation *in vivo*. *Journal of the American Society of Nephrology*, **3**, 599 (abstract).

Knight, J.F. (1990). The rheumatic poison: a survey of some published investigations of the immunopathogenesis of Henoch–Schönlein purpura. *Pediatric Nephrology*, **4**, 533–41.

Kobayashi, K., Shibata, T., and Sugisaki, T. (1993). Aggravation of rat Masugi nephritis by heterologous anti-rat myeloperoxidase (MPO) antibody. *Clinical and Experimental Immunology*, **93**(suppl.1), 20 (abstract).

Lauque, D., Courtin, J.P., Fournie, B., Oksman, F., Pourrat, J., and Carles, P. (1990). Pneumorenal syndrome induced by d-Penicillamine: Goodpasture's syndrome or microscopic polyarteritis? *Revue Médecine Interne*, **11**, 168–71.

Le Roux, G., Wautier, M.P., Guillevin, L., and Wautier, J.L. (1986). IgG binding to endothelial cells in systemic lupus erythematosus. *Thrombosis and Haemostasis*, **56**, 144–6.

Leung, D.Y., Collins, T., Lapierre, L.A., Geha, R.S., and Pober, J.S. (1986). Immunoglobulin M antibodies present in the acute phase of Kawasaki syndrome lyse cultured vascular endothelial cells stimulated by gamma interferon. *Journal of Clinical Investigation*, **77**, 1428–35.

Leung D.Y.M., Cotran, R.S., Kurt-Jones, E., Burns, J.C., Newburger, J.W., and Pober, J.S. (1989). Endothelial cell activation and high interleukin-1 secretion in the pathogenesis of acute Kawasaki disease. *Lancet*, **2**, 1298–302.

Levo, Y., Gorevic, P.D., Kassab, H.J., Zucker-Franklin, D., and Franklin, E.C. (1977). Association between hepatitis B virus and essential mixed cryoglobulinemia. *New England Journal of Medicine*, **296**, 1501–4.

Macarron, P., Garcia Diaz, J.E., Azofra, J.A. *et al.* (1992). D-penicillamine therapy associated with rapidly progressive glomerulonephritis. *Nephrology Dialysis Transplantation*, **7**, 161–4.

Mader, R., and Keystone, E.C. (1992). Infections that cause vasculitis. *Current Opinion in Rheumatology*, **4**, 35–8.

Marcellin, P., Calmus, Y., Takahashi, H. *et al.* (1991). Latent hepatitis B virus (HBV) infection in systemic necrotizing vasculitis. *Clinical and Experimental Rheumatology*, **9**, 23–8.

Mathieson, P.W., Thiru, S., and Oliveira, D.B. (1992). Mercuric chloride treated brown Norway rats develop widespread tissue injury including necrotizing vasculitis. *Laboratory Investigation*, **67**, 121–9.

Mayet, W.J., Csernok, E., Szymkowiak, C., Gross, W.L., and Meyer zum Buschenfelde, K.H. (1993*a*). Human endothelial cells express proteinase 3, the target antigen of anticytoplasmic antibodies in Wegener's granulomatosis. *Blood*, **82**, 1221–9.

Mayet, W.J., and Meyer zum Buschenfelde, K.H. (1993*b*). Antibodies to proteinase 3 increase adhesion of neutrophils to human endothelial cells. *Clinical and Experimental Immunology*, **94**, 440–6.

McMahon, B.J., Heyward, W.L., Templin, D.W., Clement, D., and Lanier, A.P. (1989). Hepatitis B-associated polyarteritis nodosa in Alaskan Eskimos: Clinical and epidemiologic features and long-term follow-up. *Hepatology*, **9**, 97–101.

McMahon, B.J., Alberts, S.R., Wainwright, R.B., Bulkow, L., and Lanier, A.P. (1990). Hepatitis B-related sequelae. Prospective study in 1400 hepatitis B surface antigen-positive Alaska native carriers. *Archives of Internal Medicine*, **150**, 1051–4.

Michalak, T. (1978). Immune complexes of hepatitis B surface antigen in the pathogenesis of periarteritis nodosa. *American Journal of Pathology*, **90**, 619–28.

Misiani, R., Bellavita, P., Fenili, D., Borelli, G., Marchesi, D., Massazza, M. *et al.* (1992). Hepatitis C virus infection in patients with essential mixed cryoglobulinemia. *Annals of Internal Medicine*, **117**, 573–7.

Mozes, E., Kohn, L.D., Hakim, F., and Singer, D.S. (1993). Resistance of MHC class I-deficient mice to experimental systemic lupus erythematosus. *Science*, **261**, 91–3.

Mulder, A.H.L., Horst, G., Limburg, P.C., and Kallenberg, C.G.M. (1993). Activation of neutrophils by anti-neutrophil cytoplasmic antibodies (ANCA) is FcR dependent. *Clinical and Experimental Immunology*, **93** (suppl.1), 16 (abstract).

Mulder, A.H., Stegeman, C.A., and Kallenberg, C.G. (1995). Activation of granulocytes by anti-neutrophil cytoplasmic antibodies (ANCA) in Wegener's granulomatosis: predominant role for the IgG3 subclass of ANCA. *Clinical and Experimental Immunology*, **101**, 227–32.

Nassberger, L., Sjoholm, A.G., and Thysell, H. (1990). Antimyeloperoxidase antibodies in patients with extracapillary glomerulonephritis. *Nephron*, **56**, 152–6.

Pascual, M., Perrin, L., Giostra, E., and Schifferli, J.A. (1990). Hepatitis C virus in patients with cryoglobulinemia type II. *Journal of Infectious Diseases*, **162**, 567–9 (letter).

Peces, R., Riera, J.R., Arboleya, L.R., and Lopez-Larrea, J.A. (1987). Goodpasture's syndrome in a patient receiving penicillamine and carbimazole. *Nephron*, **45**, 316–20.

Perl, A., Gorevic, P.D., Ryan, D.H., Condemi, J.J., Ruszkowski, R.J., and Abraham, G.N. (1989). Clonal B cell expansions in patients with essential mixed cryoglobulinaemia. *Clinical and Experimental Immunology*, **76**, 54–60.

Porges, A.J., Redecha, P.B., Csernok, E., Gross, W.L., and Kimberly, R.P. (1993). Monoclonal ANCA (anti-MPO and anti-PR3) engage and activate neutrophils via Fc gamma receptor IIA. *Clinical and Experimental Immunology*, **93** (suppl.1), 18 (abstract).

Ravnskow, U., Lundstrom, S., and Norden, A. (1983). Hydrocarbon exposure and glomerulonephritis: evidence from patients' occupations. *Lancet*, **ii**, 121–16.

Rees, A.J., Peters, D.K., Compston, D.A., and Batchelor, J.R. (1978). Strong association between HLA-DRw2 and antibody-mediated Goodpasture's syndrome. *Lancet*, **i**, 966–8.

Rees, A.J., Peters, D.K., Amos, N., Welsh, K.I., and Batchelor, J.R. (1984). The influence of HLA-linked genes on the severity of anti-GBM antibody-mediated nephritis. *Kidney International*, **26**, 444–50.

Savage, C.O., Pottinger, B.E., Gaskin, G., Lockwood, C.M., Pusey, C.D., and Pearson, J.D. (1991). Vascular damage in Wegener's granulomatosis and microscopic polyarteritis: presence of anti-endothelial cell antibodies and their relation to anti-neutrophil cytoplasm antibodies. *Clinical and Experimental Immunology*, **85**, 14–19.

Savage, C.O., Pottinger, B.E., Gaskin, G., Pusey, C.D., and Pearson, J.D. (1992). Autoantibodies developing to myeloperoxidase and proteinase 3 in systemic vasculitis stimulate neutrophil cytotoxicity toward cultured endothelial cells. *American Journal of Pathology*, **141**, 335–42.

Sergent, J.S., Lockshin, M.D., Christian, C.L., and Gocke, D.J. (1976). Vasculitis with hepatitis B antigenemia: Long term observations in nine patients. *Medicine*, **55**, 1–18.

Shoenfeld, Y., Rauch, J., Massicotte, H., Datta, S.K., Andre-Schwartz, J., and Stollar, B.D. *et al.* (1983). Polyspecificity of monoclonal lupus antibodies produced by human-human hybridomas. *New England Journal of Medicine*, **308**, 414–20.

Simpson, I.J., Skinner, M.A., Guersen, A., Peake, J.S., Abott, W.G., Fraser, J.D. *et al.* (1995). Peripheral blood T lymphocytes in systemic vasculitis: increased T cell receptor V beta 2 gene usage in microscopic polyarteritis. *Clinical and Experimental Immunology*, **101**, 220–6.

Smeenk, R., Brinkman, K., van den Brink, H., Termaat, R.M., Berden, J., Nossent, H. *et al.* (1990). Antibodies to DNA in patients with systemic lupus erythematosus. Their role in the diagnosis, the follow-up and the pathogenesis of the disease. *Clinical and Experimental Rheumatology*, **9** (suppl.1), 100–10.

Sturfelt, G., Nived, O., and Sjoholm, A.G. (1992). Kinetic analysis of immune complex solubilization: complement function in relation to disease activity in SLE. *Clinical and Experimental Rheumatology*, **10**, 241–7.

Takemura, T., Yoshioka, K., Akano, N., Miyamoto, H., Matsumoto, K., and Maki, S. (1987). Glomerular deposition of cross-linked fibrin in human kidney diseases. *Kidney International*, **32**, 102–11.

Tanaka, M., Fujisawa, S., and Okuda, R. (1969). Anaphylactoid purpura in childhood: III. Follow-up study of serum levels of immunoglobulins (G,M,A). *Annals of Paediatrics (Japan)*, **15**, 19–26.

Van de Wiel, B.A., Dolman, K.M., van der Meer Gerritsen C.H., Hack, C.E., von dem Borne, A.E., and Goldschmeding, R. (1992). Interference of Wegener's granulomatosis autoantibodies with neutrophil proteinase 3 activity. *Clinical and Experimental Immunology*, **90**, 409–14.

Vargunam, M., Adu, D., Taylor, C.M. *et al.* (1992). Endothelium myeloperoxidase-antimyeloperoxidase interaction in vasculitis. *Nephrology Dialysis Transplantation*, **7**, 1077–81.

Varagunam, M., Nwosu, A.C., Adu, D. *et al.* (1993). Little evidence for anti-endothelial-cell antibodies in microscopic polyarteritis and Wegener's granulomatosis. *Advances in Experimental Medicine and Biology*. **336**, 419–22.

Vogt, B.A., Kim, Y., Jennette, J.C., Falk, R.J., Burke, B.A., and Sinaiko, A. (1994). ANCA-positive crescentic glomerulonephritis as a complication of propylthiouracil treatment. *Journal of Pediatrics*, **986–8**.

Wieslander, J., Bygren, P., and Heinegard D. (1984a). Isolation of the specific glomerular basement membrane antigen involved in Goodpasture syndrome. *Proceedings of the National Academy of Science USA*, **81**, 1544–8.

Wieslander, J., Barr, J.F., Butkowski, R.J., Edwards, S.J., Bygren, P., Heinegard, D. *et al.* (1984b). Goodpasture antigen of the glomerular basement membrane: localization to noncollagenous regions of type IV collagen. *Proceedings of the National Academy of Science USA*, **81**, 3828–42.

Wieslander, J., Langeveld, J., Butkowski, R., Jodlowski, M., Noelken, M., and Hudson, B.G. (1985). Physical and immunochemical studies of the glomerular domain of type IV collagen. Cryptic properties of the Goodpasture antigen. *Journal of Biological Chemistry*, **260**, 8564–70.

Yang, J.J., Jennette, J.C., Falk, R.J. (1994). Immune complex glomerulonephritis is induced in rats immunized with heterologous myeloperoxidase. *Clinical and Experimental Immunology*, **97**, 466–73.

Yoshioka, K., Michael, A.F., Velosa, J., and Fish, A.J. (1985). Detection of hidden nephritogenic antigen determinants in human renal and nonrenal basement membranes. *American Journal of Pathology*, **121**, 156–65.

7
Clinical aspects of systemic vasculitis
Gillian Gaskin and Charles D. Pusey

Necrotizing inflammation of small blood vessels is the hallmark of the primary systemic vasculitides associated with rapidly progressive glomerulonephritis. Other primary vasculitic syndromes affect larger vessels, and vasculitis may also occur as a variable accompaniment to other systemic diseases, including rheumatoid arthritis, systemic lupus erythematosus, and infective endocarditis. This chapter will deal principally with the small vessel vasculitides, Wegener's granulomatosis and microscopic polyangiitis.

Classification of vasculitic syndromes

Historical descriptions

Systemic vasculitis was first described in 1866 by Kussmaul and Maier, who reported 'periarteritis nodosa' in a patient with fever, muscle, intestinal and renal disease, nodular swellings along the course of medium-sized arteries, and inflammatory changes within and around the vessel wall. The term 'polyarteritis nodosa' was later adopted, with the realization that the arterial wall itself was the target of inflammation (Rose and Spencer 1957). In the years that followed, vasculitic illnesses were increasingly recognized, and several other distinctive patterns emerged.

Wegener's granulomatosis, defined by the triad of destructive respiratory tract lesions, granulomata, and glomerulonephritis, was initially described by Klinger, but fully characterized by Wegener (1936/1987), and by the comprehensive studies of Fahey *et al.* (1954) and Godman and Churg (1954). An anatomically limited form of Wegener's granulomatosis, sparing the kidneys, was reported by Carrington and Liebow in 1966.

Microscopic polyarteritis was first identified by Davson and coworkers in 1948, who reported patients with a systemic vasculitis, initially labelled as polyarteritis nodosa, with extensive glomerular changes: patchy fibrinoid necrosis of glomerular tufts with varying degrees of crescent formation. Currently, with the realization that capillaries and venules may also be affected in such patients, the term 'microscopic polyangiitis' is preferred to 'microscopic polyarteritis'.

Churg and Strauss (1951) gave their name to another variant of polyarteritis nodosa, which was characterized by fever, asthma, eosinophilia, cardiac failure, peripheral neuropathy, and gastrointestinal and renal disease. The pathological findings included necrotizing arteritis, eosinophil-rich inflammation, and a tendency to granuloma formation. The typical renal abnormalities included intrarenal arteritis and arteriolitis, and interstitial nephritis; eosinophils were prominent in these lesions. Segmental glomerular lesions were common but rarely severe.

Diagnosis and classification

By the 1970s, with the increasing effectiveness of treatment for systemic vasculitis, it was no longer possible to examine a full range of tissues at the end of the natural history of the disease. Clinical and pathological criteria were therefore adapted to permit a diagnosis during life, exemplified by the pragmatic approach of Lanham *et al.* (1984) to the diagnosis of Churg–Strauss syndrome. In the past five years, attention has focused on the development of consistent criteria for the classification of vasculitic syndromes, to facilitate clinical and scientific studies. Two recent approaches merit comment.

ACR 1990 criteria for the classification of vasculitis

The American College of Rheumatologists (Hunder *et al.* 1990) identified the clinical features most commonly and most specifically associated with certain vasculitic syndromes, and proposed combinations of features which would identify patients with these syndromes. Unfortunately, the criteria did not differentiate the patient with small vessel vasculitis reflected by focal necrotizing glomerulonephritis from the patient with classical polyarteritis nodosa without nephritis, and intense discussion followed.

Chapel Hill consensus criteria for the nomenclature of vasculitis

An international meeting at Chapel Hill, North Carolina, led to consensus proposals for an alternative nomenclature (Jennette *et al.* 1994) and the salient features are illustrated in Table 7.1. The distinction between syndromes depends chiefly on the size of vessel affected, taking into account the presence or absence of certain specific features. A syndrome is classified by the smallest vessel affected. Thus, although a diagnostic label of Wegener's granulomatosis (typically a small vessel vasculitis) may be given to a patient who also has involvement of muscular arteries, a diagnosis of polyarteritis nodosa may not be given to a patient with necrotizing glomerulonephritis. The Chapel Hill terminology will be used throughout this chapter.

The Chapel Hill classification does not include 'idiopathic rapidly progressive glomerulonephritis' (i.e. idiopathic focal necrotizing and crescentic glomerulonephritis without anti-glomerular basement membrane antibodies). This is now widely considered to be part of the small vessel vasculitis spectrum, and is sometimes described as 'renal-limited vasculitis', since there is no clinical evidence of extrarenal angiitis. However, it is worth emphasizing that Harrison *et al.* (1964) described patients from the pre-treatment era who were diagnosed

Table 7.1   The Chapel Hill consensus on the nomenclature of systemic vasculitis

Syndromes affecting small vessels (capillaries, venules, and arterioles)	
Wegener's granulomatosis	Granulomatous inflammation in the respiratory tract;necrotizing vasculitis affecting small- to medium-sized vessels.
Churg-Strauss syndrome	Eosinophil-rich and granulomatous inflammation in the respiratory tract; necrotizing vasculitis affecting small- and medium-sized vessels; asthma and eosinophilia.
Microscopic polyangiitis	Necrotizing vasculitis, with few or no immune deposits, affecting small vessels.
Henoch–Schönlein purpura	Vasculitis, with IgA-dominant immune deposits, affecting small vessels.
Essential cryoglobulinaemic vasculitis	Vasculitis, with cryoglobulin deposits, affecting small vessels, and associated with circulating cryoglobulins.
Cutaneous leucocytoclastic angiitis	Isolated cutaneous leucocytoclastic angiitis without systemic vasculitis or glomerulonephritis.
Syndromes affecting medium-sized vessels	
Polyarteritis nodosa	Necrotizing inflammation of medium-sized or small arteries without glomerulonephritis or vasculitis in arterioles, capillaries, or venules.
Kawasaki disease	Arteritis involving large, medium-sized, and small arteries; associated with mucocutaneous lymph node syndrome.
Syndromes affecting large vessels	
Giant cell arteritis	Granulomatous arteritis of the aorta and its major branches, with a predilection for the extracranial branches of the carotid artery.
Takayasu arteritis	Granulomatous inflammation of the aorta and its major branches.

as having isolated nephritis on renal biopsy, but who were found at autopsy to have more widespread disease. Additional supporting evidence that idiopathic rapidly progressive glomerulonephritis is a variant of small vessel vasculitis includes similar age at presentation, similar non-specific constitutional symptoms, identical renal histology, a similar response to steroids and immunosuppressive therapy, and occasional progression to a generalized vasculitis. Furthermore, antineutrophil cytoplasmic antibodies (ANCA) have been reproducibly detected in both conditions. In this chapter, ANCA-associated idiopathic rapidly progressive glomerulonephritis will be regarded as renal-limited vasculitis.

Association with antineutrophil cytoplasmic antibodies (ANCA)

In the past 10 years, the discovery of autoantibodies directed against components of neutrophil cytoplasm in certain vasculitic syndromes has significantly altered the clinical approach. Although Davies *et al.* (1982) were the first to describe these autoantibodies, Van der Woude *et al.* (1985) were the first to appreciate the link with vasculitis when reporting a close association with Wegener's granulomatosis. Much subsequent work focused on defining the spectrum of diseases associated with ANCA and the nature of the target antigens (reviewed by Kallenberg *et al.* 1994). ANCA are not unique to Wegener's granulomatosis, but are also closely associated with microscopic polyangiitis (Savage *et al.* 1987), and isolated focal necrotizing glomerulonephritis (Falk and Jennette 1988; Cohen Tervaert *et al.* 1989; Niles *et al.* 1991; Sinico *et al.* 1994), although in these conditions the findings are more heterogeneous. Patients with Churg–Strauss syndrome usually have ANCA (Cohen Tervaert *et al.* 1991; Gaskin *et al.* 1991*a*; Guillevin *et al.* 1993), whereas patients with polyarteritis nodosa, as defined by the Chapel Hill criteria, rarely do so (Guillevin *et al.* 1993). Thus, the presence of ANCA identifies the primary vasculitis syndromes with prominent renal involvement. Larger vessel vasculitides, such as giant cell arteritis and Takayasu's arteritis are not generally associated with ANCA.

Two neutrophil primary granule enzymes are the target of the majority of ANCA in systemic vasculitis. ANCA directed against proteinase-3 (Goldschmeding *et al.* 1989; Niles *et al.* 1989; Ludemann *et al.* 1990) are strongly associated with Wegener's granulomatosis and produce a cytoplasmic staining pattern (c-ANCA) in a standard indirect immunofluorescence assay on ethanol-fixed neutrophils (Wiik 1989). ANCA directed against myeloperoxidase (Falk and Jennette, 1988; Cohen Tervaert *et al.* 1990*a*) usually produce a perinuclear staining pattern (p-ANCA). ANCA in vasculitis may occasionally be directed against other neutrophil proteins, including elastase, alpha-enolase, lactoferrin, bactericidal/permeability increasing protein (BPI, also known as CAP57), and h-lamp-2, although the importance of these reactivities is unclear (Esnault *et al.* 1994; Kain *et al.* 1995). The possible role of ANCA in the pathogenesis of vasculitis is discussed in Chapter 6.

ANCA binding to diverse neutrophil proteins, but only rarely to proteinase 3 or myeloperoxidase, have also been detected in patients with non-vasculitic diseases, including inflammatory bowel disease and primary sclerosing cholangitis (reviewed by Peter *et al.* 1993). 'False positive' ANCA are also reported occasionally in other diseases including certain infections (Davenport *et al.* 1994; Efthimiou *et al.* 1991; Wagner *et al.* 1991; Pudifin *et al.* 1994). Confirmation of ANCA positivity by both indirect immunofluorescence and ELISA against purified proteinase-3 or myeloperoxidase increases the likelihood of a diagnosis of vasculitis and this combination of assay methodologies is advised (Hagen *et al.* 1995*c*).

Many recent publications have combined the clinical syndromes of Wegener's granulomatosis, microscopic polyangiitis and renal-limited vasculitis as 'ANCA-associated vasculitis and glomerulonephritis'. However, since assays for ANCA have not yet been perfected, nor the full clinical implications of a given ANCA specificity determined, this chapter will categorize patients when possible according to their clinical characteristics rather than the autoantibody specificity.

Epidemiology of systemic vasculitis

Incidence

The primary systemic vasculitides are uncommon diseases, but their incidence appears to be increasing (Andrews *et al.* 1990). In 1982, Scott and coworkers estimated an incidence of 4.6 new cases per year of systemic vasculitis of the polyarteritis type per million population, based on the number of patients treated in a district hospital in the UK over a period of 8 years. Current estimates are nearer 15 per million per year (Watts *et al.* 1995).

Primary systemic vasculitis is predominantly a disease of adult life. Both Wegener's granulomatosis and microscopic polyangiitis present most commonly in the fifth or sixth decade; they are rare in childhood, and often atypical in this age group. In our experience there is a slight male predominance, which is present in most series of patients with both Wegener's granulomatosis (Fauci *et al.* 1983; Luqmani *et al.* 1994*a*) and microscopic polyangiitis (Savage *et al.* 1985; Coward *et al.* 1986; Adu *et al.* 1987).

The majority of patients affected by small vessel vasculitis are European Caucasoids; 97% of the 158 patients with Wegener's granulomatosis reported from the United States National Institutes of Health were White (Hoffman *et al.* 1992*a*). Nonetheless, cases have also been reported in Indian Caucasians. There is an impression that microscopic polyangiitis is more common in Southern Europe, and Wegener's granulomatosis more prevalent in Northern Europe, but this has not been formally documented.

Genetic factors

Familial vasculitis is recognized, although rare. The literature includes families with a mixture of vasculitic syndromes, familial antimyeloperoxidase ANCA-associated vasculitis, and siblings with Wegener's granulomatosis. In one report (Knudsen *et al.* 1988) the illness developed in siblings after they had lived apart for 25 years, suggesting a genetic predisposition rather than shared environmental exposure. We know of two sisters with Wegener's granulomatosis and two siblings with polyarteritis nodosa but have also studied monozygotic twins discordant for vasculitis. Recent studies, using accurate genotyping methods, have failed to demonstrate a consistent HLA association with systemic vasculitis (Spencer *et al.* 1992; Zhang *et al.* 1995; Hagen *et al.* 1995*b*). There is a possible association with polymorphisms of the C3 component of complement. In one study (Finn *et al.* 1994) there was an increased frequency of the rarer C3F allele in vasculitis patients; the relative risk of developing vasculitis was 2.6 in heterozygotes and 5.1 in homozygotes.

An association with certain polymorphisms of α-1-antitrypsin, the major phys-iological inhibitor of the ANCA antigen, proteinase-3, has also been reported. The frequency of deficient 'Z' alleles appears to be increased in vasculitis patients with ANCA directed against proteinase-3 (Esnault *et al.* 1993; Elzouki *et al.* 1994). There appears in addition to be an increase in frequency of the 'S' allele in patients with myeloperoxidase-specific ANCA (Griffith *et al.* 1995). The pathogenetic significance of these findings is not known.

Environmental factors

Various reports suggest a link between small vessel vasculitis and infection. Davies *et al.* (1982) first reported ANCA in patients with vasculitis-like illnesses accompanying serological evidence of Ross River virus infection. Falk *et al.* (1990) and Geffriaud-Ricouard *et al.* (1993) noted a seasonal variation in present-ation. There are reports of an association, in limited numbers of cases, with the human immunodeficiency virus (Calabrese *et al.* 1989) and with parvovirus B19 infection (Corman and Dolson 1992). An association between hepatitis B infect-ion and polyarteritis nodosa (but not small vessel vasculitis) is well recognized (Gocke *et al.* 1970). There are also reports of vasculitis presenting and relapsing shortly after vaccinations.

Certain drugs are associated with the development of a vasculitis-like illness, including D-penicillamine (reviewed in Devogelaer *et al.* 1987) and hydralazine (first reported by Björck *et al.* 1985). Silica exposure has been postulated as a risk factor for the development of vasculitis. Arnalich *et al.* (1989) reported a patient with silicosis who developed systemic vasculitis; subsequent case-control studies have suggested an increased frequency of silica exposure in patients with ANCA-associated crescentic glomerulonephritis and Wegener's granulomatosis.

Finally, it is important to remember that vasculitis may occur in association with malignancy; this possibility should always be considered in the presence of atypical features or the absence of ANCA.

Clinical features

Blood vessels in any part of the body may be affected by the inflammatory process; however, certain organ systems are more commonly involved. How and why the vasculitis preferentially localizes to certain organs is not known. The clinical fea-tures of patients treated at Hammersmith Hospital are summarized in Fig. 7.1.

Features unique to Wegener's granulomatosis

By definition, certain features are specific to Wegener's granulomatosis, including granulomatous inflammation and vasculitis in the respiratory tract.

Upper airways involvement

Upper airways disease occurs in over 90% of patients (Fauci *et al.* 1983; Hoffman *et al.* 1992*a*), and may cause epistaxis, rhinorrhoea, nasal discomfort,

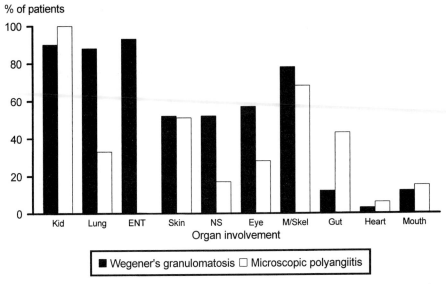

Fig. 7.1 Organ involvement in patients with small vessel vasculitis treated at Hammersmith Hospital, 1974–88.

blockage of the paranasal sinuses or nasolacrimal duct, conductive deafness, haemoptysis, or hoarseness. Destruction of nasal cartilage may follow soft tissue necrosis and leads to the characteristic saddle-nose deformity, but gross destruction of bone or skin is unusual and suggests an alternative diagnosis, such as lethal midline granuloma or other malignancy. Upper airway inflammation may be insidious, and sometimes reveals itself only when critical subglottic stenosis occurs. Pulmonary function tests, with analysis of the inspiratory limb of a flow–volume loop, are helpful in early diagnosis. The characteristic histological features of vasculitis and necrotizing, loosely formed, granulomata are demonstrated in only a minority of head and neck biopsies (Devaney *et al.* 1990).

Pulmonary involvement

Granulomatous inflammation in the lung is apparent at presentation in around 90% of patients. The symptoms are non-specific, including dyspnoea, cough, haemoptysis, and chest pain. Parenchymal granulomas produce rounded lesions on radiography, often with cavitation, and if diagnostic features of Wegener's granulomatosis in other organs are lacking, biopsy may be required to confirm the diagnosis and exclude neoplasms. Granulomata can also be found in the bronchi, often as an incidental finding at bronchoscopy; bronchial stenosis may follow. An ominous, although not specific, manifestation of disease in the lungs is alveolar haemorrhage (Haworth *et al.* 1985). Some patients simply have ill-defined infiltrates apparent on chest radiography which are not readily classifiable as either granuloma or haemorrhage, and some have pleural effusions. One detailed histological study of the lung in Wegener's granulomatosis (Travis *et al.* 1991) revealed a variety of lesions, both specific and non-specific. In 87 open lung biopsies, the three major findings were parenchymal necrosis, vasculitis of arteries, veins and capillaries, and poorly formed granulomas, accompanied by a mixed inflammatory infiltrate. Minor findings were interstitial fibrosis, alveolar haemorrhage, tissue eosinophilia, and bronchial and bronchiolar lesions.

Granulomatous inflammation outside the respiratory tract

Granulomatous inflammation can affect many parts of the body. In the kidney, interstitial granulomata may be demonstrated unequivocally in only a minority of biopsies (Ronco *et al.* 1983). A granulomatous reaction round the glomerulus is more common, but may not be specific to Wegener's granulomatosis, and may simply follow severe necrotizing inflammation and crescent formation. Other reported sites include the orbit, brain, pituitary, prostate, salivary glands, skin, gingiva ('strawberry gums'), and vertebrae. Inflammatory masses have also been reported in unusual sites such as the retroperitoneum, mediastinum, and breast.

Generalized versus limited Wegener's granulomatosis

Not all reports of Wegener's granulomatosis describe the same spectrum or severity of disease. Early studies described a disseminated disease progressing relentlessly to death from renal and respiratory failure. Even though effective treatment is now available, nephrologists often see patients with advanced renal and extrarenal disease. In contrast, other specialists may treat patients with mild and anatomically limited disease: the 'limited Wegener's granulomatosis' without overt renal involvement first reported by Carrington and Liebow (1966) and recently re-examined by Luqmani *et al.* (1994*a*). The absence of renal involvement does not necessarily imply a benign course; pulmonary involvement may itself be life-threatening, as may vasculitis in other organs recruited later in the course of the disease. A stepwise progression from localized respiratory disease to generalized disease is not the invariable pattern, and in some patients disease is extensive at presentation. Renal disease may even be the first manifestation of Wegener's granulomatosis, with typical respiratory lesions following several years later.

Features of generalized small vessel vasculitis

These are not specific to Wegener's granulomatosis, and also occur in microscopic polyangiitis and Churg–Strauss syndrome.

Constitutional and musculoskeletal symptoms

Many patients with Wegener's granulomatosis and microscopic polyangiitis report malaise, weight loss or fever and flu-like symptoms at presentation. Arthralgia and myalgia are also common and arthritis has been reported (Savage *et al.* 1985; Noritake *et al.* 1987).

Renal disease

The characteristic finding is a necrotizing glomerulonephritis, which is initially focal and segmental, becoming diffuse and crescentic as the disease progresses. Microscopic haematuria, proteinuria, and granular and red cell casts will suggest the presence of nephritis, even before renal function is impaired. However, without intervention, function will often decline to the point of oliguria and dialysis-dependence in only a few weeks. Macroscopic haematuria and heavy proteinuria occur infrequently (Bindi *et al.* 1993; Geffriaud Ricouard *et al.* 1993) and hypertension is present in fewer than half the patients (Adu *et al.* 1987; Savage *et al.* 1985; Coward *et al.* 1986; Bindi *et al.* 1993; Geffriaud Ricouard *et al.* 1993). When hypertension occurs, fluid overload and the presence of long-standing renal disease may be important contributory factors.

The pathological features of the characteristic glomerulonephritis are described in detail in Chapter 4. Lesions and crescents of varying ages may coexist; there may be a mixture of normal glomeruli, glomeruli showing active necrosis or crescent formation, and glomeruli that are segmentally or globally sclerosed. This contrasts with the appearances in anti-glomerular basement membrane disease, where a diffuse glomerulonephritis with lesions of similar age is the rule. An interstitial infiltrate of inflammatory cells is common in Wegener's granulomatosis and microscopic polyangiitis, and includes T lymphocytes; it may rarely be the predominant finding (Cameron 1991). Vasculitis can affect interlobular arteries and arterioles (Novak *et al.* 1982), but it is not detected in the majority of biopsies (Savage *et al.* 1985; Hoffman *et al.* 1992a). Immunofluorescence microscopy shows absent or scanty immune deposits, hence the description 'pauci-immune' glomerulonephritis. Low levels of immunoglobulin and complement deposition are seen particularly in necrotic or sclerotic lesions. Electron microscopy only rarely shows immune deposits (Ronco *et al.* 1983; Jennette *et al.* 1989).

Eye involvement

The spectrum of eye involvement is greatest in Wegener's granulomatosis, where it includes conjunctivitis, episcleritis, corneal ulceration, uveitis, retinal vasculitis, and optic neuropathy, as well as orbital involvement and obstruction of the nasolacrimal duct due to granulomatous masses. It affects up to 50% of patients and carries a significant ocular morbidity (Bullen *et al.* 1983). Episcleritis also occurs in microscopic polyangiitis, and affected 24% of patients in one series (Savage *et al.* 1985).

Nervous system involvement

Vasculitis affecting the nervous system has a variety of presentations (reviewed by Cohen Tervaert and Kallenberg 1993). Peripheral lesions typically cause an asymmetrical mononeuritis multiplex, or occasionally a distal sensory neuropathy; cranial nerves may also be affected, singly or multiply. Cerebral vasculitis may lead to major neurological deficits when large arteries are involved or haemorrhage occurs. More subtle abnormalities occur when small vessels are affected, including alteration of conscious level and seizures; metabolic abnormalities enter the differential diagnosis in patients with renal failure. Cerebrospinal fluid analysis may reveal a raised protein or pleocytosis, and imaging of the brain by computerized tomography or magnetic resonance imaging may be helpful, although there are no changes that are pathognomonic of small vessel vasculitis.

Cutaneous involvement

Cutaneous manifestations are frequent, and may be widespread or isolated. Typical lesions are palpable purpura, nailbed infarcts, and splinter haemorrhages. Soft tissue infarction of the extremities may also occur if larger vessels are involved. Pauci-immune necrotizing leucocytoclastic vasculitis is the most common finding on biopsy (Barksdale *et al.* 1995; Jennette *et al.* 1989), and may affect small arteries, veins, or capillaries. The clinical presentation may be similar to cryoglobulinaemic vasculitis or Henoch–Schönlein purpura; immunofluorescence studies make the distinction.

Gastrointestinal tract vasculitis

Gut vasculitis occurs in both Wegener's granulomatosis and microscopic polyangiitis, and may present with abdominal pain, diarrhoea, or gastrointestinal bleeding (Camilleri *et al.* 1983). Complications include major bleeding and bowel perforation through ulcerating lesions. Severe ulceration of the oral mucosa occurs in a number of patients.

Alveolar haemorrhage

Systemic vasculitis is now the most common cause of Goodpasture's syndrome, the combination of pulmonary haemorrhage and rapidly progressive glomerulonephritis. The diagnosis of alveolar haemorrhage is made in the context of haemoptysis, dyspnoea, anaemia, hypoxia, and diffuse alveolar shadowing on radiography and may be confirmed by demonstration of an increased transfer factor for carbon monoxide. Histology reveals pauci-immune alveolar capillaritis (Bosch *et al.* 1994) but biopsy is only obligatory if an important differential diagnosis requires exclusion. The early mortality is high.

Cardiac involvement

Cardiac involvement is relatively unusual, except in Churg Strauss syndrome, although dysrhythmias, cardiac failure, dilated cardiomyopathy, and pericarditis have all been reported. Valvular lesions have also been described in Wegener's granulomatosis.

Relationship between clinical features and ANCA specificity

Clinical features segregate to some extent with ANCA specificity. c-ANCA specific for proteinase-3 are particularly associated with sinus disease and granulomatous lung vasculitis (Cohen Tervaert *et al.* 1990*a*; Jennette *et al.* 1989), and therefore with a diagnosis of Wegener's granulomatosis (Venning *et al.* 1990; Weber *et al.* 1992). p-ANCA specific for myeloperoxidase are associated with renal-limited vasculitis (Falk and Jennette, 1988; Ulmer *et al.* 1992), microscopic polyangiitis (Geffriaud Ricouard *et al.* 1993), and Churg–Strauss syndrome (Cohen Tervaert *et al.* 1991; Gaskin *et al.* 1991*a*). The distinction is not absolute, but interpretation of published data is obscured by the use of differing diagnostic criteria. In our experience, around 90% of patients with Wegener's granulomatosis, diagnosed using Chapel Hill consensus criteria, had antibodies to proteinase-3, whereas fewer than 5% had antibodies to myeloperoxidase. Both ANCA specificities were found, with approximately equal frequency, in the patients with microscopic polyangiitis and renal-limited vasculitis.

A minority of patients with small vessel vasculitis have ANCA of specificities other than proteinase-3 and myeloperoxidase, including BPI (CAP57) and elastase, but there are no clear associations with particular clinical characteristics.

Confirmation of diagnosis

Ultimately, this depends on proof by histology, but many other investigations, including assays for ANCA, can yield supporting evidence.

Haematology and biochemistry

The typical haematological features are anaemia, usually with a normocytic normochromic pattern, neutrophil leucocytosis, and thrombocythaemia. Eosinophilia is a feature of Churg–Strauss syndrome, but slight eosinophilia has also been reported in other forms of vasculitis (Ronco *et al.* 1983). Erythrocyte sedimentation rate (Fauci *et al.* 1983) and C-reactive protein will usually be increased (Hind *et al.* 1984); the latter is more specific in renal failure and more sensitive to changes in disease activity. Other biochemical abnormalities include low albumin (even in the absence of significant albuminuria), raised alkaline phosphatase, and hyperglobulinaemia. Serum urea and creatinine concentrations are usually increased, but values in the normal range do not exclude the presence of nephritis. Renal involvement is usually revealed by urinary abnormalities: proteinuria (rarely in the nephrotic range), red cells, and granular and red cell casts. In some cases, the urine sediment understates the histological severity of nephritis.

Immunology

Assays for ANCA

The internationally validated indirect immunofluorescence assay (Wiik 1989) is the most widely used test for ANCA, and is able to differentiate c-ANCA and p-ANCA. It is robust (Hagen *et al.* 1993), but requires a skilled observer and can be difficult to quantify. Importantly, it may not achieve adequate specificity as a single test; a p-ANCA pattern may be mimicked by antinuclear antibodies and produced by antibodies to a variety of neutrophil components which are not strongly associated with vasculitis. Indeed, when large numbers of sera are screened for ANCA, p-ANCA without antimyeloperoxidase reactivity may predominate (Ulmer *et al.* 1992).

To overcome these disadvantages, numerous solid-phase assays have been designed, variously using crude neutrophil extracts, purified neutrophil granules, and, most recently, purified antigens. A recent international standardization effort (Hagen *et al.* 1995*c*) concluded that immunofluorescence assays should be combined with solid-phase assays using purified proteinase-3 and myeloperoxidase to achieve sufficiently high assay specificity. With this approach, a positive ANCA in the setting of suspected vasculitis is highly suggestive that the diagnosis is correct (Niles *et al.* 1991; Hagen *et al.* 1995*c*). A negative ANCA in the setting of limited Wegener's granulomatosis is common, and negative ANCA has been reported in a very small proportion of cases with generalized small vessel vasculitis (Bindi *et al.* 1993).

Most ANCA assays are designed to detect IgG, although certain authors have also suggested a particular importance for ANCA of IgM isotype. An initial report suggested an association of ANCA of IgM class only with pulmonary haemorrhage (Jayne *et al.* 1989), although a later study detected coexisting IgG and IgM ANCA in such patients (Esnault *et al.* 1992), and others have not confirmed the association (Kokolina *et al.* 1994).

Other immunological abnormalities

The concentrations of circulating complement components are usually normal or raised. Rheumatoid factors are common, but not specific for vasculitis. Immunoassays using cultured endothelial cells, which currently have no place in routine clinical practice, have identified anti-endothelial cell antibodies in the sera of patients with systemic vasculitis (see Savage *et al.* 1991), but these are not invariably present (Varagunam *et al.* 1993) and are also detectable in other rheumatological disorders.

Radiology

The application of a variety of imaging techniques may assist in initial diagnosis, definition of disease extent, and procurement of a diagnostic biopsy.

Pulmonary imaging

In Wegener's granulomatosis, the specific radiological findings are rounded opacities corresponding to granulomata; computerized tomography may reveal additional lesions (Cordier *et al.* 1990). A diffuse alveolar filling pattern may indicate alveolar haemorrhage due to small vessel vasculitis, although the differential diagnoses of pulmonary oedema and severe infection must always be considered.

Upper airways imaging

In Wegener's granulomatosis, sinus abnormalities on plain radiographs are very common. Magnetic resonance imaging of the upper airways is more sensitive, and detects abnormalities in up to 90% of patient's with Wegener's granulomatosis (Muhle *et al.* 1993). It offers an alternative modality to image the laryngeal region (Hoffman *et al.* 1992a).

Renal ultrasound

This is not diagnostic, but should be performed to exclude other causes of renal dysfunction, and to guide renal biopsy.

Angiography

Involvement of medium-sized arteries is compatible with a diagnosis of microscopic polyangiitis or Wegener's granulomatosis (Jennette *et al.* 1994), although it is neither diagnostic nor common. Visceral angiography is not, therefore, part of routine investigation when these diagnoses are suspected, although it may be warranted in the light of certain symptoms and may demonstrate the presence of aneurysms or, less specifically, irregularities of calibre and arterial occlusions.

Radiolabelled leucocyte scanning

Areas affected by vasculitis, including the gut (Reuter *et al.* 1993), may be identified by their uptake of Indium-labelled leucocytes.

Histopathology

Histology remains the gold standard for diagnosis. However, in each case the clinician must decide which is the most productive site to biopsy, which is the safest, and whether the invasiveness of the procedure is justified. For example, biopsy of a single kidney may not be justified in the context of a highly suggestive clinical picture, supportive radiology, and a positive ANCA.

Diagnosis of small vessel vasculitis is usually most readily obtained from a renal biopsy showing a pauci-immune focal necrotizing glomerulonephritis with crescent formation. Biopsy from other organs, such as skin or intestine, may confirm the presence of a vasculitis. Firm diagnosis of Wegener's granulomatosis is more difficult, requiring demonstration of necrotizing granulomata. Biopsy of the upper airways is relatively easy, but frequently not diagnostic; transbronchial biopsies are similarly often too small and fragmented. Open-lung biopsy is more reliable, but invasive. Our practice is to confirm necrotizing glomerulonephritis by renal biopsy, and to consider the presence of clinical and radiological evidence of granulomatous disease in the upper and lower respiratory tracts as sufficient evidence for the diagnosis of Wegener's granulomatosis, if biopsy of nasal lesions is not confirmatory. Open-lung biopsy is performed only if there is no other route to diagnosis, or if it is necessary to exclude lung malignancy.

Investigations and differential diagnosis

Other investigations will often be needed to exclude other diagnoses, the most important of which are outlined below.

Anti-glomerular basement membrane disease (see Chapter 5)

Rapidly progressive glomerulonephritis, with or without lung haemorrhage, should provoke a search for anti-glomerular basement membrane (anti-GBM) antibodies, although a clinical picture of widespread systemic disease favours small vessel vasculitis. Infrequently, there is clinical evidence of both diseases.

ANCA coexisting with anti-GBM antibodies are now well recognized (Jayne *et al.* 1990), and current data suggest that ANCA may be detected in 10–20% of patients with anti-GBM disease, while anti-GBM antibodies specific for the α3 chain of type IV collagen may be found in 2–3% of patients with ANCA. ANCA specificity in these cases is usually for myeloperoxidase (Niles *et al.* 1991; Bosch *et al.* 1991). Patients with both ANCA and anti-GBM antibodies may have evidence of renal vasculitis (Weber *et al.* 1992), frequently have disease outside the kidneys and lungs (Jayne *et al.* 1990), and respond to treatment in a way more typical of vasculitis than of anti-GBM disease, particularly if ANCA titre is high (Bosch *et al.* 1991). Furthermore, like vasculitis patients they are at significant risk of relapse (Jayne *et al.* 1990).

Systemic lupus erythematosus (SLE) (see Chapter 8)

The combination of arthralgia and clinical evidence of nephritis is compatible with both lupus and primary systemic vasculitis. Although the age, gender, and ethnic background of the patient might favour one syndrome rather than the other, the final distinction must be made by solid-phase assays for ANCA, anti-nuclear and anti-double stranded DNA antibodies, estimation of serum complement, and renal biopsy with immunohistology. Although patients with SLE may have detectable ANCA on screening assay, the specificities recognized are distinct from those in primary systemic vasculitis (Schnabel *et al.* 1995).

Other vasculitic syndromes

Differentiation of Wegener's granulomatosis from Churg–Strauss syndrome can occasionally be difficult, since in some cases there may be marked tissue eosinophilia without peripheral blood eosinophilia or asthma. Symptoms resulting from nasal polyps in Churg–Strauss syndrome may cause initial confusion.

Mixed essential cryoglobulinaemia and Henoch–Schönlein purpura also enter the differential diagnosis of small vessel vasculitis with glomerulonephritis, but may be distinguished by the nature and extent of immune deposits on renal biopsy; detectable cryoglobulins and hypocomplementaemia point to a diagnosis of mixed essential cryoglobulinaemia.

Infective endocarditis (see Chapter 9)

There are reports of detectable ANCA (by screening assay) in patients with endocarditis and glomerulonephritis (Wagner *et al.* 1991; Soto *et al.* 1994) and, clinically, the features may be very similar to those of systemic vasculitis. Current experience suggests that further investigations, including repeated blood cultures, trans-oesophageal echocardiography, serum complement estimation, purified antigen ANCA assays, and renal biopsy with immunohistology are advisable.

Treatment

Historical aspects

Wegener's granulomatosis

Historically, the prognosis of untreated Wegener's granulomatosis was bleak, with a mean survival of only five months. The presence of renal failure was a particularly ominous sign before dialysis was generally available, although death from respiratory failure was also common. Corticosteroids were the first agents to make an impact on outcome, but the benefit was not sustained and the disease eventually became refractory. The addition of alkylating agents was a major advance, and initial reports described benefit from intravenous nitrogen mustard and chlorambucil. Cyclophosphamide was introduced in the 1970s, and rapidly became the mainstay for therapy for Wegener's granulomatosis (Fauci *et al.* 1983).

Polyarteritis

The earliest attempts to treat microscopic polyangiitis and classical polyarteritis used oral corticosteroids alone; cytotoxic agents were subsequently added in more severe cases. Five-year survival improved from 12% in untreated patients, to 53% in patients treated with steroids alone, and 80% in those treated with a combination of steroids and cytotoxic agents (typically azathioprine) (Leib *et al.* 1979). In later reports of patients with microscopic polyangiitis (Savage *et al.* 1985; Coward *et al.* 1986; Adu *et al.* 1987) and focal segmental necrotizing glomerulonephritis (Serra *et al.* 1984; Fuiano *et al.* 1988), a combination of steroids and cytotoxic agents was used in the majority.

The NIH steroid and cyclophosphamide regimen

In 1983, Fauci and coworkers reported the treatment of 85 patients with Wegener's granulomatosis at the US National Institutes of Health (Fauci *et al.* 1983). Their regimen has been widely copied and has been viewed as the gold standard against which to compare other approaches.

Initial therapy comprised daily oral cyclophosphamide (2 mg/kg) and daily oral prednisolone (1 mg/kg); the starting doses were doubled in fulminant disease. The steroids were converted to an alternate day regimen over a period of 1–2 months and reduced to a dose of 20 mg on alternate days by 6–12 months. They were subsequently tailed off, provided there was no evidence of disease activity. The cyclophosphamide was continued at the starting dose until the patient had been in complete remission for at least one year, and then reduced by 25 mg every two to three months. In some patients it was withdrawn completely; in others it was maintained at a dose below which disease activity recurred. Throughout the period of treatment, the cyclophosphamide dose was adjusted to keep the total white cell count above $3000–3500/mm^3$; patients who could only tolerate low doses were given additional prednisolone.

Complications of the NIH regimen

This regimen, although initially highly successful, was associated with significant long-term morbidity due to the effects of corticosteroids, cyclophosphamide, and the disease itself (Hoffman *et al.* 1992*a*). The more severe steroid-related manifestations included induction of diabetes (in 8%), cataracts (in 21%), bony fractures (in 11%), and aseptic bone necrosis (in 3%). Significant infections occurred during follow-up in 46% of the patients; half of the serious bacterial, pneumocystis, and fungal infections occurred during the period of daily steroid therapy. In our series, Cohen *et al.* (1982) identified the dose of steroids as the most important factor predisposing to infection in patients treated for immune-mediated renal diseases.

Major adverse effects attributable to cyclophosphamide included haemorrhagic cystitis, occurring in 43% of the patients reported by Hoffman *et al.* (1992*a*), and 15% of a similar group of patients reported by Stillwell *et al.* (1988), in which the risk was related to cumulative dose. Bladder cancer developed in approximately 2.5% of the patients in each series, demonstrating a 33-fold increase in risk. Infertility was a major concern with this regimen; Fauci *et al.* (1983) reported severe oligospermia in two men and Hoffman *et al.* (1992*a*) noted that after one year of the drug, 57% of women between 18 and 35 were amenorrhoeic, unable to conceive, or had evidence of ovarian failure. Long-term haematological abnormalities attributed to cyclophosphamide include persistent hypogammaglobulinaemia, myelodysplastic syndromes, and haematological malignancies. Hoffman *et al.* (1992*a*) calculated that the risk of lymphoma was increased 11-fold.

Current approaches to initial therapy

Adaptations of the NIH regimen

Most strategies retain cyclophosphamide and corticosteroids to induce remission, but aim to avoid the long-term risks of cyclophosphamide by using lower total doses, often turning to other drugs for maintenance of remission and treatment of relapse.

The regimen we have used during the past 20 years, for both Wegener's granulomatosis and microscopic polyangiitis, is outined in Table 7.2. The most important departure from the NIH regimen is the switch from cyclophosphamide to azathioprine for maintenance therapy, after approximately three months, to reduce the risk of cyclophosphamide toxicity. Many groups have used a similar approach (Coward *et al.* 1986; Adu *et al.* 1987; Serra *et al.* 1984; Fuiano *et al.* 1988). A comparison of this approach with the use of one year's cyclophosphamide is currently the subject of a trial, co-ordinated by a European Community-sponsored group of researchers (Rasmussen *et al.* 1995). Two variants of our protocol are worthy of comment. First, we reduce the dose of cyclophosphamide in older patients, who appear to be especially prone to leucopenia; in patients aged over 55 years we limit the starting dose of cyclophosphamide to 2 mg/kg. Second, we use additional therapy in all patients with fulminant disease; this is discussed in detail below.

Table 7.2   Treatment regimens used at Hammersmith Hospital, London

Induction	Prednisolone	60 mg daily for most adults
	Cyclophosphamide	2–3 mg/kg daily
		(2 mg/kg if age > 55 years)
Fulminant disease	Standard induction drug therapy	
	plus	
	Plasma exchange	3–4 litres daily for albumin
		(5–10 days)
	or	
	Methylprednisolone	500 mg IV × 3
		(if plasma exchange not possible)
Maintenance	Prednisolone	Tapering daily dose
	Azathioprine	1–2 mg/kg daily until remission
		> 1 year
		(unless relapse on treatment,
		when cyclophosphamide is used)

Pulsed cyclophosphamide

There has been increasing interest in the use of pulsed intravenous cyclophosphamide, which offers two potential advantages: a reduction in the total dose administered (provided the course of therapy is not unusually long), and the easy concomitant use of MESNA to prevent bladder toxicity. Pulsed cyclophosphamide has now been used in Wegener's granulomatosis (Hoffman *et al.* 1990; Haubitz *et al.* 1991; Reinhold Keller *et al.* 1994; Guillevin *et al.* 1995), ANCA-associated glomerulonephritis and vasculitis (Falk *et al.* 1990; Haubitz *et al.* 1995), and mixed primary vasculitic disorders (Adu *et al.* 1993). It has most frequently been used in first-line therapy, although Hoffman *et al.* (1990) used it for relapse and salvage therapy. Dose intervals in the published reports varied from 2 weeks (initially) to 2 months; typical pulse size was 0.5–0.75g/m^2, with adjustments for renal failure, age, and leucopaenia. Pulses were usually, but not invariably (Gordon *et al.* 1993), given intravenously.

In over half of the studies listed above, pulsed cyclophosphamide produced an initial improvement equal to that achieved with oral cyclophosphamide. This was maintained during follow-up in the studies by Falk *et al.* (1990), Haubitz *et al.* (1991), and the Birmingham group in the UK (Adu *et al.* 1997), but not in the study of Guillevin *et al.* (1995), who reported a higher relapse rate (62% vs 28%) in pulse-treated patients. Haubitz *et al.* (1995) reported an equivalent response in the majority of subgroups, but an inferior rate of recovery from dialysis dependence (1/7 vs 4/6), despite the routine addition of pulsed methylprednisolone.

The best initial results were reported in studies using doses initially at two or three week intervals. The least satisfactory results from pulse therapy were reported by Hoffman *et al.* (1990), when it was used chiefly for relapse or salvage, and Reinhold-Keller *et al.* (1994), whose patients mostly had non-renal Wegener's granulomatosis. Adverse effects were significant in the study by Hoffman *et al.* (1990), who used doses of 1 g/m^2, but the same or less than those of continuous oral therapy in the remainder.

Overall, the current evidence still favours daily oral cyclophosphamide if control of disease is critical; pulsed therapy may be preferred if avoidance of side-effects is particularly important. It is unclear whether continuous or pulsed therapy is the better choice for patients newly presenting with moderately severe disease. Further studies are needed to define the optimal size and spacing of pulse doses.

Methotrexate

Weekly methotrexate has recently been tried as an alternative to cyclophosphamide in patients with Wegener's granulomatosis (Hoffman *et al.* 1992*b*; Sneller *et al.* 1995), although it is unlikely to have a place in the routine treatment of patients with moderate or severe renal impairment because of the increased risk of toxicity. It was used in combination with oral corticosteroids and administered orally at a dose of 0.3 mg/kg/week, increasing gradually until a mean stable weekly dose of 20 mg was reached. Remission was achieved in 30/41 patients studied, at a median of 4.2 months, and patients were then treated for a further year. Eleven patients relapsed: seven during methotrexate and four following withdrawal. Side-effects included abnormal liver enzymes necessitating a dose reduction (in 25%) and reversible methotrexate-induced pneumonitis (in 7%). Two patients died from *Pneumocystis carinii* when taking methotrexate and high-dose oral steroids; the overall incidence of opportunist infections was 9.5%.

Cyclosporin

Responses to cyclosporin are documented in a number of case reports, suggesting that it may prove valuable in selected cases. It is increasingly used in vasculitis therapy in children (M. Dillon, personal communication).

Intravenous immunoglobulin

Another immunomodulatory treatment which has been used with some success in vasculitis is intravenous immunoglobulin. Jayne *et al.* (1991) used Sandoglobulin™ 0.4g/kg/day for 5 days, in conjunction with varying regimens of steroids and cytotoxic agents. Clinical improvement was noted in all six patients with small vessel vasculitis, and complete remission was achieved in five. Progressive renal impairment stabilized in one patient, and despite the theoretical risk of renal toxicity of high-dose immunoglobulin, renal function did not change in the remaining patients. Relapse occurred in three patients during follow-up, at 2, 6, and 9 months. No adverse effects were noted. Less satisfactory results were reported by Richter *et al.* (1993), although a different preparation of immunoglobulin was used. Further studies are required to determine whether the optimal role of intravenous immunoglobulin is as an adjunctive agent for induction therapy, as a sole therapy for selected patients, or as a second-line agent when other treatments are problematic.

Cotrimoxazole

This has been used in the treatment of Wegener's granulomatosis (DeRemee 1988), although it is not recommended as a first-line agent in severely ill patients, or as a single agent for maintenance therapy of generalized disease. There are no data on its use in microscopic polyangiitis. Successes were initially reported in the treatment of Wegener's granulomatosis predominantly affecting the respiratory tract, and benefit in similar patients was confirmed more recently. In maintenance of remission it has proved unsatisfactory as a sole agent in generalized disease (Reinhold-Keller *et al.* 1993), but promising as an adjunct to conventional therapy (Stegeman *et al.* 1995).

Adjunctive therapy for severe glomerulonephritis

Two therapies, used in addition to conventional drugs, have gained considerable acceptance. They are plasma exchange and pulsed intravenous methylprednisolone. There are many reports of benefit attributed to these therapies in uncontrolled studies, and in addition, a number of more systematic analyses. Proponents of the two strategies also report beneficial effects on other manifestations of severe vasculitis, including lung haemorrhage and neurological vasculitis, although these have not been subjected to randomized trials.

Two controlled trials pointed to a benefit of adjunctive plasma exchange in severe rapidly progressive glomerulonephritis (RPGN). Pusey *et al.* (1991) randomized patients to receive at least five 4-litre exchanges in addition to oral steroids, cyclophosphamide, and azathioprine; 10/11 dialysis-dependent patients treated with plasma exchange discontinued dialysis, while only 3/8 patients in the control group did so. Cole *et al.* (1992) randomized patients to receive 10 exchanges, each of one plasma volume, in addition to a regimen of intravenous methylprednisolone, prednisone, and azathioprine; 3/4 dialysis-dependent patients treated with plasma exchange discontinued dialysis, while only 2/7 in the control group did so. Neither study demonstrated an additional benefit of plasma exchange in patients with lesser degrees of renal impairment at presentation. Two earlier studies of plasma exchange did not demonstrate a convincing effect, but neither study rigidly separated those who received plasma exchange from those who did not and both included patients with RPGN associated with systemic diseases other than vasculitis (Thysell *et al.* 1982; Glockner *et al.* 1988).

Pulsed intravenous methylprednisolone has been used widely as an adjunct to conventional immunosuppression for severe RPGN. The doses used and outcomes reported vary. Bolton and Sturgill (1989) used three pulses of 30 mg/kg in addition to oral prednisolone and reported discontinuation of dialysis in 16/23 patients, in contrast to 0/9 of those not given the additional therapy. Falk *et al.* (1990) used lower doses (7 mg/kg) added to varying regimens of prednisolone and cyclophosphamide, and reported that 6/12 patients were able to discontinue dialysis. Andrassy *et al.* (1991) used 250 mg pulses of methylprednisolone as one component of a variety of protocols; of 12 dialysis-dependent patients who did not also receive plasma exchange, 11 recovered renal function, and this was maintained during follow-up in 8 patients.

A randomized controlled comparison of plasma exchange and methylprednisolone is in progress (Rasmussen *et al.* 1995). In uncontrolled comparisons, McLelland *et al.* (1989), Bruns *et al.* (1989), and Levy and Winearls (1994) found plasma exchange and intravenous methylprednisolone to be equally effective, although in the latter study, interpretation of the results was complicated by the fact that many of the patients studied received both therapies. Both treatments have disadvantages; plasma exchange is expensive, mainly due to the cost of albumin replacement solutions, and carries the risks of allergic reactions, transfer of infection, bleeding due to anticoagulation, and depletion of clotting factors. Methylprednisolone is cheaper, and more widely available, but may be associated with an increased risk of infection and with the increased likelihood of long-term corticosteroid toxicity, including avascular necrosis of bone. Combination of the two therapies has been used successfully (Levy and Winearls 1994) although it is unclear whether this conferred additional benefit. Others (Adu *et al.* 1987; Rondeau *et al.* 1989) have drawn attention to the risk of sepsis in patients in whom multiple immunosuppressive strategies are combined.

Treatment of refractory disease

A minority of patients with vasculitis will show relentless progression of disease, in spite of aggressive therapy, or will continue to show disease activity for such prolonged periods that toxicity of conventional treatment becomes limiting. Therapeutic agents used in this situation include anti-T lymphocyte antibodies (Mathieson *et al.* 1990; Lockwood *et al.* 1993; Hagen *et al.* 1995a; Lockwood *et al.* 1996), and this strategy, together with other experimental approaches, is discussed in detail in Chapter 11.

Maintenance therapy

There are wide variations in the policies adopted to maintain a remission induced with corticosteroids and cyclophosphamide. In a recent survey of 15 European centres (Rasmussen *et al.* 1995), eight different drug combinations were used in the first year. There was even greater variability in the second year, and by this time, patients in four centres were off therapy completely. In the 1970s, most of our patients discontinued therapy during the first year; 25% had relapsed by 12 months. Our treatment period has progressively lengthened, and the relapse rate has fallen to 11% at 1 year, and from 53% to 22% at 5 years (Gaskin and Pusey 1995). The majority of our patients are now still taking a cytotoxic agent, which is usually azathioprine, in the third year. Other groups emphasize that relapse is a major problem during follow-up (Gordon *et al.* 1993), and suggest that early discontinuation of therapy is associated with recurrence of disease (Coward *et al.* 1986).

Our maintenance regimen comprises prednisolone and azathioprine, with azathioprine substituted dose-for-dose for oral cyclophosphamide once remission is achieved, typically at about three months. Typical doses at different time points are illustrated in Fig. 7.2. Azathioprine is usually well tolerated, is safer than

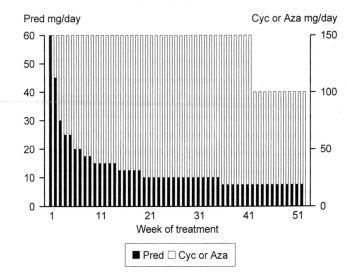

Fig. 7.2 Typical schedule of treatment reduction in the first year in a 60 kg patient with small vessel vasculitis treated at Hammersmith Hospital. Prednisolone (Pred) is progressively reduced. Cyclophosphamide (Cyc) is replaced by azathioprine (Aza) at 3 months.

cyclophosphamide and satisfactorily maintains remission in many patients. A minority of patients require reversion to cyclophosphamide for relapse. However, in our experience, relapse in patients on treatment is rarely severe and if diagnosed promptly, permanent renal damage is unusual.

The optimal duration of therapy is unknown. Relapse can occur years after initial presentation and, even at a late stage, may have devastating consequences. Conversely, a policy of life-long treatment in all patients would subject many of them to unacceptable toxicity. Our current impression is that patients with persisting ANCA, irrespective of specificity (Gaskin *et al.* 1991*b*; De'Oliviera *et al.* 1995), and patients whose disease was initially associated with proteinase-3-specific ANCA, are at greatest risk of relapse and merit continuing low-dose immunosuppression.

Treatment of relapse

Minor relapses can often be managed by a temporary increase in the baseline steroid and/or azathioprine dose, whereas relapses affecting the function of vital organs are usually treated with higher-dose steroids and cyclophosphamide. Adjunctive therapy may occasionally be required, for severe renal or neurological relapse or alveolar hameorrhage, although we rarely see relapses of this severity in patients still on maintenance immunosuppression. In the unusual event of severe relapse in a patient on maximal therapy, or in a patient intolerant of standard drugs, the more experimental treatments outlined in Chapter 11 should be considered.

Assessment of disease activity and risk of relapse to guide therapy

It is clear from the above discussion that the ability to diagnose active disease, and to identify patients at risk from relapse is critically important.

Assessment of disease activity

This depends in part on clinical findings, and on routine investigations such as the blood count, renal function, urinary sediment, and chest radiograph. It is worth remembering that the clinical manifestations of relapse often differ from the presenting illness (Gordon *et al.* 1993). For example, features of extrarenal vasculitis may develop in patients who initially had isolated renal disease. We have also treated a patient with features of microscopic polyangiitis at presentation, who developed necrotizing pulmonary granulomas 12 years later.

The ESR is slow to reflect changes in disease activity, and estimations of C-reactive protein are more reliable (Hind *et al.* 1984; Jayne *et al.* 1995). Nonetheless, these markers are not specific, and sometimes reflect the presence of infection rather than active vasculitis. Objective assessment of disease activity, which is essential for clinical trials, is a difficult task. Scoring systems have been designed to assign a numerical value to disease activity (see, for example, Luqmani *et al.* 1994*b*).

Prediction of relapse

The abnormalities described above tend to coincide with relapse, and have little predictive value. Recent reports suggest that useful information can be gained from serial estimations of ANCA, whether specific for proteinase-3 or myeloperoxidase. Immunofluorescence titres correlate in general with disease activity (Van der Woude *et al.* 1985; Nolle *et al.* 1989; Egner and Chapel 1990) although some authors find the association too weak to be prognostically useful (Kerr *et al.* 1993). Persisting ANCA point to risk of relapse (Gaskin *et al.* 1991*b*) and rising titres may precede relapse (Cohen Tervaert *et al.* 1989; Jayne *et al.* 1995). The interval is typically 1–3 months, but occasionally much greater (Hoffman *et al.* 1992*a*; De'Oliviera *et al.* 1995); ANCA sometimes persist for long periods at high titre without evidence of relapse.

Cohen Tervaert *et al.* (1990*b*) advocated additional treatment in patients with a rising ANCA titre. The recommendation was based on a controlled trial in Wegener's granulomatosis; patients were randomized to receive additional therapy if a fourfold rise in immunofluorescence titre was detected. Currently, few clinicians place this degree of reliance on changing ANCA concentrations; our own policy is to avoid reductions in maintenance therapy in the presence of a persisting or rising ANCA, and to monitor closely for signs of relapse.

Outcome

Control of disease

Induction of remission

The recent literature suggests that although a response to first-line therapy is seen in 90% of patients, complete resolution of disease activity is achieved in only 70–80% (Hoffman *et al.* 1992*a*; Gordon *et al.* 1993; Sneller *et al.* 1995). Many clinicians are familiar with the patient with 'grumbling' disease.

Maintenance of remission

Between one-third and one-half of patients with small vessel vasculitis will relapse during follow-up (Hoffman *et al.* 1992*a*; Gordon *et al.* 1993). Relapse occurs in both Wegener's granulomatosis and microscopic polyangiitis; our data suggest that the relapse rate is higher in those with proteinase-3-specific ANCA. The consequences may be severe. Gordon *et al.* (1993) reported that of 42 relapses, 2 led to the death of the patient and 2 to the need for chronic dialysis. Our own experience with a larger group of patients is similar; 4/139 relapses led to death and 10/139 to chronic dialysis, and the most severe relapses occurred in patients no longer taking immunosuppressive therapy (Gaskin and Pusey 1995).

Relapse can occur at any time during follow-up; Hoffman *et al.* (1992*a*) reported relapses occurring from 3 months to 16 years after induction of complete remission. Our data indicate that the majority of relapses occur in patients no longer receiving combined steroid and cytotoxic therapy (Gaskin and Pusey 1995) and this accords with other reports of relapse after reduction or discontinuation of immunosuppressive therapy (Fauci *et al.* 1983; Coward *et al.* 1986; Geffriaud Ricouard *et al.* 1993). Consequently, withdrawal of treatment should be gradual, only performed when there is no sign of disease activity, and accompanied by close monitoring for early signs of relapse. Infection may also precipitate relapse. Unfortunately, a minority of patients relapse despite continuing therapy, at comparable doses to those who remain in remission (Gordon *et al.* 1993), and with no other explanation apparent.

Improvement in renal function

Patients with vasculitis may recover from severe initial renal failure. We have treated 80 patients with a creatinine greater than 500 μmol/l with a combination of oral steroids, cyclophosphamide, and five or more plasma exchanges; 73% were alive with improved renal function two months after presentation. Figure 7.3 illustrates the response to treatment in one such patient. Other studies confirm that recovery from dialysis-dependence is common, even when the biopsy shows a high percentage of crescents (Andrassy *et al.* 1991). In this respect, the rapidly progressive nephritis of small vessel vasculitis differs from that of anti-GBM disease (see Chapter 5) and usually justifies aggressive immunotherapy. Although renal recovery may occasionally take several months (Coward *et al.* 1986), our impression is that late recovery is usually incomplete.

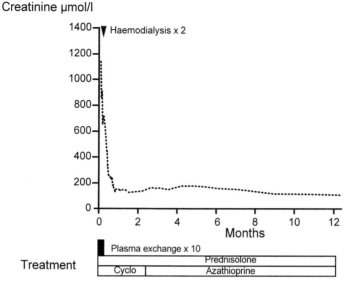

Creatinine µmol/l

Fig. 7.3 Response to treatment in a patient with Wegener's granulomatosis treated with prednisolone, cyclophosphamide, and plasma exchange.

A proportion of the patients with independent renal function after initial therapy later progress to end-stage renal failure. Some have a long history of untreated or partially treated disease, and have extensive glomerular sclerosis and interstitial damage on initial renal biopsy (Andrassy *et al.* 1991; Bindi *et al.* 1993). Others sustain further renal damage during relapse. In contrast, patients who make a good response to initial therapy, and who remain in remission, usually maintain stable and independent renal function during long-term follow-up (our data and Coward *et al.* 1986; Adu *et al.* 1987; Grotz *et al.* 1991; Andrassy *et al.* 1991).

Mortality

Figure 7.4 illustrates survival data from our series of patients treated for small vessel vasculitis; other published experience is similar. Around 10% of patients die in the early stages of treatment (Adu *et al.* 1987; Coward *et al.* 1986). Early deaths are typically due to uncontrolled disease, and often due to pulmonary haemorrhage, which may be compounded by superimposed infection. A small number of deaths occur later in the first year, with a significant contribution from opportunist infections, especially in patients still on high doses of corticosteroids, or with lymphopenia induced by cyclophosphamide. *Pneumocystis carinii* is one of the most commonly reported opportunist infections (Sneller *et al.* 1995; Guillevin *et al.* 1995). One-year survivals are generally around 80% (Levy and Winearls 1994; Coward *et al.* 1986). Causes of late deaths include relapse and the

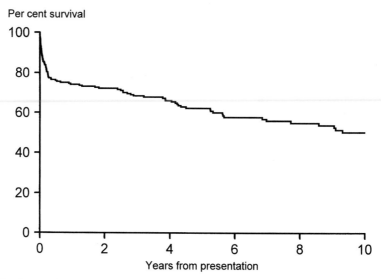

Fig. 7.4 Actuarial survival of patients treated for small vessel vasculitis at Hammersmith Hospital, 1974–95.

adverse effects of therapy, including haematological malignancy in patients treated for prolonged periods with cyclophosphamide. The remainder are attributable to unrelated causes in a predominantly elderly population. Prognosis has improved with early recognition of relapse and the more judicious use of immunosuppression; five-year survivals of 55–75% are the norm (Coward *et al.* 1986; Gordon *et al.* 1993), even when many of the patients present with advanced renal impairment.

There are certain subgroups in whom a fatal outcome is more likely, including those with oliguria and advanced renal failure at presentation (ten Berge *et al.* 1985; Serra *et al.* 1984). Indeed, mortality is higher in patients with renal disease than those without (Luqmani *et al.* 1994*a*). Failure to achieve independent renal function with initial therapy also carries an increased mortality, although this is no higher than that of patients with end-stage renal failure due to other causes (Nissensen and Port 1990). Older patients fare less well in many series, with a higher incidence of fatal infections. However, our experience is that these can be minimized by modification of immunosuppressive regimens. One systemic manifestation clearly associated with a high early mortality is the presence of lung haemorrhage.

Morbidity

Patients responding to initial therapy do not invariably remain in good health during follow-up. Irreversible organ damage from vasculitis affected 86% of the patients reported by Hoffman *et al.* (1992*a*) and 42% suffered long-term adverse effects from treatment. Patients may describe poor health which interferes with their regular activities.

Outcome on renal replacement therapy

Coward *et al.* (1986) noted no special problems related to either haemodialysis or chronic ambulatory peritoneal dialysis (CAPD). A review of outcome of end-stage renal disease due to rare causes by Nissenson and Port (1990) showed a survival in the polyarteritis group of illnesses comparable to that in control populations: 62% at three years.

Patients with vasculitis have been transplanted successfully once the disease is in remission (Hoffman *et al.* 1992a), and have even successfully completed pregnancy thereafter, but the optimal time for transplantation is uncertain. Yang *et al.* (1994) performed transplantation three months after presentation in a patient without severe extrarenal vaculitis. A period of six months in remission would seem a sensible recommendation. Patients who are still ANCA-positive have been transplanted successfully and, provided that the concentration is not rising rapidly, their continued presence is not a bar to transplantation (Noel *et al.* 1993). Clearly, such patients will receive immunosuppressive therapy and should be closely monitored.

Relapse may still occur in patients on long-term dialysis and after transplantation (Schmitt *et al.* 1993). There is a risk that because relapse in dialysis patients is uncommon (Gordon *et al.* 1993), the diagnosis may be delayed or missed. We have seen pulmonary haemorrhage misdiagnosed as fluid overload and intestinal vasculitis with perforation treated as CAPD peritonitis; the true diagnoses were revealed at autopsy. Relapse has occurred in two of our patients following cadaveric transplantation. One developed necrotizing glomerulonephritis in the graft, as reported previously by Turney *et al.* (1986). Relapse after transplantation may be even be the first indicator of the cause of the underlying renal failure (Stegeman *et al.* 1994).

Renal involvement in other vasculitic disorders

Churg–Strauss syndrome

This disorder is a vasculitis of small and medium sized vessels, frequently associated with ANCA, in which necrotizing glomerulonephritis may occur (Churg and Strauss 1951), although less commonly than in Wegener's granulomatosis or microscopic polyangiitis. The characteristic clinical features (Lanham *et al.* 1984) are asthma, eosinophilia exceeding $1.5 \times 10^9/l$, and a necrotizing vasculitis affecting particularly the heart, skin, bowel, and the musculoskeletal and nervous systems. Pulmonary infiltrates, allergic rhinitis, and nasal polyps occur frequently. As in other forms of small vessel vasculitis, life-threatening alveolar haemorrhage may occur, although this is rare.

Histological changes in the kidney were clearly described in the post-mortem study of Churg and Strauss, but have been detected less frequently in life. For example, Chumbley *et al.* (1977) reported 30 patients with the condition, of whom only 1 had 'renal failure', and 3 had slight elevations of urea and creatinine. Clutterbuck *et al.* (1990) described renal disease in 16 of 19 patients treated in our unit, reflecting the nature of our referral practice. Nephrotic syndrome occurred in 3 patients and serum creatinine concentration was greater than 500 μmol/l in 4 patients. The dominant histological pattern was a focal segmental glomerulonephritis; overt vasculitis and eosinophilic infiltration were less common.

Corticosteroids have been the mainstay of therapy in most reported series (Chumbley *et al.* 1977; Lanham *et al.* 1984), but when severe renal disease is present a strategy which is similar to the treatment of rapidly progressive glomerulonephritis in microscopic polyangiitis is usually employed. The prognosis is generally good; 10 of 19 patients in Clutterbuck's series had a normal serum creatinine at 2–10 years after diagnosis.

Polyarteritis nodosa

This is a necrotizing vasculitis involving medium-sized muscular arteries and leading to aneurysm formation. Significant renal impairment may result from renal infarction or ischaemia, or occasionally from accelerated phase hypertension. The Chapel Hill criteria preclude a diagnosis of polyarteritis nodosa in patients with rapidly progressive glomerulonephritis.

Giant cell arteritis

This condition is predominantly a disease of the elderly and typically affects the branches of the carotid artery. Rarely, it can involve intrarenal vessels, or lead to widely disseminated visceral arteritis (Lie 1978). Exceptionally, patients with otherwise typical temporal arteritis have been reported to develop focal necrotizing glomerulonephritis (see Pascual *et al.* 1994 for a recent example). The distinction between giant cell arteritis and other vasculitides more frequently associated with renal disease is not always clear-cut, since there are reports of temporal artery involvement in Churg–Strauss syndrome and in Wegener's granulomatosis.

Takayasu's arteritis

This is typically a disease of young women which causes inflammation in large arteries, particularly the aorta and its main branches. The main renal arteries are frequently involved but glomerular disease is rare. Focal segmental necrotizing glomerulonephritis with crescent formation has been described in one case, which responded to treatment with pulse methylprednisolone (Hellman *et al.* 1987).

Behçet's syndrome

This disease is characterized clinically by ocular inflammation, oral and genital ulceration, and variable thrombotic, neurological, pulmonary, and rheumatic features. Pathologically there is a leucocytoclastic vasculitis chiefly involving veins, venules, and capillaries. Patients with Behçet's syndrome have been reported to develop necrotizing or crescentic glomerulonephritis, but it is sometimes difficult to be certain from the descriptions whether most of these patients really had microscopic polyangiitis or Wegener's granulomatosis. Yang *et al.* (1993) reported a patient meeting criteria for the diagnosis of Behçet's syndrome, who also had cutaneous vasculitis, and renal failure associated with globally and segmentally sclerosed glomeruli, with c-ANCA by immunofluorescence. Other reported patterns of renal pathology in Behçet's syndrome include IgA nephropathy, minimal change nephrotic syndrome with renal vein thrombosis, and AA amyloidosis. Renal dysfunction may also result from the nephrotoxicity of cyclosporin or FK506 used in treatment.

Relapsing polychondritis

This disease is characterized by episodic inflammation and destruction of cartilaginous structures, with diverse clinical manifestations including features of systemic vasculitis in some patients. Recently, ANCA have been detected (Geffriaud Ricouard *et al.* 1993). Necrotizing glomerulonephritis is well recognized, perhaps affecting 20% of patients, and may follow a rapidly progressive course with crescent formation (Chang-Miller and *et al.* 1987). Cytotoxic therapy in addition to corticosteroids is advocated for patients with glomerular disease.

Conclusion

Rapidly progressive glomerulonephritis is a prominent feature of the ANCA-associated diseases, Wegener's granulomatosis and microscopic polyangiitis, and may rarely occur in other vasculitic conditions. The high mortality of these conditions without therapy has been transformed by the use of immunosuppressive regimens. Indeed, patients may recover from severe renal failure, provided that irreversible renal scarring has not supervened.

Unfortunately, longer-term outcome is marked by morbidity due to residual organ damage, disease relapse, and drug side-effects. This is a major focus of current endeavours; treatments of lower toxicity are being tested, and improved ANCA assays are being used to facilitate early diagnosis, and to inform decisions about long-term drug therapy. In the future, knowledge of the pathogenesis of vasculitis should permit the rational design of specific therapeutic agents, which, singly or in combination, have a greater efficacy and a lower toxicity than those in current use.

References

Adu, D., Howie, A.J., Scott, D.G.I., Bacon, P.A., McGonigle, R.J.S., and Michael, J. (1987). Polyarteritis and the kidney. *Quarterly Journal of Medicine*, **62**, 221–37.

Adu, D., Pall, A., Luqmani, R.A., Richards, N.T., Howie, A.J., Guery, P. *et al.* (1997). Controlled trial of pulse versus continuous prednisolone and cyclophosphamide in the treatment of systemic vasculitis. *Quarterly Journal of Medicine*, **90**, 401–10.

Andrassy, K., Erb, A., Koderisch, J., Waldherr, R., and Ritz, E. (1991). Wegener's granulomatosis with renal involvement: patient survival and correlations between initial renal function, renal histology, therapy and renal outcome. *Clinical Nephrology*, **35**, 139–47.

Andrews, M., Edmunds, M., Campbell, A., Walls, J., and Feehally, J. (1990). Systemic vasculitis in the 1980s—is there an increasing incidence of Wegener's granulomatosis and microscopic polyarteritis? *Journal of the Royal College of Physicians London*, **24**, 284–8.

Arnalich, F., Lahoz, C., Picazo, M.L., Monereo, A., Arribas, J.R., Martinez Ara, J. *et al.* (1989). Polyarteritis nodosa and necrotizing glomerulonephritis associated with long-standing silicosis. *Nephron*, **51**, 544–7.

Barksdale, S.K., Hallahan, C.W., Kerr, G.S., Fauci, A.S., Stern, J.B., and Travis, W.D. (1995). Cutaneous pathology in Wegener's granulomatosis. A clinicopathologic study of 75 biopsies in 46 patients. *American Journal of Surgical Pathology*, **19**, 161–72.

Bindi, P., Mougenot, B., Mentre, F., Noel, L., Peraldi, M. Vanhille, P. *et al.* (1993). Necrotizing crescentic glomerulonephritis without significant immune deposits: a clinical and serological study. *Quarterly Journal of Medicine*, **86**, 55–68.

Björck, S., Svalander, C., and Westberg, G. (1985). Hydralazine-associated glomerulonephritis. *Acta Medica Scandinavica*, **218**, 261–9.

Bolton, W.K. and Sturgill, B.C. (1989). Methylprednisolone therapy for acute crescentic rapidly progressive glomerulonephritis. *American Journal of Nephrology*, **9**, 368–75.

Bosch, X., Mirapeix, E., Font, J., Borrellas, X., Rodriguez, R., Lopez Soto, A. *et al.* (1991). Prognostic implication of anti-neutrophil cytoplasmic autoantibodies with myeloperoxidase specificity in anti-glomerular basement membrane disease *Clinical Nephrology*, **36**, 107–113.

Bosch, X., Lopez-Soto, A., Mirapeix, E., Font, J., Ingelmo, M., and Urbano-Marquez, A. (1994). Antineutrophil cytoplasmic autoantibody-associated alveolar capillaritis in patients presenting with pulmonary haemorrhage. *Archives of Pathological Laboratory Medicine*, **118**, 517–22.

Bruns, F.J., Adler, S., Fraley, D.S., and Segel, D.P. (1989). Long-term follow-up of aggressively treated idiopathic rapidly progressive glomerulonephritis. *American Journal of Medicine*, **86**, 400–6.

Bullen, C.L., Liesegang, T.J., McDonald, T.J., and DeRemee, R.A. (1983). Ocular compliations of Wegener's granulomatosis. *Ophthalmology*, **90**, 279–90.

Calabrese, L.H., Estes, M., Yen-Lieberman, B., Proffitt, M.R., Tubbs, R., Fishleder, A.J. *et al.* (1989). Systemic vasculitis in association with human immunodeficiency virus infection. *Arthritis and Rheumatism*, **32**, 569–76.

Cameron, J.S. (1991). Renal vasculitis: microscopic polyarteritis and Wegener's granuloma. In *Renal involvement in systemic vasculitis. Contributions to nephrology*, (ed. A. Sessa, M. Meroni, and G. Battini) Vol. 94, pp. 58–65. Karger, Basel.

Camilleri, M., Pusey, C.D., Chadwick, V.S., and Rees, A.J. (1983). Gastrointestinal manifestations of systemic vasculitis. *Quarterly Journal of Medicine*, **52**, 141–9.

Carrington, C.B. and Liebow, A. (1966). Limited forms of angiitis and granulomatosis of Wegener's type. *American Journal of Medicine*, **41**, 497–527.

Chang-Miller, A. Okamura, M., Torres, V.E., Michet, C.J., Wegener, R.D., Donadio, J.V.Jr., Offord, K.P., Holley, K.E. *et al.* (1987). Renal involvement in relapsing polychondritis. *Medicine*, **66**, 202–17.

Chumbley, L.C., Harrison, E.G., and DeRemee, R.A. (1977). Allergic granulomatosis and angiitis (Churg–Strauss syndrome). Report and analysis of 30 cases. *Mayo Clinic Proceedings*, **52**, 477–84.

Churg, J. and Strauss, L. (1951). Allergic granulomatosis, allergic angiitis and periarteritis nodosa. *American Journal of Pathology*, **27**, 277–301.

Clutterbuck, E.J., Evans, D.J., and Pusey, C.D. (1990). Renal involvement in Churg–Strauss syndrome. *Nephrology Dialysis Transplantation*, **5**, 161–7.

Cohen Tervaert, J.W. and Kallenberg, C. (1993). Neurologic manifestations of systemic vasculitides. *Rheumatic Disease Clinics of North America*, **19**, 913–40.

Cohen Tervaert, J.W., van der Woude, F.J., Fauci, A.S., Ambrus, J.L., Velosa, J., Keane, W.F. *et al.* (1989). Association between active Wegener's granulomatosis and anticytoplasmic antibodies. *Archives of Internal Medicine*, **149**, 2461–5.

Cohen Tervaert, J.W., Goldschmeding, R., Elema, J.D., van der Giessen, M., Huitema, M.G., van der Hem, G.K. *et al.* (1990*a*). Autoantibodies against myeloid lysosomal enzymes in cresentic glomerulonephritis. *Kidney International*, **37**, 799–806.

Cohen Tervaert, J.W., Huitema, M.G., Hene, R.W., Sluiter, W.J., The, T.H., van der Hem, G.K. *et al.* (1990*b*). Prevention of relapses in Wegener's granulomatosis by treatment based on antineutrophil cytoplasmic antibody titre. *Lancet*, **336**, 709–11.

Cohen Tervaert, J.W., Goldschmeding, R., Elema, J.D., von dem Borne, A.E., and Kallenberg, C.G. (1991). Antimyeloperoxidase antibodies in Churg–Strauss syndrome. *Thorax*, **46**, 70–1.

Cohen, J., Pinching, A.J., Rees, A.J., and Peters, D.K. (1982). Infection and immunosuppression. A study of the infective complications of 75 patients with immunologically-mediated renal disease. *Quarterly Journal of Medicine*, **51**, 1–15.

Cole, E., Cattran, D., Magil, A., Greenwood, C., Churchill, D., Sutton, D. *et al.* and the Canadiar. Apheresis Study Group (1992). A prospective randomized trial of plasma exchange as additive therapy in idiopathic crescentic glomerulonephritis. *American Journal of Kidney Diseases*, **20**, 261–9.

Cordier, J.F., Valeyre, D., Guillevin, L., Loire, R., and Brechot, J.M. (1990). Pulmonary Wegener's granulomatosis. A clinical and imaging study of 77 cases. *Chest*, **97**, 900–12.

Corman, L.C. and Dolson, D.J. (1992). Polyarteritis nodosa and parvovirus B19 infection. *Lancet*, **339**, 491.

Coward, R.A., Hamdy, N.A.T., Shortland, J.S., and Brown, C.B. (1986). Renal micropolyarteritis: a treatable condition. *Nephrology Dialysis Transplantation*, **1**, 31–7.

Davenport, A., Lock, R.J., and Wallington, T.B. (1994). Clinical relevance of testing for antineutrophil cytoplasm antibodies (ANCA) with a standard indirect immunofluorescence ANCA test in patients with upper or lower respiratory tract symptoms. *Thorax*, **49**, 213–17.

Davies, D.J., Moran, J.E., Niall, J.F., and Ryan, G.B. (1982). Segmental necrotising glomerulonephritis with antineutrophil antibody: possible arbovirus aetiology? *British Medical Journal*, **285**, 606.

Davson, J., Ball, J., and Platt, R. (1948). The kidney in periarteritis nodosa. *Quarterly Journal of Medicine*, **17**, 175–202.

De'Oliviera, J.G., Gaskin, G., Dash, A., Rees, A.J., and Pusey, C.D. (1995). Relationship between disease activity and ANCA concentration by ELISA in long-term management of systemic vasculitis. *American Journal of Kidney Diseases*, **25**, 380–9.

DeRemee, R.A. (1988). The treatment of Wegener's granulomatosis with trimethoprim/sulfamethoxazole: illusion or vision? *Arthritis and Rheumatism*, **31**, 1068–72.

Clinical aspects of systemic vasculitis

Devaney, K.O., Travis, W.D., Hoffman, G., Leavitt, R., Lebovics, R., and Fauci, A.S. (1990). Interpretation of head and neck biopsies in Wegener's granulomatosis: a pathologic study of biopsies in 70 patients. *American Journal of Surgical Pathology*, **14**, 555–64.

Devogelaer, J., Pirson, Y., Vandenbroucke, J., Cosyns, J., Brichard, S., and Nagant de Deuxchaisnes, C. (1987). D-penicillamine induced crescentic glomerulonephritis: report and review of the literature. *Journal of Rheumatology*, **14**, 1036–41.

Efthimiou, J., Spickett, G., Lane, D., and Thompson, A. (1991). Antineutrophil cytoplasmic antibodies, cystic fibrosis, and infection. *Lancet*, **337**, 1037–8.

Egner, W. and Chapel, H.M. (1990). Titration of antibodies against neutrophil cytoplasmic antigens is useful in monitoring disease activity in systemic vasculitides. *Clinical and Experimental Immunology*, **82**, 244–9.

Elzouki, A.N., Segelmark, M., Wieslander, J., and Eriksson, S. (1994). Strong link between the alpha 1-antitrypsin PiZ allele and Wegener's granulomatosis. *Journal of Internal Medicine*, **236**, 543–48.

Esnault, V.L.M., Soleimani, B., Keogan, M.T., Brownlee, A.A., Jayne, D.R.W., and Lockwood, C.M. (1992). Association of IgM with IgG ANCA in patients presenting with pulmonary haemorrhage. *Kidney International*, **41**, 1304–10.

Esnault, V.L.M., Testa, A., Audrain, M., Roge, C., Hamidou, M., Barrier, J.H. Sesboue, R., Martin, J.P., Lesavre, P. (1993). Alpha 1-antitrypsin genetic polymorphism in ANCA-positive systemic vasculitis. *Kidney International*, **43**, 1329–32.

Esnault, V.L., Short, A.K., Audrain, M.A., Jones, S.J., Martin, S.J., Skehel, J.M., and Lockwood, C.M. (1994). Autoantibodies to lactoferrin and histone in systemic vasculitis identified by anti-myeloperoxidase solid phase assays. *Kidney International*, **46**, 153–60.

Fahey, J.L., Leonard, E., Churg, J., and Godman, G. (1954). Wegener's granulomatosis. *American Journal of Medicine*, **17**, 168–79.

Falk, R.J. and Jennettee, J.C. (1988). Anti-neutrophil cytoplasmic autoantibodies with specificity for myeloperoxidase in patients with systemic vasculitis and idiopathic necrotizing and crescentic glomerulonephritis. *New England Journal of Medicine*, **318**, 1651–7.

Falk, R.J., Hogan, S., Carey, T.S., and Jennette, J.C. (1990). Clinical course of anti-neutrophil cytoplasmic autoantibody-associated glomerulonephritis and systemic vasculitis. *Annals of Internal Medicine*, **113**, 656–63.

Fauci, A.S., Haynes, B.F., Katz, P., and Wolff, S. (1983). Wegener's granulomatosis: prospective clinical and therapeutic experience with 85 patients over 21 years. *Annals of Internal Medicine*, **98**, 76–85.

Finn, J.E., Zhang, L., Agrawal, S., Jayne, D.R.W., Oliveira, D.B.G., and Mathieson, P.W. (1994). Molecular analysis of C3 allotypes in patients with systemic vasculitis. *Nephology Dialysis Transplantation*, **9**, 1564–7.

Fuiano, G., Cameron, J.S., Raftery, M., Hartley, B.H., Williams, D.G., and Ogg, C.S. (1988). Improved prognosis of renal microscopic polyarteritis in recent years. *Nephology Dialysis Transplantation*, **3**, 383–91.

Gaskin, G. and Pusey, C.D. (1995). Evolution of a policy to prevent vasculitis relapse. *Clinical and Experimental Immunology*, **101**(suppl.1), 46 (abstract).

Gaskin, G., Clutterbuck, E.J., and Pusey, C.D. (1991a). Renal disease in Churg–Strauss syndrome: diagnosis, management and outcome. In *Renal involvement in systemic vasculitis. Contributions to nephrology*, (ed. A. Sessa, M. Meroni, and G. Battini) Vol. 94, pp. 58–65. Karger, Basel.

Gaskin, G., Savage, C.O.S., Ryan, J.J., Jones, S., Rees, A.J., Lockwood, C.M. *et al.* (1991*b*). Anti-neutrophil cytoplasmic antibodies and disease activity during long-term follow-up of 70 patients with systemic vasculitis. *Nephrology Dialysis Transplantation*, 6, 689–94.

Geffriaud Ricouard, C., Noel, L.H., Chauveau, D., Houhou, S., Grunfeld, J.P., and Lesavre, P. (1993). Clinical spectrum associated with ANCA of defined antigen specificities in 98 selected patients. *Clinical Nephrology*, 39, 125–6.

Glockner, W., Sieberth, H.G., Wichmann, H.E., Backes, E., Bambauer, R., Boesken, W.H. *et al.* (1988). Plasma exchange and immunosuppression in rapidly progressive glomerulonephritis: a controlled multi-centre study. *Clinical Nephrology*, 29, 1–88.

Gocke, D.J., Hsu, K., Morgan, C., Bombardieri, S., Lockshin, M., and Christian, C.L. (1970). Association between polyarteritis and Australia antigen. *Lancet*, ii, 1149–53.

Godman, G.C. and Churg, J. (1954). Wegener's granulomatosis: pathology and review of the literature. *Archives of Pathology*, 58, 533–53.

Goldschmeding, R., van der Schoot, C.E., ten Bokkel Huinink, D., Hack, C.E., van den Ende, M.E., Kallenberg, C.G.M. *et al.* (1989). Wegener's granulomatosis autoantibodies identify a novel diisopropylfluorophosphate-binding protein in the lysosomes of normal human neutrophils. *Journal of Clinical Investigation*, 84, 1577–87.

Gordon, M., Luqmani, R.A., Adu, D., Greaves, I., Richards, N., Michael, J. *et al.* (1993). Relapses in patients with a systemic vasculitis. *Quarterly Journal of Medicine*, 86, 779–89.

Griffith, M.E., Lovegrove, J., Gaskin, G., Whitehouse, D., and Pusey, C.D. (1996). C-ANCA positivity in systemic vasculitis is associated with the Z allele of α1 AT and P-ANCA positivity with the S allele. *Nephology Dialysis Transplantation*, 11, 438–43.

Grotz, W., Wanner, C., Keller, E., Bohler, J., Peter, H.H., Rohrbach, R. *et al.* (1991). Crescentic glomerulonephritis in Wegener's granulomatosis: morphology, therapy, outcome. *Clinical Nephrology*, 35, 243–51.

Guillevin, L., Visser, H., Noel, L.H., Pourrat, J., Vernier, I., Gayraud, M. *et al.* (1993). Antineutrophil cytoplasm antibodies in systemic polyarteritis nodosa with and without hepatitis B virus infection and Churg–Strauss syndrome—62 patients. *Journal of Rheumatology*, 20, 1345–9.

Guillevin, L., Lhote, F., Jarrousse, B., Cohen, P., Jacquot, C., Lesavre, P. *et al.* (1995). Treatment of severe Wegener's granulomatosis (WG): a prospective trial comparing prednisone (CS), pulse cyclophosphamide (CY) versus CS and oral CY *Clinical and Experimental Immunology*, 101(suppl.1), 43 (abstract).

Hagen, E.C., Andrassy, K., Chernok, E., Daha, M.R., Gaskin, G., Gross, W. *et al.* (1993). The value of indirect immunofluorescence and solid phase techniques for ANCA detection. A report on the first phase of an international cooperative study on the standardization of ANCA assays. EEC/BCR Group for ANCA Assay Standardization. *Journal of Immunological Methods*, 159, 1–16.

Hagen, E.C., de Keizer, R.J.W., Andrassy, K., van Boven, W.P.L., Bruijn, J.A., van Es, L.A. *et al.* (1995*a*). Compassionate treatment of Wegener's granulomatosis with rabbit anti-thymocyte globulin. *Clinical Nephrology*, 43, 351–9

Hagen, E.C., Stegeman, C.A., D'Amaro, J., Schreuder, G.M.T., Lems, S.P.M., Cohen Tervaert, J.W. *et al.* (1995*b*). Decreased frequency of HLA-DR13DR6 in Wegener's granulomatosis. *Kidney International*, 48, 801–5.

Hagen, E.C. for the EC/BCR project for ANCA assay standardization (1995*c*). Development and standardization of solid-phase assays for the detection of anti-neutrophil cytoplasmic antibodies (ANCA) for clinical application: report of a large clinical evaluation study. *Clinical and Experimental Immunology*, **101**(suppl.1), 29.

Harrison, C.V., Loughridge, L.W., and Milne, M.D. (1964). Acute oliguric renal failure in acute glomerulonephritis and polyarteritis. *Quarterly Journal of Medicine*, **129**, 39–55.

Haubitz, M., Frei, U., Rother, U., Brunkhorst, R., and Koch, K.M. (1991). Cyclophosphamide pulse therapy in Wegener's granulomatosis. *Nephrology Dialysis Transplantation*, **6**, 531–5.

Haubitz, M., Brunkhorst, R., Schellong, S., Gobel, U., Schurek, H.J., and Koch, K.M. (1995). A prospective randomised study comparing daily oral versus monthly i.v. cyclophosphamide application in patients with ANCA-associated vasculitis and renal involvement (preliminary results). *Clinical and Experimental Immunology*, **101** (suppl.1), 43 (abstract).

Haworth, S.J., Savage, C.O.S., Carr, S., Hughes, J.M.B., and Rees, A.J. (1985). Pulmonary haemorrhage complicating Wegener's granulomatosis and microscopic polyarteritis. *British Medical Journal*, **290**, 1775–8.

Hellman, D.B., Hardy, K., Lindenfield, S., and Ring, E. (1987). Takayasu's arteritis associated with crescentic glomerulonephritis. *Arthritis and Rheumatism*, **30**, 451–4.

Hind, C.R.K., Winearls, C.G., Lockwood, C.M., Rees, A.J., and Pepys, M.B. (1984). Objective monitoring of activity in Wegener's granulomatosis by measurement of serum C-reactive protein concentration. *Clinical Nephrology*, **21**, 341–5.

Hoffman, G.S., Leavitt, R.Y., Fleisher, T.A., Minor, J.R., and Fauci, A.S. (1990). Treatment of Wegener's granulomatosis with intermittent high dose intravenous cyclophosphamide. *American Journal of Medicine*, **89**, 403–10.

Hoffman, G.S., Kerr, G.S., Leavitt, R.Y., Hallahan, C.W., Lebovics, R.S., Travis, W.D. *et al.* (1992a). Wegener granulomatosis: an analysis of 158 patients. *Annals of Internal Medicine*, **116**, 488–98.

Hoffman, G.S., Leavitt, R.Y., Kerr, G.S., and Fauci, A.S. (1992b). The treatment of Wegener's granulomatosis with glucocorticoids and methotrexate. *Arthritis and Rheumatism*, **35**, 1322–9.

Hunder, G.G., Arends, W.P., Bloch, D.A., Calabrese, L.H., Fauci, A.S., Fries, J.S. *et al.* (1990). The American College of Rheumatology 1990 criteria for the classification of vasculitis. *Arthritis and Rheumatism*, **33**, 1065–145.

Jayne, D.R.W., Jones, S.J., Severn, A., Shaunak, S., Murphy, J., and Lockwood, C.M. (1989). Severe pulmonary haemorrhage and systemic vasculitis in association with circulating anti-neutrophil cytoplasm antibodies of IgM class only. *Clinical Nephrology*, **32**, 101–6.

Jayne, D.R.W., Marshall, P.D., Jones, S.J., and Lockwood, C.M. (1990). Autoantibodies to GBM and neutrophil cytoplasm in rapidly progressive glomerulonephritis. *Kidney International*, **37**, 965–70.

Jayne, D.R., Davies, M.J., Fox, C.J., Black, C.M., and Lockwood, C.M. (1991). Treatment of systemic vasculitis with pooled intravenous immunoglobulin. *Lancet*, **337**, 1137–9.

Jayne, D.R.W., Gaskin, G., Pusey, C.D., and Lockwood, C.M. (1995). ANCA and prediction of relapse in systemic vasculitis. *Quarterly Journal of Medicine*, **88**, 127–33.

Jennette, J.C., Wilkman, A.S., and Falk, R.J. (1989). Anti-neutrophil cytoplasmic autoantibody-associated glomerulonephritis and vasculitis. *American Journal of Pathology*, **135**, 921–30.

Jennette, J.C., Falk, R.J., Andrassy, K., Bacon, P.A., Churg, J., Gross, W.L. *et al.* (1994). Nomenclature of systemic vasculitides. Proposal of an international consensus conference. *Arthritis and Rheumatism*, 37, 187–92.

Kain, R., Matsui, K., Exner, M., Binder, S., Schaffner, G., Sommer, E.M. *et al.* (1995). A novel class of autoantigens of anti-neutrophil cytoplasmic antibodies in necrotizing and crescentic glomerulonephritis: the lysosomal membrane glycoprotein h-lamp-2 in neutrophil granulocytes and a related protein in glomerular endothelial cells. *Journal of Experimental Medicine*, 181, 585–97.

Kallenberg, C.G., Brouwer, E., Weening, J.J., and Tervaert, J.W. (1994). Anti-neutrophil cytoplasmic antibodies: current diagnostic and pathophysiological potential. *Kidney International*, 46, 1–15.

Kerr, G.S., Fleisher, T.A., Hallahan, C.W., Leavitt, R.Y., Fauci, A.S., and Hoffman, G.S. (1993). Limited prognostic value of changes in antineutrophil cytoplasmic antibody titer in patients with Wegener's granulomatosis *Arthritis and Rheumatism*, 36, 365–71.

Knudsen, B.B., Joergensen, T., and Munch-Jensen, B. (1988). Wegener's granulomatosis in a family. *Scandinavian Journal of Rheumatology*, 17, 225–7.

Kokolina, E., Noel, L.H., Nusbaum, P., Geffriaud, C., Grunfeld, J.P., Halbwachs Mecarelli, L. *et al.* (1994). Isotype and affinity of anti-myeloperoxidase autoantibodies in systemic vasculitis. *Kidney International*, 46, 177–84.

Lanham, J.G., Elkon, K.B., Pusey, C.D., and Hughes, G.R. (1984). Systemic vasculitis with asthma and eosinophilia: a clinical approach to the Churg–Strauss syndrome. *Medicine*, 63, 65–81.

Leib, E.S., Restivo, C., and Paulus, H.E. (1979). Immunosuppressive and corticosteroid therapy of polyarteritis nodosa. *American Journal of Medicine*, 67, 941–5.

Levy, J.B. and Winearls, C.G. (1994). Rapidly progressive glomerulonephritis: what should be first-line therapy? *Nephron*, 67, 402–7.

Lie, J.T. (1978). Disseminated giant cell arteritis. Histopathological description and differentiation from other granulomatous vasculitides. *American Journal of Clinical Pathology*, 69, 299–305.

Lockwood, C.M., Thiru, S., Isaacs, J.D., Hale, G., and Waldmann, H. (1993). Long-term remission of intractable systemic vasculitis with monoclonal antibody therapy. *Lancet*, 341, 1620–2.

Lockwood, C.M., Thiru, S., Stewart, S., Hale, G., Isaacs, J., Wraight, P. *et al.* (1996). Treatment of refractory Wegener's granulomatosis with humanized monoclonal antibodies. *Quarterly Journal of Medicine*, 89, 903–12.

Ludemann, J., Utecht, B., and Gross, W.L. (1990). Anti-neutrophil cytoplasm antibodies in Wegener's granulomatosis recognize an elastinolytic enzyme. *Journal of Experimental Medicine*, 171, 357–62.

Luqmani, R.A., Bacon, P.A., Beaman, M., Scott, D.G.I., Emery, P., Lee, S.J. *et al.* (1994*a*). Classical versus non-renal Wegener's granulomatosis. *Quarterly Journal of Medicine*, 87, 161–7.

Luqmani, R.A., Bacon, P.A., Moots, R.J., Janssen, B.A., Pall, A., Emery, P. *et al.* (1994*b*). Birmingham Vasculitis Activity Score (BVAS) in systemic necrotizing vasculitis. *Quarterly Journal of Medicine*, 87, 671–8.

Mathieson, P.W., Cobbold, S.P., Hale, G., Clark, M.R., Oliveira, D.B., Lockwood, C.M. *et al.* (1990). Monoclonal antibody therapy in systemic vasculitis. *New England Journal of Medicine*, 323, 250–4.

McClelland, P., Williams, P.S., Stevens, M.E., and Bone, J.M. (1989). Aggressive immuno-suppression in glomerulonephritis *Nephrology Dialysis Transplantation*, **4**, 917–8.

Muhle, C., Koltze, H., Splelman, R.P., Reinhold-Keller, E., Richter, C., Beigel, A. *et al.* (1993). MRI of the head in Wegener's granulomatosis—results of a prospective study, *Clinical and Experimental Immunology*, **93** (suppl. 1), 36 (abstract).

Niles, J.L., McCluskey, R.T., Ahmad, M.F., and Amin Arnaout, M. (1989). Wegener's granulomatosis autoantigen is a novel neutrophil serine proteinase. *Blood*, **74**, 1888–93.

Niles, J.L., Pan, G.L., Collins, A.B., Shannon, T., Skates, S., Fienberg, R. *et al.* (1991). Antigen-specific radioimmunoassays for anti-neutrophil cytoplasmic antibodies in the diagnosis of rapidly progressive glomerulonephritis. *Journal of the American Society of Nephrology*, **2**, 27–36.

Nissensen, A.R. and Port, F.K. (1990). Outcome of end-stage renal disease in patients with rare causes of renal failure: III. Systemic/vascular disorders. *Quarterly Journal of Medicine*, **74**, 65–74.

Noel, L., Morin, M.P., Thervet, E., Legendre, C., Vandapel, O., Kreis, H. *et al.* (1993). Successful kidney transplantation in a patient with microscopic polyarteritis and positive ANCA. *Clinical and Experimental Immunology*, **93**(suppl.1), 43 (abstract).

Nolle, B., Specks, U., Ludemann, J., Rohrbach, M.S., DeRemee, R.A., and Gross, W.L. (1989). Anticytoplasmic autoantibodies: their immunodiagnostic value in Wegener's granulomatosis. *Annals of Internal Medicine*, **111**, 28–40.

Noritake, D.T., Weiner, S.R., Bassett, L.W., Paulus, H.E., and Weisbart, R. (1987). Rheumatic manifestations of Wegener's granulomatosis. *Journal of Rheumatology*, **14**, 949–51.

Novak, R.F., Christiansen, R.G., and Sorensen, E.T. (1982). The acute vasculitis of Wegener's granulomatosis in renal biopsies. *American Journal of Clinical Pathology*, **78**, 367–71.

Pascual, J., Quereda, C., Lia no, F., García-Villanueva, M.J., Mampaso, F., and Ortuno, J. (1994). Endstage renal disease after necrotising glomerulonephritis in an elderly patient with temporal arteritis. *Nephron*, **66**, 236–7.

Peter, H.H., Metzger, D., Rump, A., and Rother, E. (1993). ANCA in diseases other than systemic vasculitis. *Clinical and Experimental Immunology*, **93** (suppl. 1), 12–14.

Pudifin, D.J., Duursma, J., Gathiram, V., and Jackson, T.F. (1994). Invasive amoebiasis is associated with the development of anti-neutrophil cytoplasmic antibody. *Clinical and Experimental Immunology*, **97**, 48–51.

Pusey, C.D., Rees, A.J., Evans, D.J., Peters, D.K., and Lockwood, C.M. (1991). Plasma exchange in focal necrotizing glomerulonephritis without anti-GBM antibodies. *Kidney International*, **40**, 757–63.

Rasmussen, N., Jayne, D.R.W., Abramowicz, D., Andrassy, K., Bacon, P.A., Cohen Tervaert, J.W. *et al.* (1995). European therapeutic trials in ANCA-associated systemic vasculitis: disease scoring, consensus regimens and proposed clinical trials. *Clinical and Experimental Immunology*, **101**(suppl.1), 29–34.

Reinhold-Keller, E., Beigel, A., Duncker, G., Heller, M., and Gross, W.L. (1993). Trimethoprim-sulphamethoxazole (T/S) in the long-term treatment of Wegener's granulomatosis. *Clinical and Experimental Immunology*, **93**(suppl.1), 38 (abstract).

Reinhold-Keller, E., Kekow, J., Schnabel, A., Schmitt, W.H., Heller, M., Beigel, A. *et al.* (1994). Influence of disease manifestation and antineutrophil cytoplasmic antibody titer on the response to pulse cyclophosphamide therapy in patients with Wegener's granulomatosis. *Arthritis and Rheumatism*, **37**, 919–24.

Reuter, H., Qasim, F.J., Wraight, P., and Lockwood, C.M. (1993). The clinical significance of 111-Indium leucocyte imaging in systemic vasculitis. *Clinical and Experimental Immunology*, **93**(suppl.1), 36 (abstract).

Richter, C., Schnabel, A., Csernok, E., Reinhold-Keller, E., and Gross, W.L. (1993). Treatment of Wegener's granulomatosis with intravenous immunoglobulin. In *ANCA-associated vasculitides: immunological and clinical aspects*, (ed. W.L. Gross) pp. 487–9. Plenum, New York

Ronco, P., Verroust, P., Mignon, F., Kourilsky, O., Vanhille, P., Meyrier, A. *et al.* (1983). Immunopathological studies of polyarteritis nodosa and Wegener's granulomatosis: a report of 43 patients with 51 renal biopsies. *Quarterly Journal of Medicine*, **52**, 212–23.

Rondeau, E., Levy, M., Dosquet, P., Ruedin, P., Mougenot, B., Kanfer, A. *et al.* (1989). Plasma exchange and immunosuppression for rapidly progressive glomerulonephritis: prognosis and complications. *Nephrology Dialysis Transplantation*, **4**, 196–200.

Rose, G.A. and Spencer, H. (1957). Polyarteritis nodosa. *Quarterly Journal of Medicine*, **26**, 43–81.

Savage, C.O.S., Winearls, C.G. Evans, D.J., Rees, A.J., and Lockwood, C.M. (1985). Microscopic polyarteritis: presentation, pathology and prognosis. *Quarterly Journal of Medicine*, **56**, 467–83.

Savage, C.O.S., Winearls, C.G., Jones, S., Marshall, P.D., and Lockwood, C.M. (1987). Prospective study of radioimmunoassay for antibodies against neutrophil cytoplasm in diagnosis of systemic vasculitis. *Lancet*, **i**, 1389–93.

Savage, C.O.S., Pottinger, B.E., Gaskin, G., Lockwood, C.M., Pusey, C.D., and Pearson, J.D. (1991). Vascular damage in Wegener's granulomatosis and microscopic polyarteritis: presence of anti-endothelial cell antibodies and their relation to anti-neutrophil cytoplasm antibodies. *Clinical and Experimental Immunology*, **85**, 14–19.

Schmitt, W.H., Mistry, N., Erbsloh-Muller, B., and Gross, W.L. (1993). Study of relapses in Wegener's granulomatosis following renal transplantation. *Clinical and Experimental Immunology*, **93**(suppl.1), 43(abstract).

Schnabel, A., Csernok, E., Isenberg, D.A., Mrowka, C., and Gross, W.L. (1995). Antineutrophil cytoplasmic antibodies in systemic lupus erythematosus: prevalence, specificities and clinical significance. *Arthritis and Rheumatism*, **38**, 633–7.

Scott, D.G.I., Bacon, P.A., Elliott, P.J., Tribe, C.R., and Wallington, T.B. (1982). Systemic vasculitis in a district general hospital 1972–1980: clinical and laboratory features, classification and prognosis of 80 cases. *Quarterly Journal of Medicine*, **51**, 292–311.

Serra, A., Cameron, J.S., Turner, D.R., Hartley, B., Ogg, C.S, Neild, G.H. *et al.* (1984). Vasculitis affecting the kidney: presentation, histopathology and long-term outcome. *Quarterly Journal of Medicine*, **53** 181–207.

Sinico, R.A., Radice, A., Pozzi, C., Ferrario, F., and Arrigo, G. (1994). Diagnostic significance and antigen specificity of antineutrophil cytoplasmic antibodies in renal diseases. A prospective multicentre study. Italian Group of Renal Immunopathology. *Nephology Dialysis Transplantation*, **9**, 505–10.

Sneller, M.C., Hoffman, G.S., Talar-Williams, C., Kerr, G.S., Hallahan, C.W., and Fauci, A.S. (1995). An analysis of forty-two Wegener's granulomatosis patients treated with methotrexate and prednisone. *Arthritis and Rheumatism*, **38**, 608–13.

Soto, A., Jorgensen, C., Oksman, F., Noel, L.H., and Sany, J. (1994). Endocarditis associated with ANCA. *Clinical and Experimental Rheumatology*, **12**, 203–4.

Spencer, S.J.W., Burns, A., Gaskin, G., Pusey, C.D., and Rees, A.J. (1992). HLA class II specificities in vasculitis with antibodies to neutrophil cytoplasmic antigens. *Kidney International*, **41**, 1059–63.

Stegeman, C.A., Tervaert, J.W., van Son, W.J., and Tegzess, A.M. (1994). Necrotizing glomerulonephritis associated with antimyeloperoxidase antibodies in a renal transplant recipient with renal failure of unknown origin. *Nephrology Dialysis Transplantation*, **9**, 839–42.

Stegeman, C.A., Cohen Tervaert, J.W., de Jong, P.E., and Kallenberg, C.G.M. (1995). Prevention of relapses of Wegener's granulomatosis by treatment with trimethoprim-sulfamethoxazole. A multi-centre placebo-controlled trial in 81 patients. *Clinical and Experimental Immunology*, **101**(suppl.1), 44(abstract).

Stillwell, T.J., Benson, R.C., DeRemee, R.A., McDonald, T.J., and Weiland, L.H. (1988). Cyclophosphamide-induced bladder toxicity in Wegener's granulomatosis. *Arthritis and Rheumatism*, **31**, 465–70.

Ten Berge, I.J.M., Wilmink, J.M., Meyer, C.J.L.M., Surachno, J., ten veen, K.H., Balk, T.G. *et al.* (1985). Clinical and immunological follow-up of patients with severe renal disease in Wegener's granulomatosis. *American Journal of Nephrology*, **5**, 21–9.

Thysell, H., Bygren, P., Bengtsson, U., Lindholm, T., Norlin, M., Jonsson, M. *et al.* (1982). Immunosuppression and the additive effect of plasma exchange in treatment of rapidly progressive glomerulonephritis. *Acta Medica Scandinavica*, **212**, 107–14.

Travis, W.D., Hoffman, G.S., Leavitt, R.Y., Pass, H.I., and Fauci, A.S. (1991). Surgical pathology of the lung in Wegener's granulomatosis: review of 87 open lung biopsies from 67 patients. *American Journal of Surgical Pathology*, **15**, 315–33.

Turney, J.H., Adu, D., Michael, J., and McMaster, P. (1986). Recurrent crescentic glomerulonephritis in renal transplant recipient treated with cyclosporin. *Lancet*, **i**, 1104.

Ulmer, M., Rautmann, A., and Gross, W.L. (1992). Immunodiagnostic aspects of auto-antibodies against myeloperoxidase. *Clinical Nephrology*, **37**, 161–8.

Van der Woude, F.J., Rasmussen, N., Lobatto, S., Wiik, A., Permin, H., van Es, L.A. *et al.* (1985). Autoantibodies against neutrophils and monocytes: tool for diagnosis and marker of disease activity in Wegener's granulomatosis. *Lancet*, **i**, 425–9.

Varagunam, M., Nwosu, Z., Adu, D., Garner, C., Taylor, C.M., Michael, J. *et al.* (1993). Little evidence for anti-endothelial antibodies in microscopic polyarteritis and Wegener's granulomatosis. *Nephrology Dialysis Transplantation*, **8**, 113–17.

Venning, M.C., Quinn, A., Broomhead, V., and Bird, A.G. (1990). Antibodies directed against neutrophils (C-ANCA and P-ANCA) are of distinct diagnostic value in systemic vasculitis. *Quarterly Journal of Medicine*, **77**, 1287–96.

Wagner, J., Andrassy, K., and Ritz, E. (1991). Is vasculitis in subacute bacterial endocarditis associated with ANCA? *Lancet*, **337**, 799–800.

Watts, R.A., Carruthers, D.M., and Scott, D.G.I. (1995). Epidemiology of systemic vasculitis: changing incidence or definition? *Seminars in Arthritis and Rheumatology*, **25**, 28–34.

Weber, M.F., Andrassy, K., Pullig, O., Koderisch, J., and Netzer, K. (1992). Antineutrophil-cytoplasmic antibodies and antiglomerular basement membrane antibodies in Goodpasture's syndrome and in Wegener's granulomatosis. *Journal of the American Society of Nephrology*, **2**, 1227–34.

Wegener, F. (1936). Über generalisierte, septische Gefasserkrankungen. *Verhandlungen der Deutschen Pathologischen Gesellschaft*, **29**, 202–10.

Wegener, F. (1987). On generalised septic vessel diseases, (trans.). *Thorax*, **42**, 918–19. (Originally published 1936).

Wiik, A. (1989). Delineation of a standard procedure for indirect immunofluorescence detection of anti-neutrophil cytoplasmic antibodies (ANCA). *APMIS*, **97**(suppl.6), 12–13.

Yang, C.W., Park T.S., Kim, S.Y., Chang, Y.S., Yoon, Y.S., Bang, B.K. *et al.* (1993). Antineutrophil cytoplasmic autoantibody associated vasculitis and renal failure in Behçet disease. *Nephrology Dialysis Transplantation*, **8**, 871–73.

Yang, C.W., Kim, Y.S., Kim, S.Y., and Bang, B.K. (1994). Renal transplantation of ANCA-positive idiopathic crescentic glomerulonephritis: two-year follow-up. *Clinical Nephrology*, **42**, 209 (letter).

Zhang, L., Jayne, D.R.W., Zhao, M.H., Lockwood, C.M., and Oliveira, D.B.G. (1995). Distribution of MHC class II alleles in primary systemic vasculitis. *Kidney International*, **47**, 294–8.

8

Crescentic nephritis in systemic lupus erythematosus

Howard A. Austin III, Dimitrios T. Boumpas and James E. Balow

Glomerulonephritis is a major determinant of the course and prognosis of systemic lupus erythematosus (SLE). Although nearly the entire spectrum of glomerular, interstitial, and vascular lesions is seen in lupus nephritis, severe crescentic glomerulonephritis, and its usual clinical counterpart, rapidly progressive glomerulonephritis, characterize a relatively small subset of patients (<10%) early in the course of SLE. In spontaneous murine lupus nephritis, the disease typically progresses through stages from mild mesangial nephropathy to severe proliferative glomerulonephritis; rapidly progressive renal failure with necrotizing-crescentic glomerulonephritis is the expected cause of death in some strains of lupus-prone mice (Theofilopoulos and Dixon 1985; Balow *et al.* 1987). Interestingly, recent evidence suggests a genetic predisposition to crescent formation among certain strains of lupus-prone mice (Kinjoh *et al.* 1993).

It is not known for certain how closely the natural history of human lupus nephritis parallels that of its murine counterpart. Historical evidence would suggest that the natural courses of the diseases may be comparably devastating, based on detailed documentation of an extremely low five-year renal survival (<30%) in patients with lupus nephritis studied during the 1950s and 1960s (Muehrcke *et al.* 1957; Pollak *et al.* 1961, 1964; Baldwin *et al.* 1970, 1977). However, modern immunosuppressive drugs and other ancillary medical therapies seem to have dramatically attenuated the renal disease of SLE. Overall, five-year renal survival in patients even with severe proliferative lupus nephritis is now greater than 75% (Wallace *et al.* 1982; Austin *et al.* 1986; Cameron 1993; Donadio and Glassock 1993). Although it is possible that the natural history of SLE or referral patterns have changed over time, our own clinical experience and analysis of renal biopsy pathology do not suggest that the improved prognosis of patients with proliferative lupus nephritis in the past three decades is related to an amelioration of SLE itself, or to a particular reduction in the severity of the renal disease.

A broad range of clinical presentations is observed among patients with lupus nephritis. Early recognition and pre-emptive treatment of that minority of individuals who are at high risk for rapid deterioration of renal function is not easily accomplished. Patients with new onset lupus nephritis and rapidly declining renal function are likely to have various combinations of extensive endocapillary proliferation (diffuse proliferative glomerulonephritis), massive subendothelial immune deposits, severe karyorrhexis and fibrinoid necrosis, and/or a substantial proportion of glomeruli surrounded by cellular crescents (Figs 8.1–8.3). Rapid deterioration of renal function may also occur in patients with less fulminant active histological changes in the setting of previously established chronic, irreversible parenchymal injury (Austin *et al.* 1994*a*). In some cases, lupus flares incited by pregnancy or intercurrent infections may lead to accelerated renal disease (Yeung *et al.* 1985).

Many clinical and pathological factors appear to converge and influence the course of lupus nephritis. The impact of various clinical features on renal prognosis, in particular, has been studied; high-risk patients have been identified according to the presence of azotaemia, hypertension, nephrotic syndrome, hypocomplementaemia, and anaemia (Kimberly *et al.* 1981*a*; Ginzler *et al.* 1982, 1993; Austin *et al.* 1994*b*; Appel *et al.* 1987; Laitman *et al.* 1989; Esdaile *et al.* 1989; Levey *et al.* 1992; McCurdy *et al.* 1992; Nossent *et al.* 1989). Several of these features have been shown to be independent predictors of renal function outcome, in that they contain prognostic information that significantly enhances predictions based on combinations of other very strong risk factors (Ginzler *et al.* 1982; Whiting-O'Keefe *et al.* 1982; Magil *et al.* 1988; Esdaile *et al.* 1989, 1991; Austin *et al.* 1994*b*).

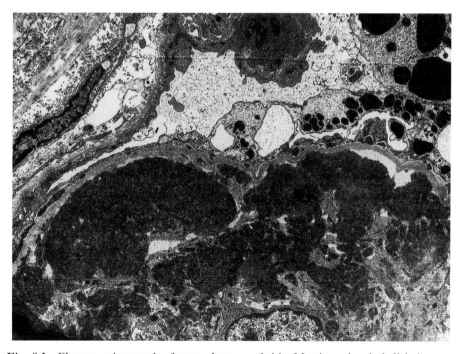

Fig. 8.1 Electron micrograph of severe lupus nephritis. Massive subendothelial electron-dense deposits are present. These large immune complexes give rise to 'wire loops' and so-called hyaline thrombi on light microscopy.

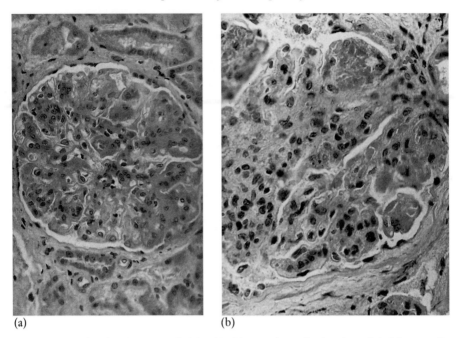

(a)   (b)

Fig. 8.2 Proliferative lupus nephritis. (a) Glomerular tuft showing global hypercellularity and capillary loop thickening (wire loop lesions), (H & E, ×300). (b) Glomerulus with severe hypercellularity and several segments with fibrinoid necrosis (H & E, ×400).

The strength of these clinical prognostic indicators is diminished somewhat by the fact that most can be modified by appropriate therapeutic interventions. Indeed, it is logical that certain clinical factors which might normally have a very profound influence on the natural history of the disease could be thwarted by effective treatment. In some cases, outcome predictions based on clinical parameters can be strengthened if the time course of critical features (such as the rate of change of renal function) is characteristic and can be ascertained accurately (Kimberly *et al.* 1981*a*).

As observed in other forms of glomerulonephritis, the renal biopsy offers a relatively direct and detailed assessment of the type and severity of lupus nephritis (Pirani and Salinas-Madrigal 1968; Grishman *et al.* 1973; Churg and Sobin 1982; Balow *et al.* 1987; Kashgarian 1994). Histological features that identify patients at high risk for accelerated renal function deterioration (subendothelial deposits, fibrinoid necrosis, and cellular crescents) will be reviewed among individuals with new onset lupus nephritis and among those with variable degrees of pre-existing irreversible pathological change. The contributions of clinical and demographic factors will also be considered.

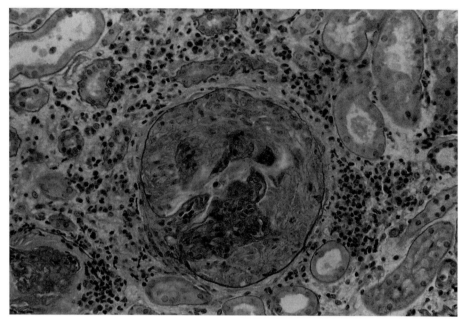

Fig. 8.3   Crescentic lupus nephritis. A circumferential crescent is causing severe compression of the glomerular tuft. Mononuclear cells are infiltrating the interstitium around Bowman's capsule. Tubular separation and atrophy are evident (PAS, ×400).

Analysis of factors affecting the severity and prognosis of lupus nephritis

Subendothelial deposits

Subendothelial immune complex deposition (Fig. 8.1) is characteristic of severe lupus nephritis (Pirani and Olesnicky 1982; Churg and Sobin 1982). Hyperactive B cells produce autoantibodies that react with DNA nucleosome complexes and other cellular components (Schwartz and Stollar 1985). Localization of the resultant immune complexes to the subendothelial region of the glomerular capillary wall, adjacent to the circulation, leads to the release of complement components, cytokines and other factors that promote inflammation, cellular injury, proliferation, and eventually, sclerosis (Couser 1990; Foster *et al.* 1993). Consequently, subendothelial immune complexes have been associated with clinical features and histological evidence of severe active lupus nephritis (Grishman *et al.* 1973; Sinniah and Feng 1976). Tateno and colleagues (1983) found that the severity of renal dysfunction, proteinuria, and hypocomplementaemia each correlated with the extent of subendothelial immune complex formation.

Subendothelial deposits have been correlated with a poor prognosis in some studies (Whiting-O'Keefe *et al.* 1982; Bhuyan *et al.* 1982; Tateno *et al.* 1983; Esdaile *et al.* 1991), but not all (Esdaile *et al.* 1989; Austin *et al.* 1984). Tateno and coworkers (1983) found that patients with massive subendothelial deposits had a very poor prognosis. The cumulative survival rate approximated 70% at one year and 40% at five years. However, the presence or extent of subendothelial deposits at study entry has not emerged as an important prognostic factor in a cohort of 166 patients followed at the National Institutes of Health (NIH) (Austin *et al.* 1994*a*). Hecht and colleagues (1976) have observed that the persistence of subendothelial deposits after a trial of immunosuppressive therapy, rather than their presence at study entry, identified patients most likely to experience a deterioration of renal function. This apparently reflects ongoing immune-mediated injury in this subset of patients because subendothelial deposits tend to resolve relatively quickly with effective immunosuppressive therapy (Pirani and Olesnicky 1982). Consequently, examination of follow-up kidney biopsy specimens for the presence and extent of subendothelial deposits may be particularly informative.

Fibrinoid necrosis

Karyorrhexis and fibrinoid necrosis (See Fig. 8.2) are indicative of a fulminant inflammatory process that disrupts the glomerular filtration surface and usually heals by scarring (Churg and Sobin 1982; Valeri *et al.* 1994; Akhtar *et al.* 1994). These kidney lesions have identified high-risk patients with lupus nephritis (Morel-Maroger *et al.* 1976; Bhuyan *et al.* 1982; Magil *et al.* 1988; McCurdy *et al.* 1992). Necrotizing lesions affecting 50% or more of glomeruli on a renal biopsy sample are particularly ominous. Of six patients in the NIH cohort with high-grade fibrinoid necrosis, three have manifested progressive deterioration of renal function within four years (Austin *et al.* 1994*a*). The occurrence of less extensive fibrinoid necrosis did not appear to influence prognosis significantly. In these cases, necrotizing lesions tended to affect one or two segments within a minority of the glomeruli sampled. Thus, if immunosuppressive therapy was effective, the destructive process and subsequent scarring appeared to be circumscribed.

Cellular crescents

These may rapidly develop, apparently as a result of gross haemorrhage from glomerular capillaries. The combination of blood clot, ingressing macrophages, and proliferating epithelial cells compresses the glomerular tuft and may obstruct the outflow of filtrate from Bowman's capsule (See Chapters 1–3). Crescent formation may thus cause extensive disruption of the glomerular architecture (Fig. 8.3) and an abrupt deterioration of renal function in many forms of glomerulonephritis (Levy *et al.* 1976; Counahan *et al.* 1977; Hind *et al.* 1983; Walker *et al.* 1985; Schmitt *et al.* 1990). In most conditions, rapidly progressive glomerulonephritis (RPGN) is associated with large cellular crescents encircling a majority of glomeruli. Extensive crescent formation is seen infrequently in patients with lupus nephritis (Cameron *et al.* 1979; McCluskey 1982; Ponticelli *et al.* 1987) and identifies patients at very high risk for catastrophic changes in renal function. Yeung and colleagues (1985) found that 16 of 27 lupus patients with acute deterioration of renal function had 50% or more of glomeruli affected by crescents. There were only 10 patients among 166 in the NIH cohort with 50% or more of glomeruli affected by cellular crescents (Austin *et al.* 1994*a*); they were significantly more likely than others to experience a doubling of serum creatinine despite intensive immunosuppressive therapy (Fig. 8.4). The probability of this adverse outcome approximated to 20% after 2 months and 50% after 30 months.

Other active and chronic pathological lesions

Although the impact of severe crescents is striking, the practical clinical utility of evaluating high-grade cellular crescents is limited by the small fraction of lupus patients that typically manifest this histological finding (Austin *et al.* 1994*a*; Bakir *et al.* 1994). Patients with severe lupus nephritis more often have cellular crescents that affect a minority of glomeruli (McCluskey 1982). Among 166 patients participating in prospective clinical trials of lupus nephritis at the NIH, 40% of biopsies had cellular crescents impinging on less than one-half of glomeruli (Austin *et al.* 1994*a*). These patients were at significantly increased risk of doubling serum creatinine when compared with those without cellular crescents. It is clear from Fig. 8.4 that the presence of a modest number of cellular crescents, considered alone, is a weak indicator of patients likely to experience a rapid deterioration of renal function. The predictive value of these histological lesions can be strengthened substantially by consideration of a combination of active and chronic, irreversible pathological features. Individual sclerosing and atrophic morphological attributes (glomerular sclerosis, tubular atrophy, and particularly, interstitial fibrosis) identify patients at increased risk for progressive renal dysfunction (Whiting-O'Keefe *et al.* 1982; Austin *et al.* 1984, 1994*a,b*; Banfi *et al.* 1985; Rush *et al.* 1986; Magil *et al.* 1988). Patients with a modest proportion of cellular crescents (< 50%) and moderate to severe interstitial fibrosis are at markedly increased risk for renal function deterioration (Fig. 8.5). For this subgroup of patients, the probability of doubling serum creatinine was approximately 20% at 12 months and 40% at 30 months. In short, the risk of renal insufficiency in patients with moderate acute and chronic histological lesions is comparable with the risk of renal function deterioration among patients with severe active lesions (i.e. >50% of glomeruli affected by cellular crescents).

Characteristics of patients with cellular crescents

Yeung and colleagues (1984) compared the clinical characteristics of lupus patients with extensive crescent formation (≥50% of glomeruli affected) with those with less severe histological change. Patients with large numbers of cellular

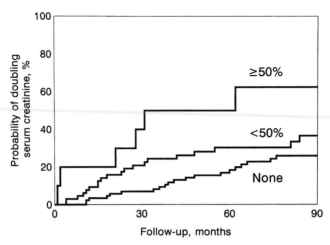

Fig. 8.4 Probability of doubling serum creatinine in 166 patients with lupus nephritis followed at the NIH with no cellular crescents (None), a modest number of cellular crescents (<50%), or extensive cellular crescents (≥50%).

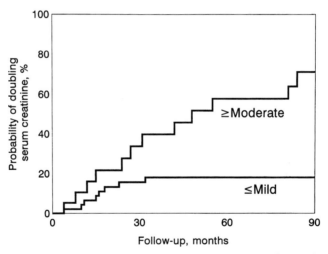

Fig. 8.5 Survival curves demonstrating the prognostic impact of a modest number of cellular crescents (<50%) plus moderate to severe interstitial fibrosis. High-risk patients had a modest number of cellular crescents and moderate to severe interstitial fibrosis (≥Moderate). Other patients had a modest number of cellular crescents and little or no interstitial fibrosis (≤Mild).

crescents were more likely than the others to manifest azotaemia and the nephrotic syndrome. Other clinical features, including hypertension and hypocomplementaemia, did not occur more frequently in the subset of patients with extensive crescents.

Clinical and laboratory features of patients seen at the NIH are shown in Figs 8.6 and 8.7; subgroups are defined according to the percentage of glomeruli manifesting cellular crescents. The presence of cellular crescents was associated with significantly increased values of serum creatinine and 24-hour urinary protein excretion, as well as significantly reduced values of haematocrit and serum albumin. Azotaemia, anaemia, and hypoalbuminaemia were particularly severe among patients with 50% or more of glomeruli manifesting cellular crescents.

Value of presenting clinical features in prediction of subsequent renal outcomes

There has been widespread interest in the predictive value of various clinical features of lupus nephritis (Appel *et al.* 1978, 1987; Kimberly *et al.* 1981*a*; Whiting-O'Keefe *et al.* 1982; Ginzler *et al.* 1982, 1993; Esdaile *et al.* 1989, 1991; Austin *et al.* 1994*b*). To illustrate this, azotaemia, anaemia, ethnic group, hypocomplementaemia, and hypertension have been associated with an increased risk of renal function deterioration among 166 patients followed at the NIH (Table 8.1). The first three clinical and demographic features emerged as particularly strong, independent predictors of progressive renal function deterioration (Austin *et al.* 1994*a*).

Azotaemia

Many investigators have reported that the initial serum creatinine is an important prognostic factor (Ginzler *et al.* 1982; Whiting O'Keefe *et al.* 1982; Magil *et al.*

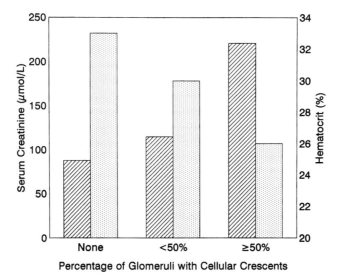

Fig. 8.6 Median values of serum creatinine (▨) and haematocrit (▨) in 166 patients with lupus nephritis in groups defined according to the number of glomeruli affected by cellular crescents.

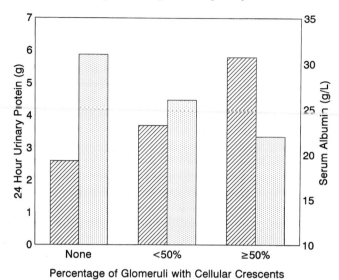

Fig. 8.7   Median values of 24-hour urine protein excretion (▨) and serum albumin (▦) in 166 patients with lupus nephritis in groups defined according to the number of glomeruli affected by cellular crescents.

Table 8.1   Predictive value of selected clinical and demographic features at study entry in 166 patients with lupus nephritis

	Probability (%) of doubling serum creatinine at:	
Variable	1 year	3 years
Serum creatinine (μmol/l)		
< 177 (2.0 mg/dl)	5	13
≥ 177	18	40
Haematocrit (%)		
≤ 26	25	45
> 26	2	12
Ethnic group		
Black	17	31
Others	3	13
C3 complement (g/l)		
≤ 0.8	9	23
> 0.8	2	9
Hypertension		
Absent	4	11
Present	9	21

1988; Esdaile *et al.* 1989, 1991; McCurdy *et al.* 1992; Levey *et al.* 1992; Austin *et al.* 1994 *a,b*). The predictive value of moderately severe azotaemia at study entry is demonstrated in Table 8.1. Among patients in the NIH cohort with a serum creatinine greater than or equal to 177 μmol/l (2.0 mg/dl), the probability of doubling serum creatinine was approximately 18% at one year and 40% at three years.

In patients with clinically active lupus nephritis, an elevated serum creatinine is probably indicative of severe, active glomerulonephritis or a combination of active and chronic histological changes. To ascertain the balance of active and chronic pathology, a kidney biopsy is frequently required. In some cases, detailed clinical information is available documenting the rate of change of renal function. For patients presenting with new-onset kidney disease, a nephritic urinary sediment, hypertension, and rapidly declining renal function, a kidney biopsy may be unnecessary (Kimberly *et al.* 1981*a*). Considering the intensity of the immunosuppressive therapy frequently recommended for patients with RPGN, it is essential that the presenting problem is defined as accurately as possible.

Anaemia

The prognostic impact of anaemia is illustrated in Table 8.1. For patients in the NIH studies with a haematocrit less than or equal to 26%, the probability of doubling serum creatinine was 25% at 12 months and 45% at 30 months.

It is interesting to note that anaemia has emerged as an important prognostic feature in several studies of lupus nephritis (Ginzler *et al.* 1982; McCurdy *et al.* 1992; Austin *et al.* 1994 *a,b*). Although anaemia is a secondary manifestation of renal insufficiency, it is also a feature of active SLE. In two large studies of prognostic factors in lupus nephritis, it was shown that anaemia was an independent predictor of renal function deterioration (Ginzler *et al.* 1982; Austin *et al.* 1994*b*). In each study, anaemia contributed prognostic information that enhanced predictions based on serum creatinine.

Ethnic group

Several investigators have observed that Black patients with lupus nephritis are at increased risk for adverse outcomes (Tejani *et al.* 1983; Austin *et al.* 1994*b*; Bakir *et al.* 1994). The risk of a progressive decline of renal function among Black patients participating in the NIH studies is shown in Table 8.1. The probability of doubling serum creatinine approximated to 17% at one year and 31% at three years. Of particular interest, ethnic group emerged as an independent predictor of renal function deterioration in a multivariate analysis that included other potentially important clinical and histological prognostic factors, including hypertension (Austin *et al.* 1994*a,b*).

Although it is difficult to identify patients at high risk for rapid deterioration of renal function employing individual clinical or histological features in isolation, it is evident from multivariate survival analysis, that evaluation of combinations of factors can enhance predictions of adverse outcome (Whiting-O'Keefe *et al.* 1982; Magil *et al.* 1988; Esdaile *et al.* 1989, 1991; Austin *et al.* 1994*a,b*). These considerations may be useful for physicians balancing the risks and potential benefits of intensive immunosuppressive therapy typically employed for patients with RPGN.

Treatment of severe lupus nephritis

Prospective randomized therapeutic trials of lupus nephritis have not focused on the treatment of crescentic glomerulonephritis or strictly defined RPGN. Two recently reported controlled clinical trials (Boumpas *et al.* 1992; Lewis *et al.* 1992) studied the treatment of patients with severe lupus nephritis identified according to many of the prognostic features described above.

There have been several reports describing a favourable short-term response to intravenous pulse methylprednisolone for patients with severe active lupus nephritis (Cathcart *et al.* 1976; Dosa *et al.* 1978; Fessel 1980; Miller 1980; Kimberly *et al.* 1981*b*; Isenberg *et al.* 1982; Ponticelli *et al.* 1982; Yeung *et al.* 1984; Ballou *et al.* 1985; Bertoni *et al.* 1994), but there is less experience employing this approach as a maintenance therapy to sustain long-term results (Liebling *et al.* 1982; Harisdangkul *et al.* 1989, Boumpas *et al.* 1992). The effectiveness and toxicity of daily high-dose oral prednisone and pulse intravenous methylprednisolone have not been rigorously compared in patients with lupus nephritis.

Immunosuppressive drug regimens that include cytotoxic drugs are more effective than prednisone alone in controlling clinical signs of active nephritis (Cameron *et al.* 1970; Steinberg *et al.* 1971; Fries *et al.* 1973; Steinberg and Decker 1974; Donadio *et al.* 1978; Dinant *et al.* 1982), in preventing renal scarring (Balow *et al.* 1984), and ultimately in reducing the risk of end-stage kidney disease (Austin *et al.* 1986; Steinberg and Steinberg 1991). Cyclophosphamide, given orally or intravenously, or in combination with azathioprine, was more efficacious than prednisone alone. Azathioprine showed only a tendency to be more effective than prednisone alone. Currently, some centres favour use of azathioprine as a maintenance therapy following initial treatment of lupus nephritis with cyclophosphamide (Cameron *et al.* 1979; Ponticelli and Banfi 1992; Donadio and Glassock 1993).

Among cytotoxic drug regimens, intermittent pulse cyclophosphamide appears to have one of the most favourable therapeutic indices (DeVita *et al.* 1991), particularly for patients with lupus nephritis at high risk for progressive renal function deterioration (Sessoms and Kovarsky 1984; Austin *et al.* 1986; McCune *et al.* 1988; Lehman *et al.* 1989; Boumpas *et al.* 1992; Eiser *et al.* 1993). Some consider that daily oral cyclophosphamide achieves more effective immunosuppression than intermittent pulse therapy; the option to use daily oral cyclophosphamide includes the recommendation to limit its use to two to three months, followed by maintenance with prednisone alone or with prednisone and azathioprine. Because our own studies (Austin *et al.* 1986) indicated that longer courses of daily cyclophosphamide were associated with increased frequencies of undesirable side-effects, we no longer use oral cyclophosphamide therapy for lupus nephritis.

A recent NIH study of severe lupus nephritis compared pulse intravenous methylprednisolone monthly for six months with two regimens of intermittent pulse cyclophosphamide. One regimen entailed monthly pulses of cyclophosphamide for six months; the second regimen included monthly pulses of cyclophosphamide for six months followed by quarterly pulses for two years. Each group received a standardized course of oral prednisone. Patients randomized to the extended course of pulse cyclophosphamide were less likely to experience a deterioration of renal function than those randomized to the six-month regimen of methylprednisolone (Fig. 8.8, upper panel); they were also less likely to experience a relapse of lupus activity than patients randomized to the six-month course of pulse cyclophosphamide (Fig. 8.8, lower panel) (Boumpas *et al.* 1992).

Of concern, an extended course of pulse cyclophosphamide may be associated with significant side-effects (Slavin *et al.* 1975; Klippel *et al.* 1990; DeVita *et al.* 1991; Fox and McCune 1994). The risk of amenorrhoea has been shown to be proportional to the number of doses of pulse cyclophosphamide and to the age of the patient under treatment (Boumpas *et al.* 1993). Haemorrhagic cystitis and bladder cancer are well-recognized risks of daily oral cyclophosphamide therapy (Plotz *et al.* 1979; Hoffman *et al.* 1992; Stillwell *et al.* 1988) and of the very high doses of pulse cyclophosphamide used in oncology practice (Pederson-Bjergaard *et al.* 1988; Devries and Freiha 1990). These lower urinary tract toxicities have not yet been observed in the doses of intravenous pulse cyclophosphamide used for treatment of lupus nephritis (Austin *et al.* 1986; McCune *et al.* 1988; Lehman *et al.* 1989; Boumpas *et al.* 1992; Valeri *et al.* 1994). Bladder complications appear to be minimized by inducing a vigorous diuresis, frequent voiding, and administration of oral or intravenous mesna (2-mercaptoethanesulphonate) to inactivate the main toxic metabolite, acrolein.

The risk of fatal opportunistic infections appears to be comparable for the various immunosuppressive regimens commonly employed for treatment of autoimmune diseases (Hellman *et al.* 1987; Bradley *et al.* 1989; Hoffman *et al.* 1989; Godeau *et al.* 1994). There are rare case reports of haematologic malignancies (Gibbons and Westerman 1988; Vasquez *et al.* 1993), as well as hepatic toxicities (Shaunak 1988; Synder 1993), and pulmonary toxicities (Sen *et al.* 1991; Queffeulou *et al.* 1994) after intravenous cyclophosphamide therapy.

There has been interest in the potential role of plasma exchange in the treatment of SLE. An important prospective controlled therapeutic trial found no advantage from the addition of plasma exchange to a regimen of prednisone and daily oral cyclophosphamide for the treatment of severe lupus nephritis (Wei *et al.* 1983; Lewis *et al.* 1992). Other investigators are evaluating the potential impact of synchronizing plasma exchange with pulse cyclophosphamide (Euler *et al.* 1994). Intravenous immunoglobulin (IV-Ig), in conjunction with plasma exchange (Euler *et al.* 1994), has been used in SLE and lupus nephritis; while IV-Ig has also been used alone for haematologic and other systemic aspects of SLE (Ballow and Parke 1989; Corvetta *et al.* 1989; Jordan 1989). The role of IV-Ig in the treatment of lupus nephritis is still considered experimental.

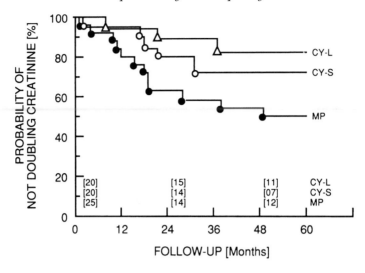

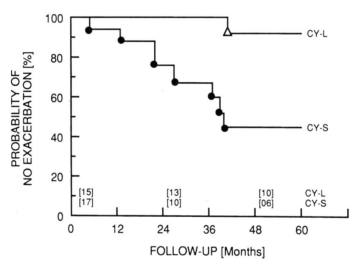

Fig. 8.8 *Upper panel*: cumulative probability of not doubling serum creatinine after treatment. MP, methylprednisolone; CY-S, short-course pulse cyclophosphamide; CY-L, long-course pulse cyclophosphamide. *Lower panel*: cumulative probabilities of no exacerbation on completion of monthly cycles in groups receiving short (CY-S) or long (CY-L) courses of pulse cyclophosphamide. (Figure reproduced with permission from Boumpas *et al.*, *Lancet*, 1992, **340**, 743.)

Cyclosporin A has received limited trials in lupus nephritis (Isenberg *et al.* 1981). Problems related to worsening hypertension and azotaemia have limited the usefulness of cyclosporin in SLE and lupus nephritis. Total lymphoid irradiation has also been studied in a small group of patients with severe lupus nephritis (Strober *et al.* 1988). To date, this approach has not been compared with other immunosuppressive regimens in a prospective study of human lupus nephritis.

Conclusion: unresolved issues and some future directions for research

There are many unanswered questions related to the pathogenesis and treatment of severe lupus nephritis. Because of the known propensity of lupus nephritis to undergo transitions from one stage to another, studies are needed to determine the benefit/risk ratio of early intervention in lupus nephritis. Experimental models provide evidence that early intervention is much more successful than later. However, given the known side-effects of currently available immunosuppressive therapies, it is mandatory to conduct prospective trials to assess directly benefit/risk in early lupus nephritis.

At the other extreme, the treatment of severe lupus nephritis, including rapidly progressive, crescentic disease, warrants continued study. In particular, the comparative benefits of pulse methylprednisolone, intermittent pulse cyclophosphamide, conventional daily cyclophosphamide, and plasma exchange (as has been suggested by Pusey *et al.* 1991 for the subset of patients with advanced microscopic polyarteritis and Wegener's granulomatosis) should be addressed in future prospective clinical trials.

The duration of therapy and use of long-term maintenance immunosuppression for lupus nephritis also warrant continued study. Based on a belief that SLE is an intrinsically episodic disease, some have argued that the courses of treatment of lupus nephritis should be limited to periods of exacerbation and recycled as often as indicated. Based on the concept that each exacerbation of lupus nephritis is associated with acquisition of chronic scarring and atrophy, others have favoured sustained, low-intensity maintenance therapy to reduce the risk of relapses. In the latter situation, some advocate quarterly pulse cyclophosphamide and others recommend conventional azathioprine; important prospective clinical trials comparing these two maintenance regimens are in progress (W.J. McCune, personal communication).

References

Akhtar, M., al-Dalaan, A., and el-Ramahi, K.M. (1994). Pauci immune necrotizing lupus nephritis: report of two cases. *American Journal of Kidney Diseases*, **23**, 320–5.

Appeal, G.B., Cohen, D.J., Pirani, C.L., Meltzer, J.I., and Este, D. (1987). Long-term follow-up of patients with lupus nephritis. A study based on the classification of the World Health Organization. *American Journal of Medicine*, **83**, 877–85.

Appel, G.B., Silva, F.G., Pirani, C.L., Meltzer, J.I., and Estes, D. (1978). Renal involvement in systemic lupus erythematosus (SLE): A study of 56 patients emphasizing histologic classification. *Medicine (Baltimore)*, **57**, 371–410.

Austin, H.A., Muenz, L.R., Joyce, K.M., Antonovych, T.T., and Balow, J.E. (1994). Diffuse proliferative lupus nephritis: Identification of specific pathologic features affecting renal outcome. *Kidney International*, **25**, 689–95.

Austin, H.A., Klippel, J.H., Balow, J.E., LeRiche, N.G.H., Steinberg, A.D., Plotz, P.H. *et al.* (1986). Therapy of lupus nephritis: Controlled trial of prednisone and cytotoxic drugs. *New England Journal of Medicine*, **314**, 614–19.

Austin, H.A., Boumpas, D.T., Vaughan, E.M., and Balow, J.E. (1994*a*). Importance of race and clinical and histological factors in 166 patients with lupus nephritis. *Journal of the American Society of Nephrology*, **5**, 346 (abstract).

Austin, H.A., Boumpas, D.T., Vaughan, E.M., and Balow, J.E. (1994*b*). Predicting renal outcomes in severe lupus nephritis: Contributions of clinical and histologic data. *Kidney International*, **45**, 544–50.

Bakir, A.A., Levy, P.S., and Dunea, G. (1994). The prognosis of lupus nephritis in African-Americans: A retrospective analysis. *American Journal of Kidney Diseases*, **24**, 159–71.

Baldwin, D.S., Lowenstein, J., Rothfield, N.F., Gallo, G., and McCluskey, R.T. (1970). The clinical course of the proliferative and membranous forms of lupus nephritis. *Annals of Internal Medicine*, **73**, 929–42.

Baldwin, D.S., Gluck, M.C., Lowenstein, J., and Gallo, G. (1977). Lupus nephritis: clinical course as related to morphologic forms and their transitions. *American Journal of Medicine*, **62**, 12–30.

Ballou, S.P., Khan, M.A., and Kushner, I. (1985). Intravenous pulse methylprednisolone followed by alternate day corticosteroid therapy in lupus erythematosus: a prospective evaluation. *Journal of Rheumatology*, **12**, 944–8.

Ballow, M. and Parke, A. (1989). The uses of intravenous immune globulin in collagen vascular disorders. *Journal of Allergy and Clinical Immunology*, **84**, 608–12.

Balow, J.E., Austin, H.A., Muenz, L.R., Joyce, K.M., Antonovych, T.T., Klippel, J.H., Steinberg, A.D. *et al.* (1984). Effects of treatment on the evolution of renal abnormalities in lupus nephritis. *New England Journal of Medicine*, **311**, 491–5.

Balow, J.E., Austin, H.A., Tsokos, G.C., Antonovych, T.T., Steinberg, A.D., and Klippel, J.H. (1987). Lupus nephritis. *Annals of Internal Medicine*, **106**, 79–94

Banfi, G., Mazzucco, G., Barbiano di Belgiojoso, G.B., Bosiso, M.B., Stratta, P., Confalonieri, R., *et al.* (1985). Morphological parameters in lupus nephritis: their relevance for classification and relationship with clinical and histological findings and outcome. *Quarterly Journal of Medicine*, **55**, 153–68.

Bertoni, M., Brugnolo, F., Bertoni, E., Salvadori, M., Romagnani, S., and Emmi, L. (1994). Long term efficacy of high-dose intravenous methylprednisolone pulses in active lupus nephritis. A 21-month prospective study. *Scandanavian Journal of Rheumatology*, **23**, 82–6.

Bhuyan, U.N., Malaviya, A.N., Dash, S.C., and Malhotra, K.K. (1982). Features of prognostic importance in the evaluation of lupus glomerulonephritis. *Indian Journal of Medical Research*, **76**, 618–27.

Boumpas, D.T., Austin, H.A., Vaughan, E.M., Klippel, J.H., Steinberg, A.D., Yarboro, C.H. *et al.* (1992). Controlled trial of pulse methylprednisone versus two regimens of pulse cyclophosphamide in severe lupus nephritis. *Lancet*, **340**, 741–5.

Boumpas, D.T., Austin, H.A., Vaughan, E.M., Yarboro, C.H., Klippel, J.H., and Balow, J.E. (1993). Risk for sustained amenorrhea in patients with systemic lupus erythematosus receiving intermittent pulse cyclophosphamide therapy. *Annals of Internal Medicine*, **119**, 366–9.

Bradley, J.D., Brandt, K.D., and Katz, B.P. (1989). Infectious complications of cyclophosphamide treatment for vasculitis. *Arthritis and Rheumatism*, **32**, 45–53.

Cameron, J.S. (1993). The long-term outcome of glomerular diseases. In *Diseases of the kidney*, 5th edn. (ed. R.W. Schrier and C.W. Gottschalk) pp. 1895–8. Little, Brown, Boston.

Cameron, J.S., Boulton-Jones, M., Robinson, R., and Ogg, C. (1970). Treatment of lupus nephritis with cyclophosphamide. *Lancet*, ii, 846–9.

Cameron, J.S., Turner, D.R., Ogg, C.S., Williams, D.G., Lessof, M.H., Chantler, C. *et al.* (1979). Systemic lupus with nephritis: A long-term study. *Quarterly Journal of Medicine*, **48**, 1–24.

Cathcart, E.S., Idelson, B.A., Scheinberg, M.A., and Couser, W.G. (1976). Benefical effects of methylprednisolone 'pulse' therapy in diffuse proliferative lupus nephritis. *Lancet*, i, 163–6.

Churg, J. and Sobin, L.H. (1982). Lupus nephritis. In *Renal disease*, pp. 127–49. Igaku-Shoin, Tokyo.

Corvetta, A., Della Bitta, R., Gabrielli, A., Spaeth, P.J., and Danieli, G. (1989). Use of high-dose intravenous immunoglobulin in systemic lupus erythematosus: report of three cases. *Clinical and Experimental Rheumatology*, **7**, 295–9.

Counahan, R., Winterborn, M.H., White, R.H.R., Heaton, J.M., Meadow, S.R., Bluett, N.H., *et al.* (1977). Prognosis of Henoch–Schönlein nephritis in children. *British Medical Journal*, **2**, 11–14.

Couser, W.G. (1990). Mediation of immune glomerular injury. *Journal of the American Society of Nephrology*, **1**, 13–29.

DeVita, S., Neri, R, and Bombardieri, S. (1991). Cyclophosphamide pulses in the treatment of rheumatic diseases: an update. *Clinical and Experimental Rheumatology*, **9**, 179–93.

Devries, C.R. and Freiha, F.S. (1990). Hemorrhagic cystitis: a review. *Journal of Urology*, **143**, 1–9.

Dinant, H.J., Decker, J.L., Klippel, J.H., Balow, J.E., Plotz, P.H., and Steinberg, A.D. (1982). Alternative modes of cyclophosphamide and azathioprine therapy in lupus nephritis. *Annals of Internal Medicine*, **96**, 728–36.

Donadio, J.V. and Glassock, R.J. (1993). Immunosuppressive drug therapy in lupus nephritis. *American Journal of Kidney Diseases*, **21**, 239–50.

Donadio, J.V., Holley, K.E., Ferguson, R.H., and Ilstrup, D.M. (1978). Treatment of diffuse proliferative lupus nephritis with prednisone and combined prednisone and cyclophosphamide. *New England Journal of Medicine*, **299**, 1151–5.

Dosa, S., Cairns, S.A., Lawler, W., Mallick, N.P., and Slotki, I.N. (1978). The treatment of lupus nephritis by methylprednisolone pulse therapy. *Postgraduate Medical Journal*, **54**, 682–32.

Eiser, A.R., Grishman, E., and Dreznin, S. (1993). Intravenous pulse cyclophosphamide in the treatment of type IV lupus nephritis. *Clinical Nephrology*, **40**, 155–9.

Esdaile, J.M., Levinton, C., Federgreen, W., Hayslett, J.P., and Kashgarian, M. (1989). The clinical and renal biopsy predictors of long-term outcome in lupus nephritis: A study of 87 patients and review of the literature. *Quarterly Journal of Medicine*, **72**, 779–833.

Esdaile, J.M., Federgreen, W., Quintal, H., Suissa, S., Hayslett, J.P., and Kashgarian, M. (1991). Predictors of one year outcome in lupus nephritis: The importance of renal biopsy. *Quarterly Journal of Medicine*, **81**, 907–18.

Euler, H.H., Schroeder, J.O., Harten, P., Zeuner, R.A., and Gutschmidt, H.J. (1994). Treatment-free remission in severe systemic lupus erythematosus following synchronization of plasmapheresis with subsequent pulse cyclophosphamide. *Arthritis and Rheumatism*, **37**, 1784–94.

Fessel, W.J. (1980). Megadose corticosteroid therapy in systemic lupus erythematosus. *Journal of Rheumatology*, **7**, 486–500.

Foster, M.H., Cizman, B., and Madaio, M.P. (1993). Nephritogenic autoantibodies in systemic lupus erythematosus: Immunochemical properties, mechanisms of immune deposition, and genetic origins. *Laboratory Investigation*, **69**, 494–507.

Fox, D.A. and McCune, W.J. (1994). Immunosuppressive drug therapy of systemic lupus erythematosus. *Rheumatic Disease Clinics of North America*, **20**, 265–99.

Fries, J.F., Sharp, G.C., McDevitt, H.O., and Holman, H.R. (1973). Cyclophosphamide therapy in systemic lupus erythematosus and polymyositis. *Arthritis and Rheumatism*, **16**, 154–62.

Gibbons, R.B. and Westerman, E. (1988). Acute nonlymphocytic leukemia following short-term, intermittent, intravenous cyclophosphamide treatment of lupus nephritis. *Arthritis and Rheumatism*, **31**, 1552–4.

Ginzler, E.M., Diamond, H.S., Weiner, M., Schlesinger, M., Fries, J.F., Wasner, C., Medsger, T.A., Jr. *et al.* (1982). A multicenter study of outcome in systemic erythematosus: I. Entry variables as predictors of prognosis. *Arthritis and Rheumatism*, **25**, 601–11.

Ginzler, E.M., Felson, D.T., Anthony, J.M., and Anderson, J.J. (1993). Hypertension increases the risk of renal deterioration in systemic lupus erythematosus. *Journal of Rheumatology*, **20**, 1694–700.

Godeau, B., Coutant-Perronne, V., Huong, D.L., Guillevin, L., Magadur, G., Bandt, M. *et al.* (1994). *Pneumocystis carinii* pneumonia in the course of connective tissue disease: report of 34 cases. *Journal of Rheumatology*, **21**, 246–51.

Grishman, E., Porush, J.G., Lee, S.L., and Churg, J. (1973). Renal biopsies in lupus nephritis. *Nephron*, **10**, 25–36.

Harisdangkul, V., Rockhold, L., and Myers, A. (1989). Lupus nephritis: Efficacy of monthly pulse therapy with intravenous methylprednisolone. *Southern Medical Journal*, **82**, 321–7.

Hecht, B., Siegel, N., Adler, M., Kashgarian, M., and Hayslett, J.P. (1976). Prognostic indices in lupus nephritis. *Medicine (Baltimore)*, **55**, 163–81.

Hellmann, D.B., Petri, M., and Whiting-O'Keefe, Q. (1987). Fatal infections in systemic lupus erythematosus: the role of opportunistic organisms. *Medicine (Baltimore)*, **66**, 341–8.

Hind, C.R.K., Paraskevakou, H., Lockwood, C.M., Evans, D.J., Peters, D.K., and Rees, A.J. (1983). Prognosis after immunosuppression of patients with crescentic nephritis requiring dialysis. *Lancet*, **i**, 263–5.

Hoffman, G.S., Leavitt, R.Y., and Fauci, A.S. (1989). Infectious complications of cyclophosphamide treatment for vasculitis. *Arthritis and Rheumatism*, **32**, 1626–7.

Hoffman, G.S., Kerr, G.S., Leavitt, R.Y., Hallahan, C.W., Lebovics, R.S., Travis, W.D. *et al.* (1992). Wegener granulomatosis: an analysis of 158 patients. *Annals of Internal Medicine*, **116**, 488–98.

Isenberg, D.A., Snaith, M.L., Morrow, J.W., Al-Khander, A.A., Cohen, S.L., Fisher, C. *et al.* (1981). Cyclosporin A for the treatment of systemic lupus erythematosus. *International Journal of Immunopharmacology*, **3**, 163–9.

Isenberg, D.A., Morrow, W.J., and Snaith, M.L. (1982). Methylprednisolone pulse therapy in the treatment of systemic lupus erythematosus. *Annals of Rheumatic Diseases*, **41**, 347–51.

Jordan, S.C. (1989). Intravenous gamma-globulin therapy in systemic lupus erythematosus and immune complex disease. *Clinical Immunology and Immunopathology*, **53**, S164–9.

Kashgarian, M. (1994). Lupus nephritis: lessons from the path lab. *Kidney International*, **45**, 928–38.

Kimberly, R.P., Lockshin, M.D., Sherman, R.L., Beary, J.F., Mouradian, J., and Cheigh, J.S. (1981*a*). 'End-stage' lupus nephritis: Clinical course to and outcome on dialysis. *Medicine (Baltimore)*, **60**, 277–87.

Kimberly, R.P., Lockshin, M.D., Sherman, R.L., McDougal, J.S., Inman, R.D., and Christian, C.L. (1981*b*). High-dose intravenous methylprednisolone pulse therapy in systemic lupus erythematosus. *American Journal of Medicine*, **70**, 817–24.

Kinjoh, K., Kyogoku, M., and Good, R.A. (1993). Genetic selection for crescent formation yields mouse strain with rapidly progressive glomerulonephritis and small vessel vasculitis. *Proceedings of the National Academy of Science USA*, **90**, 3413–17.

Klippel, J.H. (1990). Systemic lupus erythematosus: treatment-related complications super-imposed on chronic disease. *Journal of the American Medical Association*, **263**, 1812–15.

Laitman, R.S., Glicklich, D., Sablay, L.B., Grayzel, A.I., Barland, P., and Bank, N. (1989). Effect of long-term normalization of serum complement levels on the course of lupus nephritis. *American Journal of Medicine*, **87**, 132–8.

Lehman, T.J.A., Snerry, D.D., Wagner-Weiner, L., McCurdy, D.K., Emery, H.M. *et al.* (1989). Intermittent intravenous cyclophosphamide therapy for lupus nephritis. *Journal of Pediatrics*, **114**, 1055–60.

Levey, A.S., Lan, S-P., Corwin, H.L., Kasinath, B.S., Lachin, J., Neilson, E.G., Hunsicker, L.G., *et al.*, and The Lupus Nephritis Collaborative Study Group (1992). Progression and remission of renal disease in the Lupus Nephritis Collaborative Study. Results of treatment with prednisone and short-term oral cyclophosphamide. *Annals of Internal Medicine*, **116**, 114–23.

Levy, M., Broyer, M., Arsan, A., Levy-Bentolila, D., and Habib, R. (1976). Anaphylactoid purpura nephritis in childhood: Natural history and immunopathology. *Advances in Nephrology*, **6**, 183–228.

Lewis, E.J., Hunsicker, L.G., Lan, S.-P., Rohde, R.D., Lachin, J.M., and The Lupus Nephritis Collaborative Study Group (1992). A controlled trial of plasmapheresis therapy in severe lupus nephritis. *New England Journal of Medicine*, **326**, 1373–9.

Liebling, M.R., McLaughlin, K., Boonsue, S., Kasdin, J., and Barnett, E.V. (1982). Monthly pulses of methylprednisolone in SLE nephritis. *Journal of Rheumatology*, **9**, 543–8.

Magil, A.B., Puterman, M.L., Ballon, H.S., Chan, V., Lirenman, D.S., Rae, A., and Sutton, R.A.L. (1988). Prognostic factors in diffuse proliferative lupus glomerulonephritis. *Kidney International*, **34**, 511–17.

McCluskey, R.T. (1982). The value of the renal biopsy in lupus nephritis. *Arthritis and Rheumatism*, **25**, 867–75.

McCune, W.J., Golbus, J., Zeldes, W., Bohlke, P., Dunne, R., and Fox, D.A. (1988). Clinical and immunologic effects of monthly administration of intravenous cyclophosphamide in severe systemic lupus erythematosus. *New England Journal of Medicine*, **318**, 1423–31.

McCurdy, D.K., Lehman, T.J.A., Bernstein, B., Hanson, V., King, K.K., Nadorra, R. *et al.* (1992). Lupus nephritis: prognostic factors in children. *Pediatrics*, **89**, 240–6.

Miller, J.J. (1980). Prolonged use of large intravenous steroid pulses in the rheumatic diseases of children. *Pediatrics*, **65**, 989–94.

Morel-Maroger, L., Méry, J.P., Droz, D., Godin, M., Verroust, P., Kourilsky, O. *et al.* (1976). The course of lupus nephritis: Contribution of serial renal biopsies. *Advances in Nephrology*, **6**, 79–118.

Muehrcke, R.C., Kark, R.M., Pirani, C.L., and Pollak, V.E. (1957). Lupus nephritis: a clinical and pathologic study based on renal biopsies. *Medicine (Baltimore)*, **36**, 1–145.

Nossent, J.C., Bronsveld, W., and Swaak, A.J. (1989). Systemic lupus erythematosus: III. Observations on clinical renal involvement and follow up of renal function: Dutch experience with 110 patients studied prospectively. *Annals of Rheumatic Diseases*, **48**, 810–16.

Pedersen-Bjergaard, J., Ersboll, J., Hansen, V.L., Sorensen, B.L., Christoffersen, K., Hou-Jensen, K. *et al.* (1988). Carcinoma of the urinary bladder after treatment with cyclophosphamide for non-Hodgkin's lymphoma. *New England Journal of Medicine*, **318**, 1028–32.

Pirani, C.L. and Olesnicky, L. (1982). Role of electronmicroscopy in the classification of lupus nephritis. *Americal Journal of Kidney Diseases*, **2**, 150–63.

Pirani, C.L. and Salinas-Madrigal, L. (1968). Evaluation of percutaneous renal biopsy. *Pathology Annual*, **3**, 249–96.

Plotz, P.H., Klippel, J.H., Decker, J.L., Grauman, D., Wolff, B., Brown, B.C. *et al.* (1979). Bladder complications in patients receiving cyclophosphamide for systemic lupus erythematosus or rheumatoid arthritis. *Annals of Internal Medicine*, **91**, 221–3.

Pollak, V.E., Pirani, C.L., and Kark, R.M. (1961). Effect of large doses of prednisone on the renal lesions and life span of patients with lupus glomerulonephritis. *Journal of Laboratory and Clinical Medicine*, **57**, 495–511.

Pollak, V.E., Pirani, C.L., and Schwartz, F.D. (1964). The natural history of the renal manifestations of systemic lupus erythematosus. *Journal of Laboratory and Clinical Medicine*, **63**, 537–50.

Ponticelli, C. and Banfi, G. (1992). Systemic lupus erythematosus (clinical). In *Oxford textbook of clinical nephrology*, (ed. J.S. Cameron, A.M. Davison, J.P. Grunfeld, D. Kerr, and E. Ritz) pp. 646–67. Oxford University Press.

Ponticelli, C., Zueehclli, P., Banfi, G., Cagnoli, L., Scalia, P., Pasquali, S. *et al.* (1982). Treatment of diffuse proliferative lupus nephritis by intravenous high-dose methyl-predinsolone. *Quarterly Journal of Medicine*, **51**, 16–24.

Ponticelli, C., Zucchelli, P., Moroni, G., Cagnoli, L., Banfi, G., and Paquali, S. (1987). Long-term prognosis of diffuse lupus nephritis. *Clinical Nephrology*, **28**, 263–71.

Pusey, C.D., Rees, A.J., Evans, D., Peters, D.K., and Lockwood, C.M. (1991). Plasma exchange in focal necrotizing glomerulonephritis without anti-GBM antibodies. *Kidney International*, **40**, 757–63.

Queffeulou, G., Ducloux, D., Faucher, C., Carnot, F., Juvin, K., Israel Biet, D. *et al.* (1994). Fatal cyclophosphamide-induced interstitial pneumonitis in a renal trans-plant patient. *Nephrology Dialysis Transplantation*, **9**, 1655–7.

Rush, P.J., Baumal, R., Shore, A., Balfe, J.W., and Schreiber, M. (1986). Correlation of renal histology with outcome in children with lupus nephritis. *Kidney International*, **29**, 1066–71.

Schmitt, H., Bohle, A., Reineke, T., Mayer-Eichberger, D., and Vogt, W. (1990). Long-term prognosis of membranoproliferative glomerulonephritis type I. Significance of clinical and morphological parameters: An investigation of 220 cases. *Nephron*, **55**, 242–50.

Schwartz, R.S. and Stollar, B.D. (1985). Origins of anti-DNA antibodies. *Journal of Clinical Investigation*, **75**, 321–7.

Sen, R.P., Walsh, T.E., Fisher, W., and Brock, N. (1991). Pulmonary complications of combination therapy with cyclophosphamide and prednisone. *Chest*, **99**, 143–6.

Sessoms, S.L. and Kovarsky, J. (1984). Monthly intravenous cyclophosphamide in the treatment of severe systemic lupus erythematosus. *Clinical and Experimental Rheumatology*, **2**, 247–51.

Shaunak, S., Munro, J.M., Weinbren, K., Walport, M.J., and Cox, J.M. (1988). Cyclophosphamide-induced liver necrosis: a possible interaction with azathioprine. *Quarterly Journal of Medicine*, **252**, 309–17.

Sinniah, R. and Feng, P.H. (1976). Lupus nephritis: correlation between light, electron microscopic and immunofluorescent findings and renal function. *Clinical Nephrology*, **6**, 340–51.

Slavin, R.E., Millan, J.C., and Mullins, G.M. (1975). Pathology of high dose intermittent cyclophosphamide therapy. *Human Pathology*, **6**, 693–709.

Snyder, L.S., Heigh, R.I., and Anderson, M.L. (1993). Cyclophosphamide-induced hepatotoxicity in a patient with Wegener's granulomatosis. *Mayo Clinic Proceedings*, **68**, 1203–4.

Steinberg, A.D. and Decker, J.L. (1974). A double-blind controlled trial comparing cyclo-phosphamide, azathioprine and placebo in the treatment of lupus glomerulonephritis. *Arthritis and Rheumatism*, **17**, 923–37.

Steinberg, A.D. and Steinberg, S.C. (1991). Long-term preservation of renal function in patients with lupus nephritis receiving treatment that includes cyclophos-phamide versus those treated with prednisone only. *Arthritis and Rheumatism*, **34**, 945–50.

Steinberg, A.D., Kaltreider, H.B., Staples, P.J., Goetzl, E.J., Talal, N., and Decker, J.L. (1971). Cyclophosphamide in lupus nephritis: a controlled trial. *Annals of Internal Medicine*, **75**, 165–71.

Stillwell, T.J., Benson, R.C., DeRemee, R.A., McDonald, T.J., and Weiland, L.H. (1988). Cyclophosphamide-induced bladder toxicity in Wegener's granulomatosis. *Arthritis and Rheumatism*, **31**, 465–70.

Strober, S., Earinas, M.C., Field, E.H., Solovera, J.J., Kiberd, B.A., Myers, B.D. *et al.* (1988). Treatment of lupus nephritis with total lymphoid irradiation. *Arthritis and Rheumatism*, **31**, 850–8.

Tateno, S., Kobayashi, Y., Shigematsu, H., and Hiki, Y. (1983). Study of lupus nephri-tis: Its classification and the significance of subendothelial deposits. *Quarterly Journal of Medicine*, **52**, 311–31.

Tejani, A., Nicastri, A.D., Chen, C-K., Fikrig, S., and Gurumurthy, K. (1983). Lupus nephritis in Black and Hispanic children. *American Journal of Disease of Children*, **137**, 481–3.

Theofilopoulos, A.N. and Dixon, F.J. (1985). Murine models of systemic lupus erythe-matosus. *Advances in Immunology*, **37**, 269–390.

Valeri, A., Radhakrishnan, J., Estes, D., D'Agati, V., Kopelman, R., Pernis, A. *et al.* (1994). Intravenous pulse cyclosphosphamide treatment of severe lupus nephritis: a prospective five-year study. *Clinical Nephrology*, **42**, 71–8.

Vasquez, S., Kavanaugh, A.F., Schneider, N.R., Wacholtz, M.C., and Lipsky, P.E. (1993). Acute nonlymphocytic leukemia after treatment of systemic lupus erythematosus with immunosuppressive agents. *Journal of Rheumatology*, **19**, 1625–7.

Walker, R.G., Scheinkestel, C., Becker, G.J., Owen, J.E., Dowling, J.P., and Kincaid-Smith, P. (1985). Clinical and morphological aspects of the management of crescentic anti-glomerular basement membrane antibody (anti-GBM) nephritis/ Goodpasture's syndrome. *Quarterly Journal of Medicine*, **54**, 75–89.

Wallace, D.J., Podell, T.E., Weiner, J.M., Klinenberg, J.R., Forouzesh, S., and Dubois, E.L. (1982). Lupus nephritis. Experience with 230 patients in a private practice from 1950 to 1980. *American Journal of Medicine*, **72**, 209–20.

Wei, N., Klippel, J.H., Huston, D.P., Hall, R.P., Lawley, T.J., Balow, J.E. *et al.* (1983). Randomized trial of plasma exchange in mild systemic lupus erythematosus. *Lancet*, **1**, 17–22.

Whiting-O'Keefe, Q., Henke, J.E., Shearn, M.A., Hopper, J., Biava, C.G., and Epstein, W.V. (1982). The information content from renal biopsy in systemic lupus erythematosus: step-wise linear regression analysis. *Annals of Internal Medicine*, **96**, 718–23.

Yeung, C.K., Wong, K.L., Wong, W.S., Ng, M.T., Chan, K.W., and Ng, W.L. (1984). Crescentic lupus glomerulonephritis. *Clinical Nephrology*, **21**, 251–8.

Yeung, C.K., Ng, W.L., Wong, W.S., Wong, K.L., and Chan, M.K. (1985). Acute deterioration in renal function in systemic lupus erythematosus. *Quarterly Journal of Medicine*, **56**, 393–402.

9

Crescentic nephritis secondary to infection, systemic disease and other glomerulopathies

J. Stewart Cameron

Since crescents occur when breaks in glomerular capillaries allow leakage of cells and plasma proteins into Bowman's space (Chapter 1–3), it is not surprising that occasional crescents have been described in most chronic renal diseases, including some that do not primarily affect the glomerulus. Widespread crescent formation, however, requires active and specific attack on glomerular capillaries; predictably, this can occur in a variety of settings (Table 9.1). Today, crescentic nephritis is categorized using a variety of clinical, morphological, immunohistological, and serological criteria. None of the systems are entirely satisfactory; largely because crescent formation is the result of a disease, rather than a disease in itself.

As emphasized in previous chapters, three broad groups of crescentic nephritis can be distinguished:

(1) anti-glomerular basement membrane (GBM) disease characterized by circulating anti-GBM antibodies and linear deposition of antibody along the GBM;

(2) renal microscopic vasculitis characterized by scanty glomerular deposits of immunoglobulin and circulating antineutrophil cytoplasmic antibodies (ANCA) with or without clinical signs of systemic vasculitis; and

(3) a more heterogeneous group, often associated with obvious granular deposits of immunoglobulin, in which crescent formation complicates an identifiable form of nephritis, usually proliferative in type.

Contemporary opinion suggests that these three varieties account for virtually all cases of crescentic glomerulonephritis (Ferrario *et al.* 1994; Angangco *et al.* 1994), and this chapter deals with the third group of patients.

In adults, including the elderly (Potvliege *et al.* 1975; Montoliu *et al.* 1981; Kingswood *et al.* 1984), anti-glomerular basement membrane (GBM) disease accounts for 10–20% of patients with severe crescentic nephritis, whilst the remainder are divided equally between vasculitis and patients with granular immunoglobulin deposits (Whitworth *et al.* 1976; Stilmant *et al.* 1979; Neild *et al.* 1983; Velosa 1987). Far fewer children with crescentic nephritis have anti-GBM disease, and a greater proportion have granular immune deposits (Jardim *et al.*

Table 9.1 Crescentic glomerulonephritis with glomerular immune aggregates

Linear (see Chapter 5)
Anti-GBM nephritis
• 'idiopathic'
• in membranous nephropathy
• in Alport's syndrome and nail-patella syndrome
• following penicillamine
Granular
Postinfectious nephritis
• streptococcal infections
• bacterial endocarditis
• jugulo-atrial shunt infections
• miscellaneous infections
  – deep abscesses
  – *mycoplasma*
  – tuberculosis
  – *legionella*
  – HIV
  – syphilis
  – hepatitis C
  – leprosy
  – Ross river virus, etc.
Complicating systemic disorders
• systemic lupus erythematosus (SLE)
• Henoch–Schönlein purpura (HSP)
• mixed connective tissue disease
• sarcoidosis
• Behçet's syndrome
• cryoglobulinaemia (hepatitis C infection)
• dermatomyositis
• rheumatoid arthritis and juvenile rheumatoid arthritis
• rheumatic fever
• Reiter's syndrome
• Sjögren's syndrome
Complicating underlying glomerulopathies
• endocapillary/mesangial proliferative glomerulonephritis
• mesangiocapillary glomerulonephritis
• IgA nephropathy
• membranous nephropathy
• Alport's syndrome
Following medicines
• penicillamine
• hydralazine
• rifampicin
• enalapril
• interleukin-2
• interferon-α
• phenylbutazone, etc.

Table 9.1   *(Continued)*

Miscellaneous
- malignant tumours
- lymphomas and leukaemias
- silicosis
- Russell viper bite
- chronic pancreatitis
- α-1-antitrypsin deficiency

Following transplantation
- recurrence (IgA, MCGN, crescentic, anti-GBM, HSP, lupus)
- *de novo*
- anti-GBM disease in Alport's

1992; Srivastava *et al.* 1992). The proportion of cases also varies at different geographical locations; in the developing world, almost certainly, crescentic nephritis is more common than in the Northern hemisphere (Zent *et al.* 1994), the extra cases mainly being forms of nephritis associated with environmental infective factors, such as ambient bacterial and possibly parasitic infections, and showing granular immune aggregates in the glomerular tuft.

Crescentic glomerulonephritis with granular glomerular immune deposits (Table 9.1)

This third group of patients with crescentic nephritis is much more heterogeneous than anti-GBM disease or vasculitis. These patients have in almost all instances obvious granular deposits of immunoglobulins in the mesangium, the capillary wall, or both. Most have identifiable forms of proliferative nephritis, sometimes against a background of infection or other systemic disease, and fall into one of three broad groups those with: (1) infections; (2) systemic immune complex disease; and (3) crescents complicating pre-existing nephritis. There are also a small number of patients who appear to have a variety of other associated conditions.

Systemic infections

These have long been associated with glomerulonephritis, sometimes with crescentic change. This remains a problem even in contemporary urban society (see review by Montseny *et al.* 1995).

Poststreptococcal nephritis

The association between streptococcal infections and nephritis was one of the cornerstones in the formation of the concept of an immunological origin for nephritis (Tresor *et al.* 1969), and although poststreptococcal nephritis has become rather rare in developed countries, in the rest of the world it remains common. The prognosis is excellent for the vast majority of patients with post-streptococcal nephritis (Cameron 1993), but occasional patients have a rapidly progressive clinical course. Typically, these patients present with severe crescentic nephritis from the outset (Löhlein 1907; Jennings and Earle 1961; McCluskey and Baldwin 1965; Lewy *et al.* 1977; Roy *et al.* 1981; Chugh *et al.* 1981; Niaudet and Lévy 1983; Southwest Pediatric Nephrology Study Group, SPNSG 1985) and form perhaps 5% of most series of poststreptococcal nephritis. In addition, occasional patients with poststreptococcal disease develop vasculitis (Ingelfinger *et al.* 1977; Chugh *et al.* 1981) and at least six cases have been described in which typical diffuse endocapillary proliferative nephritis evolved into severe crescentic disease over periods from 10 days to 5 weeks (Morel-Maroger *et al.* 1974; Gill *et al.* 1977; Ferraris *et al.* 1983; Old *et al.* 1984; Modai *et al.* 1985; Fairley *et al.* 1987). One of these patients also developed anti-tubular basement membrane antibodies (Morel-Maroger *et al.* 1974).

Renal biopsies in poststreptococcal crescentic nephritis usually show severe endocapillary infiltration and proliferation, with immune aggregates of C3 and sometimes IgG distributed in a coarse, punctate, but diffuse distribution. These large immune aggregates correspond to the appearance of extracapillary 'humps' on electron microscopy.

Because of the small numbers involved, the *natural history* of crescentic post-streptococcal nephritis is much less clearly documented than that of either anti-GBM disease or renal microscopic polyangiitis. There were strong suggestions from early series that complete recovery and resolution of crescents occurred in some patients given supportive treatment only, possibly as many as 50% (Nakamoto *et al.* 1965; Leonard *et al.* 1970; Anand *et al.* 1975; Whitworth *et al.* 1976). Even so, the mortality was high but it is unclear whether this would have been reduced with modern supportive treatment. More recent studies have confirmed that severely affected patients can recover renal function spont-aneously (Niaudet and Lévy 1983; SPNSG 1985; Roy *et al.* 1981).

Similarly, in Lewy *et al.*'s (1977) study, of 46 children with sporadic post-streptococcal glomerulonephritis, only 4 patients died, all showing extensive crescent formation in their biopsies. Two children still showed proteinuria after 5 years' follow-up, one of whom had crescents in his initial biopsy; only 3 patients were lost to follow-up. The presence of subepithelial 'humps' on electron micro-scopy, or obvious immune deposits on immunohistology, also appears to carry a better prognosis (Hinglais *et al.* 1974; Sonsino *et al.* 1976; Neild *et al.* 1983). Postinfectious nephritis, even when crescents are present, has a reputation of being more benign than comparable idiopathic disease; the apparently good prog-nosis in poststreptococcal nephritis is, however, the result—at least in part—of the inclusion in published data of patients with relatively minor degrees of crescent formation. In Heaf *et al.*'s (1983) analysis, only 51% of patients in the infection-related group had more than 80% of glomeruli affected by crescents, compared with 69% in the anti-GBM group and 65% in the 'idiopathic' group. It must be emphasized again that the prognosis for recovery only becomes less than evens when the number of glomeruli affected by occluding crescents reaches or exceeds 60%. The literature on poststreptococcal crescentic nephritis is particularly poor in its definitions of 'extensive crescent formation'. Thus, the prognosis for postinfectious nephritis with true extensive crescent formation may not be as benign as supposed in the past.

Many, but not all, of these patients have received corticosteroids, or other forms of immunosuppressive therapy. Even so, substantial recovery has occurred spontaneously in some children with severe renal failure and over 80% crescents. In fact, Roy *et al.* (1981) could demonstrate no difference in outcome, irrespective of whether patients were given supportive measures, or were treated with a 'quintuple' immunosuppressive regimen. Similar spontaneous recoveries have been reported by the SPNSG (1985). Follow-up biopsies from these patients showed various combinations of normal, partially, or completely sclerosed glomeruli and some fibrosed crescents. Nevertheless, the proportion of intact and largely intact glomeruli suggested that many of the crescents had resolved completely (Roy *et al.* 1981). This accords with previous observations on children with poststreptococcal nephritis (Faarup *et al.* 1978; McCluskey and Baldwin 1963).

Small numbers of patients develop progressive deterioration of renal function many months after the initial recovery (Niaudet and Lévy 1983; Roy *et al.* 1981). Repeat biopsies in these patients show glomerular and interstitial scarring, presumptively related to the severity of the original injury.

It is not certain whether the relatively good prognosis in children with poststreptococcal nephritis can be extrapolated to the much rarer adults' syndrome or the patients in whom acute endocapillary nephritis evolves to crescentic glomerulonephritis over a period of weeks (Morel-Maroger *et al.* 1974; Gill *et al.* 1977; Ferraris *et al.* 1983; Old *et al.* 1984; Modai *et al* 1985; Fairley *et al.* 1987). Certainly these patients have been reported to improve immediately after the introduction of immunosuppressive therapy, but too few have been reported to know what the natural history would have been if they had been left untreated. It would be interesting to know whether the endocapillary injury and the crescentic phase have the same pathogenesis, or alternatively whether the original glomerular injury provokes a second, presumably autoimmune, phase as appeared to be the case in the patient described by Morel-Maroger *et al.* (1974) who developed anti-tubular basement membrane antibodies.

Given the present uncertainties it seems reasonable to control the streptococcal infection first, and then give a brief course of high-dose oral corticosteroids or methylprednisolone to patients presenting with severe crescentic poststreptococcal nephritis, and to reserve full immunosuppressive regimens for those patients whose crescentic disease evolves more slowly towards renal failure. There are no data to support or deny value for plasma exchange.

Infective endocarditis

Typically, infective endocarditis is associated with a focal or a diffuse proliferative nephritis (Gutman *et al.* 1972; Neugarten *et al.* 1984; Eknoyan 1985) which usually manifests itself as proteinuria and haematuria, although occasional patients may develop a full nephrotic syndrome. The epidemiology of this condition has changed dramatically in recent years in many centres, cases associated with drug abuse and *Staphylococcus aureus* replacing those associated with dental extractions and *Streptococcus viridans*. The role of antiglobulins in the pathogenesis of the nephritis has been much debated, and many patients show cryoglobulinaemia. Hypocomplementaemia is common, and continued low levels of C3 may be associated with progressive renal failure (Neugarten *et al.* 1984). Griffin *et al.* (1989) reported a patient who developed pulmonary haemorrhage, mimicking anti-GBM disease, in association with *Mycoplasma pneumoniae* pneumonia and endocarditis. The renal biopsy, however, did not show crescents.

Rarely endocarditis may be associated with severe renal failure, but even in this situation there are usually few or no crescents (Boulton-Jones *et al.* 1974; Beaufils *et al.* 1976; Eknoyan 1985), although 13/22 had some epithelial proliferation in the series of Neugarten *et al.* (1984). However, exceptional patients develop severe crescentic nephritis requiring dialysis (Beaufils *et al.* 1976; Neugarten *et al.* 1984; Rovzar *et al.* 1986).

So far as *treatment* of crescentic nephritis complicating endocarditis is concerned, the situation is very similar to that found in poststreptococcal disease. Control of infection is paramount, and may necessitate early valve replacement as well as antimicrobial agents. There is insufficient evidence to be dogmatic about the role of immunosuppressive drugs. The three patients with crescentic disease who were included in the review by Neugarten *et al.* (1984) all developed renal failure. Rovzar *et al.* (1986) treated a patient with immunosuppressive drugs and plasma exchange with apparent benefit. This seems a reasonable approach to the most severely affected patients, following control of sepsis.

Infected jugulo-atrial shunts

Renal biopsies from patients with shunt nephritis usually show a pattern of mesangiocapillary glomerulonephritis, often with prominent deposition of IgM, but occasionally this is complicated by severe crescentic disease (SPNSG 1985; Niaudet and Lévy 1983; Wakabayashi *et al.* 1985). There is usually severe persistent hypocomplementaemia, and removal of the infected shunt and its replacement with a peritoneal shunt is almost always necessary. There are no data on the use of immunosuppressive agents, and probably these are unecessary, since dramatic recoveries of function may be seen with control of infection. Wakabayashi *et al.* (1985) summarize published data on serial biopsies, including their own case of crescentic nephritis affecting 15/18 glomeruli, in which dramatic histological recovery took place with antimicrobials and shunt removal only.

Visceral abcesses

Crescentic nephritis has been reported in patients with deep-seated infections other than endocarditis (Whitworth *et al.* 1976; Beaufils *et al.* 1976; Connelly and Gallacher 1987), but it is difficult to know whether infections were responsible for the nephritis, or whether they merely exacerbated it non-specifically as described by Rees *et al.* (1977). Four of the eight patients described by Beaufils *et al.* (1976) had pure extracapillary proliferation, three had membranoproliferative glomerulonephritis, and one focal proliferative nephritis. In retrospect, it seems likely that three of the patients may have had Wegener's granulomatosis (three had pulmonary abscesses and another sinusitis) which can also be exacerbated by intercurrent infection (Rees *et al.* 1977) (see Chapter 2).

Again, whether immunosuppressive treatment has anything to offer over clearance and control of the infection is doubtful.

Other infections

A long list of infections have been reported as associated with glomerulonephritis (Davison 1992; Montseng *et al.* 1995) but in general the nephritis is mild, or if diffuse and severe, is of endocapillary type. However, crescentic nephritis has been reported during the course of a number of other viral and bacterial infections, usually with immune aggregates visible on electron microscopy or immunohistology within the glomerulus. These include Ross River Virus (Davies *et al.* 1982), *Legionella* (Wegmuller *et al.* 1985), syphilis (Walker *et al.* 1984), *Mycoplasma* (Campbell *et al.* 1991), and leprosy (Singhal *et al.* 1977; Nigham *et al.* 1986. A number of these patients were treated with immunosuppression as well as antibiotics, with variable results. Crescentic nephritis has also been attributed to rifampicin during treatment for tuberculosis (Hirsch *et al.* 1983; Murray *et al.* 1987), and to the tuberculosis itself (Sopeña *et al.* 1991). This patient was treated with immunosuppression as well as antituberculous therapy, and dialysis could be discontinued.

HIV infection

HIV has been associated with a variety of renal complications (Bourgognie 1990; Glassock 1990), but it is often difficult to evaluate the role of the virus itself separately from superadded infections or medicaments. Glomerular disease, when present, has usually been of a focal sclerosing pattern, often of the 'collapsing' variety, but IgA-associated crescentic nephritis has been described (Jindal *et al.* 1991).

Systemic immune diseases

Systemic lupus erythematosus (SLE) (see Chapter 8)

Generally, some crescents are found in patients with underlying class IV nephropathy with extensive glomerular proliferation, but cases of almost pure membranous nephropathy later complicated by extensive crescents are well recognized (Williams *et al.* 1985). Small numbers of segmental crescents are found in biopsies from many patients with focal proliferative nephritis, but it is those with underlying class IV diffuse proliferative glomerulonephritis, often referred to as WHO class IV (b), who tend to have a larger proportion of glomeruli affected. Usually these are segmental, and only rarely are a substantial proportion of glomeruli (>60%) affected. This type of lupus nephritis has been described in detail by Yeung *et al.* (1984) in 10 patients, and also by Leaker *et al.* (1987) in 18 out of 135 patients.

Surprisingly few other observers, amongst the many papers on the histological features of lupus nephritis, have addressed the question of how frequent extensive crescent formation is, and whether the presence of crescents affects prognosis. Banfi *et al.* (1985) noted 6 of 147 patients with more than 60% glomeruli affected by crescents, three of whom entered renal failure and one of whom died from extra-renal lupus. Survival in Leaker's 18 cases was better, but still poorer than in the case of class IV patients in general; 74% were still alive with renal function at 5 years, but only 47% at 10 years. In Magil's (1988) proportional hazards analysis, crescents conferred a 4.6-fold risk (95% confidence limits 1.29–14.70) of renal failure, but in a study group of only 45 patients.

There is no information on the treatment of this specific subgroup, patients receiving in general identical treatment to those with severe lupus nephritis but without extensive crescents.

Henoch–Schönlein purpura (HSP)

Moderate numbers of crescents are commonly found in renal biopsies from many patients with HSP, and the implications they have for prognosis are discussed by Haycock (1992). These crescents are often minor and segmental, and in contrast to most forms of crescentic nephritis, in which the extent of the glomerular involvement and the proportion of glomeruli are roughly proportional (Morel-Maroger 1976), in HSP there may be a high proportion of glomeruli affected by minor crescents. Prognosis, as expected, worsens the greater the numbers of glomeruli affected by large crescents, but not to a major extent until more than 50% of glomeruli are involved.

Conversely, small numbers of patients with HSP nephritis are included in most large paediatric series of patients with crescentic nephritis, especially in children and adolescents (Niaudet and Lévy 1983; Neild *et al.* 1983; SPNSG 1985, and see Chapter 10). The clinical picture and poorer prognosis of the very small number of adult patients with HSP and crescentic nephritis is similar to that in children.

The treatment of these patients has been discussed by Haycock and Cameron (1991). The usual combination of immunosuppression and plasma exchange appears to be effective on an anecdotal basis, but it must be emphasized that there is no evidence that this regimen influences the outcome of the underlying glomerular changes; it is the crescents for which the treatment is being given, and in only a tiny minority of patients will this be necessary, even in referral centres. Öner *et al.* (1993) reported excellent results in all but one of 10 children with more than 60% of glomeruli affected by crescents using intravenous methylprednisolone and cytotoxic agents, but without the use of plasma exchange.

Monoclonal gammopathies

Monoclonal synthesis of immunoglobulins can cause renal disease in a variety of ways. *Mixed 'essential' cryoglobulinaemia* is now generally recognized to be a manifestation of hepatitis C infection (D'Amico 1993), and is usually associated with a form of mesangiocapillary glomerulonephritis. Occasionally, however, it may be associated with severe crescentic disease (Weber *et al.* 1985). More recently, it has been appreciated that monoclonal gammopathies without these special properties can also be associated with crescentic nephritis. Some of these patients have had *myeloma* (Kaplan and Kaplan 1970; Dhar *et al.* 1977; Lapenas *et al.* 1983; Meyrier *et al.* 1984; Kebler *et al.* 1985; Cadnapaphornchai and Sillix 1989), whereas others have had *Waldenstrom's macroglobulinaemia* (Meyrier *et al.* 1984; Ogami *et al.* 1989). *Light chain nephropathy* may occasionally be complicated by 10–15% of glomeruli affected by crescents (Confalonieri *et al.* 1988), but true extensive crescent formation seems not to have been described. Possibly related, are the patients with *familial Mediterranean fever* (Said *et al.* 1989) and *amyloidosis* who have developed crescentic nephritis (Panner 1980; Harada *et al.* 1984; Vernier *et al.* 1987). There are almost no data on which to base statements as to how the rare patients with cryglobulinaemia and crescentic nephritis should be treated. Weber *et al.*'s case died in renal failure despite treatment with immunosuppression and plasma exchange.

Other systemic immune diseases

Polymyositis Two patients, one a child, have been reported from Japan in whom polymyositis was associated with crescentic glomerulonephritis (Kamata *et al.* 1982; Tsunemi *et al.* 1993). Immunosuppressive treatment was given, but it is difficult to see what effect it may have had.

Behçet's syndrome Glomerulonephritis of any type is very rare as a component of Behcet's syndrome, but urinary abnormalities have been frequently reported (Rosenthal *et al.* 1978). However, cases of crescentic nephritis have been noted from time to time (Olsson *et al.* 1988; Landwehr *et al.* 1980). Tietjen and Moore (1990) reported a patient with Behçet's syndrome and reviewed another eight cases from the literature; patients with up to 100% glomerular involvement with crescents have been reported. In 6/9 patients there were immune aggregates within the glomeruli, but 3 were negative for all reactants. All but two patients were treated with immunosuppression; 7 were judged to have improved, although most remained in renal failure with nephrotic range proteinuria.

Rheumatoid arthritis Rheumatoid vasculitis is not normally associated with glomerulonephritis, but a handful of patients has been described in whom diffuse crescentic nephritis was noted (Breedveld *et al.* 1985). On immunohistology, there was coarse deposition of all the usual immune reactants, except C4, along the capillary walls. Methylprednisolone and oral immunosuppression was given with good results and resolution of the nephrotic syndrome. In another case, recurrent pulmonary haemorrhage was a prominent feature (Naschitz *et al.* 1989). One case of crescentic nephritis associated with juvenile rheumatoid arthritis (Still's disease) has been reported (Becker *et al.* 1995). More recently, Harper *et al.* (1997) described 10 patients with rheumatoid arthritis and focal segmental necrotizing glomerulonephritis, nine of whom had crescents.

Sarcoidosis   Glomerular involvement in sarcoidosis is rare, and when it does occur the pattern is usually one of membranous nephropathy (Kenouch and Méry 1992). However, other patterns have been described, including a few patients with crescentic nephritis (Taylor *et al.* 1979; Vanhille *et al.* 1986).

Relapsing polychondritis   This is discussed in Chapter 7, together with vasculitis, and will not be considered here.

Rheumatic fever   Glomerulonephritis of any type is extremely rare in association with rheumatic fever, but a single case report of a patient who developed crescentic nephritis in this setting is available (Mustonen *et al.* 1983).

Mixed connective tissue disease   Usually the kidney is not involved in mixed connective tissue disease, but cases of nephritis are seen, usually with membranous or mesangial patterns, but including some with crescent formation (Kitridou *et al.* 1986).

Sjögren's syndrome   Although the glomeruli are usually spared in this condition, a case in whom crescentic nephritis was present has been described (Dussol *et al.* 1994).

Reiter's syndrome   A single patient with Reiter's syndrome, together with keratoderma blenorrhagica, developed in addition a crescentic nephritis with strong mesangial deposits of IgA (Inglis *et al.* 1994).

Chronic glomerulonephritis

IgA-associated nephropathy

Biopsies taken from patients with mesangial IgA disease frequently contain small numbers of crescents (or glomeruli with extracapillary proliferation), especially when macroscopic haematuria is present. Severe nephritis has been described regularly in series selected because they had IgA disease (Nicholls *et al.* 1984; Boyce *et al.* 1986; Lai *et al.* 1987) including papers dealing specifically with crescentic IgA disease (Abuelo *et al.* 1984; D'Amico *et al.* 1981; Welch *et al.* 1988). They have also been reported in series of patients selected because of crescentic nephritis (Whitworth *et al.* 1976; Morrin *et al.* 1978; Neild *et al.* 1983; Niaudet and Lévy 1983); a small number of patients with underlying IgA nephropathy are described.

In the large single-centre series of D'Amico *et al.* (1985), 116 of 374 patients (31%) showed at least one crescent in their renal biopsy, usually segmental. In 65 of this 116, fewer than 10% of glomeruli were involved. Only 9 patients showed between 31% and 62% affected glomeruli, and another 9 had between 21% and 30%. In the large childhood series (<15 years of age) described by Lévy *et al.* (1985) of 91 children, 20 (22%) had crescents. Only 4 children had large circumferential crescents affecting most glomeruli.

Abe and colleagues (1986) examined the apparent effect on prognosis of the presence of crescents in their adult patients. Of 205 patients, 92 had no crescents, 54 less than 25%, 34 25–50%, and 25 more than 50% of glomeruli affected. Twenty-six patients developed end-stage renal failure, 17 in the group with more than 50% glomeruli affected, and 6 of those with 25–50%; no patient without crescents developed terminal renal failure within the mean follow-up of 7.9 years.

In most patients with IgA nephropathy, the crescents are already found at first biopsy. However, Martini *et al.* (1981) described a 13-year-old boy who developed severe crescentic nephritis within a month of initial biopsy showing only mesangial lesions.

There are no good data on how these rather rare patients with IgA nephropathy and extensive crescent formation should be treated, but most clinicians in both adult and paediatric medicine have thought it useful to use the types of treatment apparently successful in other forms of crescentic nephritis. Hené *et al.* (1982) treated one patient with plasma exchange and corticosteroids, as did Coppo *et al.* (1985) in three patients, and Boobes *et al.* (1990) a further patient. Isaacs *et al.* (1990) treated one patient post-partum with disease during pregnancy. Nicholls *et al.* (1990) described the use of plasma exchange in rapidly progressive IgA nephropathy. All these authors felt that their patients had benefited from this intervention, but it is not possible to analyse which component of multiple therapy may have been important.

Mesangiocapillary glomerulonephritis (MCGN)

Between 10% and 15% of patients with mesangiocapillary or membranoproliferative nephritis have crescents on renal biopsies and they can affect large numbers of glomeruli in a small proportion of patients (McCoy *et al.* 1975; Davis *et al.* 1979; Chapman *et al.* 1980; Cameron 1983; Neild *et al.* 1983; Niaudet and Lévy 1983; SPNSG 1985; Korzets and Bernheim 1987). This is now almost universally regarded as having a bad prognosis; when Barbiano di Belgiojoso *et al.* (1977) first suggested that the presence of crescents was an adverse feature, we (Cameron *et al.* 1983) and the Parisian study (Habib 1983) confirmed this. Schmitt *et al.* (1990) performed a more elaborate analysis of the glomerular histology, with five grades, the last of which included crescent formation; these patients did worst of all.

The general consensus has been that, in adults at least, no treatment favourably affects the underlying glomerular changes in MCGN. Therefore, any strategy of treatment in crescentic nephritis is aimed principally or entirely at the crescents themselves, and one would expect progression of the glomerular changes after perhaps temporary improvement of crescent formation. In children, favourable effects have been claimed for alternate-day high-dose corticosteroid treatment (McEnery *et al.* 1985), and also 'cocktail' treatment employing combined immunosuppression and anticoagulation (Chapman *et al.* 1980). However, none of nine patients reported by Niaudet and Lévy (1983) recovered despite treatment with various combinations of steroids, alkylating agents, anticoagulants, and plasma exchange. Four of the six patients reported by Neild *et al.* (1983) had improved renal function after treatment with 'quadruple therapy' with steroids, azathioprine, anticoagulants, and dipyramidole. Even so, all but one went into renal failure later (Cameron, unpublished observations). A few patients have been subjected to plasma exchange but the results are not clear. Patients with severe crescentic MCGN of either type show a striking tendency to recurrence in allografts (Eddy *et al.* 1984) (see below).

Membranous nephropathy

At least 13 patients have been described with membranous nephropathy which was complicated by crescentic nephritis late in the course of the disease (Klassen *et al.* 1974; Nicholson *et al.*. 1975; Moorthy *et al.* 1976; Hill *et al.* 1978; Taylor *et al.* 1979; Tateno *et al.* 1981; Mitas *et al.* 1983; Kurki *et al.*1984; Koethe *et al.* 1986; Abreo *et al.* 1986; Nguyen *et al.* 1988; Kwan *et al.* 1991). Interestingly, three of the patients also had anti-GBM antibodies. One patient, without anti-GBM antibodies, developed recurrent crescentic nephritis in a renal transplant. (Hill *et al.* 1978). None of these 13 cases recovered renal function, irrespective of the presence of anti-GBM antibodies, and despite the use of immunosuppressive treatment regimens.

Alport's syndrome

Harris *et al.* (1978) reported a patient with Alport's syndrome who developed crescentic nephritis, together with some details of a relative who had behaved similarly. These patients are of great interest because of the dozen or more cases (reviewed in Cameron 1992 and below) of anti-GBM crescentic nephritis developing in normal kidneys transplanted into recipients with Alport's syndrome. There is also a report of a patient with the nail-patella syndrome who developed anti-GBM crescentic nephritis (Curtis *et al.* 1976).

Hypersensitivity to drugs

Many drugs may cause vasculitis, and in a small proportion of these crescentic nephritis may be present as part of the drug-induced syndrome. These drug-induced vasculitides are discussed in Chapter 7, whereas here, only the relatively rare crescentic nephritides without vasculitis are considered.

Penicillamine

This drug is a common cause of nephrotoxicity and is the only drug to have been shown unequivocally to cause crescentic nephritis. A related drug, bucillamine has also been reported as causing crescentic nephritis (Yoshida *et al.* 1992). Penicillamine has been associated with crescentic nephritis in patients in whom it has been used to treat rheumatoid arthritis (Banfi *et al.* 1983; Gibson *et al.* 1976; Gavaghan *et al.* 1981; Swainson *et al.* 1982; Devogelaer *et al.* 1987; Peces *et al.* 1987; Sadjadi *et al.* 1985; Macarron *et al.* 1992), primary biliary cirrhosis (Matloff and Kaplan 1980) and systemic sclerosis (Ntoso *et al.* 1986). It is of interest that no cases have been reported from widespread use of the drug in a non-immunological disease, cystinuria, although a case has been reported whose primary problem was Wilson's disease (Sternleib *et al.* 1975). Many of the affected patients have had the syndrome of pulmonary haemorrhage and crescentic nephritis without anti-GBM antibodies and, clinically, are indistinguishable from microscopic polyarteritis. Penicillamine is known to activate B cells polyclonally, and provoke synthesis of pathogenic autoantibodies. Gaskin *et al.* (1995) studied a patient with penicillamine-induced nephritis in whom antimyeloperoxidase antibodies with perinuclear ANCA were detectable. Thus, it is possible that crescentic nephritis is another reflection of the propensity of penicillamine to provoke autoantibody synthesis.

Other drugs

There are several reports suggesting that *hydralazine* may provoke crescentic nephritis (Björck *et al.* 1985, Mason and Lockwood 1986; Nässberger *et al.* 1991; Almroth *et al.* 1992), but the data are too preliminary to allow definite conclusions to be drawn. There have been single case reports apparently implicating *phenylbutazone* (Leung *et al.* 1985), *enalapril* (Bailey and Lynn 1986), and a few descriptions following *rifampicin* (Hirsch *et al.* 1983; Murray *et al.* 1987; Köhler *et al.* 1994). Crescentic nephritis has also been attributed to the use of *streptokinase* (Murray *et al.* 1986), but the development of acute renal failure in this context is not necessarily associated with crescentic change (Davies *et al.* 1990).

Chan *et al.* (1991) reported a patient in whom crescentic nephritis developed after recombinant *interleukin-2* therapy, Durand *et al.* (1995) following *interferon-α2b*, and Parker *et al.* (1995) another case who had received both treatments; immunoglobulins were absent and ANCA and anti-GBM antibodies not detected. This paper reviews three further cases associated with nephritis who had received *interferon-α2b*, but none had crescentic nephritis. All these patients also had malignancies (see below).

Miscellaneous causes

Malignancy

A small number of patients in most large series of patients with crescentic nephritis have had, or have later developed, malignant disease (Whitworth *et al.* 1976; Bierne *et al.* 1987; Neild *et al.* 1983; Dussol *et al.* 1992). However, it is difficult to be sure there is a causal link because many of the patients are relatively elderly, although the association with renal carcinoma seems secure (Neild *et al.* 1983). There are grounds for suspicion of a genuine causal link in the case of other carcinomas (Biava *et al.* 1984) and especially for lymphoid malignancies (Petzel *et al.* 1979; Pollock *et al.* 1988; Majdan *et al.* 1994).

Other possible associations

It has been suggested that *silicosis* may predispose to crescentic nephritis (Bolton *et al.* 1981; Arnalich *et al.* 1989; Sherson and Jorgenson 1989) possibly as a form of IgA nephropathy (Bonnin *et al.* 1987). *Alpha-1-antitrypsin deficiency* has also been described in two patients with crescentic nephritis (Lévy 1986; Lewis *et al.* 1985), and in another deficient patient, but in whom *phenylbutazone* appeared to be the precipitating factor (Leung *et al.* 1985). Dickmeyer *et al.* (1977) described an interesting patient with recurrent attacks of nephritis in association with *relapsing pancreatitis*; renal biopsy showed a crescentic nephritis with 70% of glomeruli affected. Finally, a case of crescentic nephritis following the bite of Russell's viper has been reported (Sitprija and Boonpucknavig 1980). This is particularly significant in view of the intense fibrin formation, leading to defibrination of circulating plasma, induced by this snake.

Crescentic nephritis following renal transplantation (see Cameron 1996)

In the majority of cases, this represents recurrence of the original disease in the allograft, but in a few patients, crescentic nephritis appears as a *de novo* phenomenon (Ihle *et al.* 1983). Boyce *et al.* (1985) noted a patient in renal failure from accelerated hypertension who developed anti-GBM nephritis in his allograft. The interesting phenomenon of crescentic nephritis appearing in recipients with Alport's syndrome transplanted with normal kidneys has been mentioned above, and is considered in more detail here.

Anti-GBM nephritis

Patients with anti-GBM disease who were transplanted, precociously developed recurrent nephritis with some frequency in the 1970s (Cameron 1982); some confusion about the relationship with the presence of anti-GBM antibodies was resolved by improvements in assays for this antibody. In patients with normal anti-GBM antibody titres, either the result of spontaneous disappearance (Flores *et al.* 1986) or, more usually, accelerated by treatment, recrudescence of antibody and recurrent disease have not been recorded except in a single isograft in a recipient who had received no immunosuppression (Almquist *et al.* 1981). Thus management centres on dialysis until antibody levels become, or are reduced to, normal levels. How long one should then wait is not clear; most clinicians wait 6–12 months and recurrent disease has not been recorded in the literature for some time. However, it is worth nothing that the presence of circulating antibody does not always lead to recurrence (Couser *et al.* 1973) and recurrence has been recorded in the apparent absence of antibody (Beliel *et al.* 1973), admittedly using the now outmoded techniques available at that time.

Mesangiocapillary nephritis (MCGN) types I and II

In type I MCGN, recurrence occurs in perhaps 25% of cases, especially those with crescent formation, but clinical nephritis or graft loss occurs in only a minority of these patients (6%). Some of these patients have had extensive crescent formation (McCoy *et al.* 1975). This is even more true of type II MCGN, in whom almost 90% show recurrence of the 'dense deposit' material within a few months, but only very rare cases develop clinical nephritis (Turner *et al.*

1974); usually, these are those with extensive crescent formation (Eddy *et al.* 1984; Sanz de Castro *et al.* 1988).

IgA nephropathy

The reappearance of IgA in the mesangium of patients with both IgA nephropathy and Henoch–Schönlein nephritis is recorded in 30–50% of subjects, appearing within days or weeks of transplantation (see Cameron 1993 for a review). However, clinical manifestations are rare, and graft loss extremely rare, at least within the first 5–10 years, although the long-term prognosis remains in doubt (Odum *et al.* 1994). The rather unusual individuals with IgA nephropathy and extensive crescent formation may be an exception, however, and show recurrence at a clinical level relatively commonly (Brensilver *et al.* 1988; Diaz-Tejeiro *et al.* 1990; Marcén *et al.* 1991), as in one of our own two patients with graft loss from IgA nephropathy. Streather and Scoble (1994) reported a patient in whom the original IgA-associated disease was indolent and scarring, whilst the recurrence revealed crescentic nephritis. Robles *et al.* (1991) reported a patient whose original biopsy showed a mesangiocapillary pattern, but without immunohistological data; crescentic (80%) nephritis with mesangial IgA developed in the allograft.

Membranous nephropathy

One patient with membranous nephropathy complicated by the appearance of diffuse crescent formation and anti-GBM antibodies had a recurrence in the allograft (Hill *et al.* 1978).

Other crescentic glomerulonephritis

In cases of crescentic nephritis with 'humps', or with granular immune aggregates within the glomerulus other than IgA, recurrence is surprisingly rare, although it has been recorded (Posborg Petersen *et al.* 1966; Porter *et al.* 1967; Richardson *et al.* 1970; Rosenfeld *et al.* 1970). Recurrence has also occurred in the presence of cyclosporin (Turney *et al.* 1986).

Vasculitis

Transplantation is generally without problems in vasculitis, even if ANCA are still present (Schmitt *et al.* 1993). However, relapse of vasculitis has been described and involves the glomeruli in a few cases (Steinman *et al.* 1980). Acute graft loss from crescentic nephritis has been recorded (Reaich *et al.* 1994). One unresolved problem is which immunosuppressive regimen to give such patients; improvement following transfer to cyclophosphamide has been recorded (Steinman *et al.* 1980) and the possibility that relapse may occur under treatment with cyclosporin has been raised.

Alport's syndrome

In the great majority of patients with Alport's syndrome the disease arises from mutations located in a gene at Xq 22 coding for an α5 non-collagenous portion of type IV collagen, found in the glomerular and other basement membranes (Barker *et al.* 1990). Thus, male Alport hemizygotes lack or have substituted a portion of the normal collagen structure, whereas allografts placed into such patients possess the normal epitope. In some patients, this seems to be sufficient to evoke an immune response with production of antibody directed against the 'new' antigen, which is capable of fixing to the allograft. However, only some patients actually showing fixation develop severe crescentic glomerulonephritis. 27 cases (Flinter 1994) have been reported since its first description in 1982 (McCoy *et al.* 1982; Milliner *et al.* 1982; Teruel *et al.* 1987; Fleming *et al.* 1988; Shah *et al.* 1988; Van der Heuvel *et al.* 1989; Rassoul *et al.* 1990; Goldman *et al.* 1990; Kashtan *et al.* 1990a; Oliver *et al.* 1991; Bach *et al.* 1992; Ding *et al.* 1994). Querin *et al.* (1986) noted linear deposition of IgG along the GBM in 5 cases of Alport's syndrome without nephritis, but no anti-GBM antibody was detectable in the serum using assays designed to detect antibodies to the $\alpha3$ chain of type IV collagen. Both they and Habib (1983), however, noted such appearances in patients with a random selection of other underlying renal diseases. All Alport allograft recipients suffering crescentic nephritis had developed renal failure early in life, and all were deaf. There was a latent period of some months after grafting before the nephritis appeared, but all grafts except one were lost to the severe nephritis, despite plasma exchange in three patients.

One puzzle is why only a few patients with Alport's syndrome—about 3.5% (Kashtan, personal communication)—develop nephritis post-transplant. For example, we have transplanted 38 children and adults with 52 grafts and never seen this complication, and at the Necker Hospital in Paris over 50 patients with Alport's have been transplanted in the adult and paediatric units without any case of *de novo* nephritis. Similarly, Göbel *et al.* (1992) did not see nephritis in 30 patients. Numbers are too small to determine risk factors, such as haploid-entity, MHC type, or closeness of tissue match. The antibodies present in different patients with recurrence seem to be directed against several different antigen specificities making a single gene mutation unlikely.

A number of groups have studied patients developing and not developing antibody and/or nephritis with probes for the COL4A5 gene which appears to be the site of disorder in the great majority—if not all—cases of true Alport's syndrome. It has emerged that patients with major deletions—amounting to complete deletion of the gene—are at the greatest risk of developing recurrent crescentic nephritis (about 1 in 3), but a few patients with point mutations or small deletions have also suffered the complication (Kashtan *et al.* 1991, Netzer *et al.* 1992; Prison *et al.* 1992); within each family the mutation appears constant, as would be expected. One unexpected feature is that three of the patients (Van der Heuvel *et al.* 1989; Ding *et al.* 1995) were female. Heterozygotes would normally be equal mosaics of normal and abnormal genes (Kashtan *et al.* 1990b) resulting from random inactivation of one of each of the pairs of X chromosomes, normal and abnormal, and thus should have tolerance of the antigen in the allograft. It could be that in some females, the great majority of cells express the abnormal chromosome and its product. However, in two patients (Ding *et al.* 1995;

Mochizuki *et al.* 1994), the inheritance was autosomal recessive and the abnormal collagen the result of a mutation in the COL4A3 gene, the chain containing the Goodpasture antigen.

References

Abe, T. *et al.* (1986) Participation of extracapillary lesions (ECL) in progression of IgA nephropathy. *Clinical Nephrology*, **25**, 7–41.

Abreo, K., Abreo, F., Mitchell, B., and Schloemer, G. (1986) Idiopathic crescentic membranous glomerulonephritis. *American Journal of Kidney Diseases*, **8**, 257–61.

Abuelo, J.G., Esparaza, A.R., Matarese, R.A., Endreny, R.G., Carvalho, J.S., and Allagra, S.R. (1984). Crescentic IgA nephropathy. *Medicine (Baltimore)*, **63**, 396–406.

Almaquist, R.D., Buckalew, V.M., Hirszel, P., Maher J.F., James, P.M., and Wilson, C.B. (1981). Recurrence of anti-glomerular basement membrane antibody mediated glomerulonephritis in an isograft. *Clinical Immunology and Immunopathology*, **18**, 54–60.

Almroth, G. *et al.* (1992). Autoantibodies and leukocyte antigens in hydralazine-associated nephritis. *Journal of Internal Medicine*, **231**, 37–42.

Anand, S.K., Trygstad, C.W., Sharma, H.M., and Northway, J.D. (1975). Extracapillary proliferative glomerulonephritis in children. *Pediatrics*, **56**, 434–42.

Angangco, R.R., Thiru, S., Esnault, V.L.M., Short, A.K., Lockwood, C.M., and Oliveira, D.G.B. (1994). Does truly 'idiopathic' crescentic glomerulonephritis exist? *Nephrology Dialysis Transplantation*, **9**, 630–6.

Arnalich, F. *et al.* (1989). Polyarteritis nodosa and necrotizing glomerulonephritis associated with long-standing silicosis. *Nephron*, **51**, 544–7.

Bach, D., Peters, A., Rowemeier, H., Degenhardt, S., Helmchen U., and Grabensee B. (1992). Antibasalmembran-Glomerulonephritis nach Verwantennierentransplantation bei hereditäre Nephropathie Alport. *Deutsche Medizinische Wochenschrift*, **116**, 1972–756.

Bailey, R.R. and Lynn, K.L. (1986). Crescentic glomerulonephritis developing in a patient taking enalapril. *New Zealand Medical Journal*, **99**, 958–9 (letter).

Banfi, G., Imbasciati, E., Guerra, L., Mihatsch, M.J., and Ponticelli, C. (1983). Extracapillary glomerulonephritis with necrotizing vasculitis in D-penicillamine-treated rheumatoid arthritis. *Nephron*, **33**, 56–60.

Banfi, G. *et al.* (1985). Morphological parameters in lupus nephritis: their relevance for classification and relationship with clinical and histological findings and outcome. *Quarterly Journal of Medicine*, **55**, 153–68.

Barbiano di Belgiojoso G. *et al.* (1977). The prognostic value of some clinical and histological parameters in membranoproliferative glomerulonephritis (MPGN). *Nephron*, **19**, 250–8.

Barker, D.F. *et al.* (1990). Identification of mutations in the COL4A5 collagen gene in Alport syndrome. *Science*, **248**, 1224–7.

Beaufils, M., Morel-Maroger, L., Sraer, J-D., Kanfer, A., Kourilsky, O., and Richet, G. (1976). Acute renal failure of glomerular origin during visceral abcesses. *New England Journal of Medicine*, **295**, 185–9.

Becker, N., Rutledge, J.C., and Avner, E.D. (1995). Clinical quiz. *Pediatric Nephrology*, **6**, 785–7

Beirne, G.J., Wagnild, J.P., Zimmerman, S.W., Mackem, P.D., and Burkholder, P.M. (1977). Idiopathic crescentic glomerueonephritis. *Medicine (Baltimore)*, **56**, 349–81.

Beliel, O.M., Coburn, J.W., Shinaberger, J.H., and Glassock, R.J. (1973). Recurrent glomerulonephritis due to anti-glomerular basement membrane antibodies in two successive allografts. *Clinical Nephrology*, **1**, 377–88.

Biava, C.G., Gonwa, T.A., Naugton, J.L., and Hopper, J., Jr. (1984). Crescentic glomerulonephritis associated with nonrenal malignancies. *American Journal of Nephrology*, **4**, 208–14.

Björck, S., Svalander, C., and Westberg, G. (1985). Hydralazine-associated glomeru lonephritis. *Acta Medica Scandinavica*, **218**, 261–9.

Bolton, W.K., Surrat, P.M., and Sturgill, B. (1981). Rapidly progressive silicon nephropathy. *American Journal of Medicine*, **71**, 823–8.

Bonnin, A., Mousson, C., Justrabo, E., Tanter, Y., Chalopin, J.M., and Rifle, G. (1987). Silicosis associated with crescentic IgA mesangial nephropathy. *Nephron*, **47**, 229–30.

Boobes Y., Baz M., Durand C., Jaber K., Goldstein P., and Berland Y. (1990). Early start of intensive therapy in malignant form of IgA nephropathy. *Nephron*, **54**, 351–3.

Boulton-Jones, J.M., Sissons, J.G.P., Evans, D.J., and Peters, D.K. (1974). Renal lesions of subacute infective endocarditis. *British Medical Journal*, **ii**, 11–14.

Bourgognie, J. (1990). Nephrology forum: renal complications of human immunodeficiency virus type I. *Kidney International*, **37**, 1571–84.

Boyce, N., Holdsworth S., Atkins R., and Dowling J. (1985). De-novo anti-GBM-antibody induced glomerulonephritis in a renal transplant. *Clinical Nephrology*, **23**, 148–51.

Boyce, N.W., Holdsworth, S.R., Thomson, N.M., and Atkins, R.C. (1986). Clinicopathological associations in mesangial IgA nephropathy. *American Journal of Nephrology*, **6**, 246–52.

Breedveld, F.C., Valentijn, R.M., Westedt, M.L., and Weening, J.J. (1985). Rapidly progressive glomerulonephritis with glomerular crescent formation in rheumatoid arthritis. *Clinical Rheumatology*, **4**, 353–9.

Brensilver, J.M., Mallat, S., Scholes, J., and McCabe, R. (1988). Recurrent IgA nephropathy in living-related donor transplantation: recurrence or transmission of familial disease? *American Journal of Kidney Diseases*, **12**, 147–51.

Cadnapaphornchai, P. and Sillix, D. (1989). Recurrence of monoclonal gammopathy-related glomerulonephritis in renal allograft. *Clinical Nephrology*, **31**, 156–9.

Cameron, J.S. (1982). Glomerulonephritis in renal transplants. *Transplantation*, **34**, 237–45.

Cameron, J.S. (1992). The nosology of crescentic nephritis. *Néphrologie*, **13**, 243–6.

Cameron, J.S. (1993). The long term outlook of glomerular disease. In *Diseases of the kidney* 5th edn., (ed. C.W. Gottschalk and R. Schrier) pp. 1895–958. Little Brown, Boston.

Cameron, J.S. (1996). Recurrent disease in transplanted kidneys. In *Transplantation biology: Cellular and molecular aspects*, (ed. N. Tilney and T.B. Strom) pp. 619–27. Raven, New York.

Cameron, J.S. *et al.* (1983). Idiopathic mesangiocapillary glomerulonephritis: comparison of types I and II in children and adults, and long term prognosis. *American Journal of Medicine*, **74**, 175–92.

Campbell, J.H., Warwick, G., Boulton-Jones, M., McLay, A., Jackson, B., and Stevenson, R.D. (1991), Rapidly progressive glomerulonephritis and nephrotic syndrome associated with *Mycoplasma pneumoniae* pneumonia. *Nephrology Dialysis Transplantation*, **6**, 518–20.

Chan, T.M., Cheng I.K.P., Wong K.L., Chan K.W., and Lai, C.L. (1991). Crescentic IgA glomerulonephritis following interleukin-2 therapy for hepatocellular carcinoma. *American Journal of Nephrology*, **11**, 493–6.

Chapman, S.J., Cameron, J.S., Chantler, C., and Turner, D. (1980). Treatment of mesangiocapillary glomerulonephritis in children with combined immunosuppression and anticoagulation. *Archives of Diseases of Childhood*, **55**, 446–51.

Chugh, K.S., Gupta, V.K., Singhal, P.C., and Sehgal, S. (1981). Case report: Poststreptococcal crescentic glomerulonephritis and pulmonary hemorrhage simulating Goodpasture's syndrome. *Annals of Allergy*, **47**, 104–6.

Confalonieri, R. *et al.* (1988). Light chain nephropathy: histological and clinical aspects in 15 cases. *Nephrology Dialysis Transplantation*, **2**, 150–6.

Connelly, C.E. and Gallacher, B. (1987). Acute crescentic glomerulonephritis as a complication of a *Staphylococcus aureus* abscess of hip joint prosthesis. *Journal of Clinical Pathology*, **40**, 1486 (letter).

Coppo, R. *et al.* (1985). Plasmapheresis in patients with rapidly progressive IgA nephropathy: removal of IgA containing circulating immune complexes and clinical recovery. *Nephron*, **40**, 488–90.

Couser, W.G., Wallace, A., Monaco, A.P., and Lewis, E.J. (1973). Successful renal transplantation in patients with circulating antibody to glomerular basement membrane: report of two cases. *Clinical Nephrology*, **1**, 381–8.

Curtis, J.J., Bhathena, D., Leach, R.P., Galla, J.H., Lucas, B.A., and Luke, R.G. (1976). Goodpasture's syndrome in a patient with the nail-patella syndrome. *American Journal of Medicine*, **61**, 401–6.

D'Amico, G. (1993). Hepatitis C virus and essential mixed cryoglobulinaemia. *Nephrology Dialysis Transplantation*, **8**, 579–81.

D'Amico, G. *et al.* (1981). IgA-mesangial nephropathy (Berger's disease) with rapid decline in renal function. *Clinical Nephrology*, **16**, 251–7.

D'Amico, G. *et al.* (1985). Idiopathic IgA mesangial nephropathy. Clinical and histological study of 374 patients. *Medicine (Baltimore)*, **64**, 49–60.

Davies, D.J., Moran, J.E., Niall, J.F., and Ryan, G.B. (1982). Segmental necrotising glomerulonephritis with antineutrophil antibody: possible arbovirus aetiology? *British Medical Journal*, **285**, 606.

Davies, K.A., Mathieson, P., Winearls, C.G., Rees, A.J., and Walport, M.J. (1990). Serum sickness and acute renal failure after Streptokinase therapy for myocardial infarction. *Clinical and Experimental Immunology*, **80**, 83–8.

Davis, C.A., McAdams, A.J., Wyatt, R.J., Forristal, J., and McEnery, P.T. (1979). Idiopathic rapidly progressive glomerulonephritis with C3 nephritic factor and hypocomplementemia. *Journal of Pediatrics*, **94**, 559–63.

Davison, A.M. (1992). Infection-associated glomerulonephritis. In *Oxford textbook of clinical nephrology*, (ed. J.S. Cameron, A.M. Davison, J-P. Grünfeld, D.N.S. Kerr, and E. Ritz) pp. 456–75. Oxford University Press.

Devogelaer, J.P., Pirson, Y., Vandenbroucke J.M., Cosyns, J.P., Brichard, S., and Nagant de Deuxchaisnes, C. (1987). D-penicillamine induced crescentic glomerulonephritis: Report and review of the literature. *Journal of Rheumatology*, **14**, 1036–41.

Dhar S.K., Smith E.C., and Fresco, R. (1977). Proliferative glomerulonephritis in monoclonal gammopathy. *Nephron*, **19**, 288–94.

Diaz-Tejeiro, R. *et al.* (1990). Loss of graft due to recurrent IgA nephropathy with rapidly progressive course: an unusual clinical evolution. *Nephron*, **54**, 431–3.

Dickmeyer, J.P., Wolfson, W., Kowell, A., and Dornfeld, L. (1977). Reversible crescentic glomerulonephritis following an acute exacerbation of chronic relapsing pancreatitis. *Archives of Internal Medicine*, **137**, 1065–7.

Ding, J., Zhou, J., Tryggvason, K., and Kashtan, C.E. (1994). COL4A5 deletions in three patients with Alport syndrome and posttransplant antiglomerular basement membrane nephritis. *Journal of the American Society of Nephrology*, **5**, 161–8.

Ding, J., Stitzel, J., Berry P., Hawkins, E., and Kashtan C.E. (1995). Autosomal recessive Alport syndrome: mutation in the COL4A3 gene in a woman with Alport syndrome and posttranplant antiglomerular basement membrane nephritis. *Journal of the American Society of Nephrology*, **5**, 1714–17.

Durand, J.M., Retornaz, F., Cietel, E., Kplanski, G., and Soubeyrand, J. (1995). Crescentic glomerulonephritis during treatment with interferon α-2b. *American Journal of Haematology*, **48**, 140–1.

Dussol, B., Berland, Y., and Casanova, P. (1992). Glomerulonéphrite a croissants diffus associée avec un carcinome gastrique. *Néphrologie*, **13**, 163–6.

Dussol, B. *et al.* (1994). Glomérulonéphrite à croissants diffus et syndrome Gougerot–Sjögren. *Néphrologie*, **15**, 295–8.

Eddy, A., Sibley, R., Mauer, S.M., and Kim, Y. (1984). Renal allograft failure due to recurrent dense intramembranous deposit disease. *Clinical Nephrology*, **21**, 305–13.

Eknoyan, G.B. (1985). Renal complications of bacterial endocarditis. *American Journal of Nephrology*, **5**, 457–69 (discussion).

Faarup, P., Norgaard, T., Elling, F., and Jensen, H. (1978). Structural changes in the kidney of patients with oliguric extracapillary glomeruonephritis during immunosuppressive therapy. *Acta Pathologia Microbiologia Scandinavica (A)*, **86**, 409–14.

Fairley, C., Mathewson, D.C., and Becker, G.J. (1987). Rapid development of diffuse crescents in post-streptococcal glomerulonephritis. *Clinical Nephrology*, **28**, 256–60.

Ferrario, F., Tadros, M.T., Napodano, P., Sinico, R.A., Fellin, G., and D'Amico, G. (1994). Critical re-evaluation of 41 cases of 'idiopathic' crescentic glomerulonephritis. *Clinical Nephrology*, **41**, 1–9.

Ferraris, J.R., Gallo, G.E., Ramirez, J., Iotti, R., and Gianantonio, C. (1983). 'Pulse' methylprednisolone therapy in the treatment of acute crescentic glomerulonephritis. *Nephron*, **34**, 207–8.

Fleming, S.J. *et al.* (1988). Antiglomerular basement membrane antibody-mediated nephritis complicating transplantation in a patient with Alport's syndrome. *Transplantation*, **46**, 857–9.

Flinter, F. (1994). Third International Workshop on Alport syndrome. *Pediatric Nephrology*, **8**, 780–2.

Flores, J.C. *et al.* (1986). Clinical and immunological evolution of oligoanuric anti-GBM nephritis treated by haemodialysis. *Lancet*, **i**, 5–8.

Gaskin, G., Thompson, E.M., and Pusey, C.D. (1995). Goodpasture-like syndrome associated with anti-myeloperoxidase antibodies following penicillamine treatment. *Nephrology Dialysis Transplantation*, **10**, 1925–8.

Gavaghan, T.E. *et al.* (1981). Penicillamine induced 'Goodpasture syndrome': successful treatment of a fulminant case. *Australian and New Zealand Journal of Medicine*, **11**, 261–5.

Gibson, T., Burry, H.C., and Ogg, C.S. (1976). Goodpasture's syndrome. *Annals of Internal Medicine*, **84**, 100–1.

Gill, D.G. *et al.* (1977). Progression of acute proliferative post-streptococcal glomerulonephritis to severe epithelial crescent formation. *Clinical Nephrology*, **8**, 449–52.

Glassock, R.J. (1990). UCLA conference: human immunodeficiency virus (HIV) infection and the kidney. *Annals of Internal Medicine*, **112**, 35–49.

Göbel, J. *et al.* (1992). Kidney transplantation in Alport's syndrome: long term outcome and allograft anti-GBM nephritis. *Clinical Nephrology*, **38**, 299–304.

Goldman, M. *et al.* (1990). Failure of two subsequent renal grafts by anti-GBM glomerulonephritis in Alport's syndrome: case report and review of the literature. *Transplant International*, **3**, 82–85.

Griffin, K.A., Schwartz, M.M., and Korbet, S.M. (1989). Pulmonary-renal syndrome of bacterial endocarditis mimicking Goodpasture's syndrome. *American Journal of Kidney Diseases*, **14**, 329–32.

Gutman, R.A., Striker, G.E., Gilliland, B.C., and Cutler, R.E. (1972). The immune complex glomerulonephritis of bacterial endocarditis. *Medicine (Baltimore)*, **51**, 1–25.

Habib, R. (1983). Glomerulonéphrite membranoproliférative. In *Néphrologie pédiatrique*, (ed. P. Royer, R. Habib, M. Mathieu, and R. Broyer) pp. 316–28. Flammarion, Paris.

Harada, A. *et al.* (1984). Renal amyloidosis associated with crescentic glomerulonephritis. *American Journal of Nephrology*, **4**, 52–5.

Harper, L., Cockwell, P., Howie, A.J., Michael, J., Richards, N.T., Savage, C.O.S. *et al.*(1997). Focal segmental necrotizing glomerulonephritis in rheumatoid arthritis. *Quarterly Journal of Medicine*, **90** 125–32.

Harris, J.P., Rakowski, T.A., Argy, W.P. Jr., and Schreiner, G.E. (1978). Alport's syndrome representing as crescentic glomerulonephritis: A report of two siblings. *Clinical Nephrology*, **10**, 245–9.

Harrison, C.V., Loughridge, L.W., and Milne, M.D. (1964). Acute oliguric renal failure in acute glomerulonephritis and polyarteritis. *Quarterly Journal of Medicine*, **129**, 39–55.

Haycock, G.B. (1992). The nephritis of Henoch-Schönlein purpura. In *Oxford textbook of clinical nephrology*, (ed. J.S. Cameron, A.M. Davison, J.-P. Grünfeld, D.N.S. Kerr, and E. Ritz) pp. 595–612. Oxford University Press.

Haycock, G.B., and Cameron, J.S. (1991). Schönlein-Henoch purpura. In *Current therapy in nephrology and hypertension*, (ed. Glassock, R.J.) pp. 129–30. Decker, Toronto.

Heaf, J.G., Jorgensen, F., and Neilsen, L.P. (1983). Treatment and prognosis of extracapillary glomerulonephritis. *Nephron*, **35**, 217–24.

Hené, R.J., Valentijn, R.M., and Kater, L. (1982). Plasmapheresis in nephropathy of Henoch Schönlein purpura and primary IgA nephropathy. *Kidney International*, **22**, 409 (abstract).

Hill, G.S., *et al.* (1978). An unusual variant of membranous nephropathy with abundant crescent formation and recurrence in the transplanted kidney. *Clinical Nephrology*, **10**, 114–20.

Hinglais, N., Garcia-Torres, R., and Kleinknecht, C. (1974). Long term prognosis in acute glomerulonephritis. The predictive value of early clinical and pathological features in 65 patients. *American Journal of Medicine*, **56**, 52–60.

Hirsch, D.J., Bia, F.J., Kashgarian, M., and Bia, M.J. (1983). Rapidly progressive glomerulonephritis during antituberculous therapy. *American Journal of Nephrology*, **3**, 7–10.

Ihle, B.U., *et al.* (1983). De novo crescentic glomerulonephritis in a renal transplant. *Transplant Proceedings*, **15**, 2147.

Ingelfinger, J.R., McCluskey, R.T., Schneeberger, E.E., and Grupe, WE. (1977). Necrotizing arteritis in acute poststreptococcal glomerulonephritis: report of a recovered case. *Journal of Pediatrics*, **91**, 228–32.

Inglis, F.G., Henderson, I., Sanders, S., and Kerr, M. (1994). Reiter's disease, keratoderma blennorhagica and rapidly progressive glomerulonephritis. *Nephrology Dialysis
Transplantation*, **9**, 824–6.

Isaacs, J.D., Evans D.J., and Pusey, C.D. (1990). Mesangial IgA disease with crescent
formation during pregnancy. Postpartum treatment with immunosuppression.
Nephrology Dialysis Transplantation, **5**, 619–22.

Jardim, H.M.P.F., Leake J., Risdon, R.A., Barratt, T.M., and Dillon M.J. (1992).
Crescentic glomerulonephritis in children. *Pediatric Nephrology*, **6**, 231–5.

Jennings, RB. and Earle, DP. (1961). Post-streptococcal glomerulonephritis: Histopathological and clinical studies of the acute, subsiding acute and early chronic latent
phase. *Journal of Clinical Investigation*, **40**, 1525–95.

Jindal, K.K., Trillo, A., Bishop, G., and Hirsch, D. (1991). Crescentic IgA nephropathy
as a manifestation of human immune deficiency virus infection. *American Journal of
Nephrology*, **11**, 147–50.

Kamata, K., Kobayashi Y., Shigematsu H., and Saito T. (1982). Childhood type
polymyositis and rapidly progressive glomerulonephritis. *Acta Pathologica Japonica*,
32, 801–6.

Kaplan, N.G. and Kaplan, M.C. (1970). Monoclonal gammopathy, glomerulonephritis,
and the nephrotic syndrome. *Archives of Internal Medicine*, **125**, 696–700.

Kashtan, C., Butkowski, R.J., Kleppel, M.M., First, M.R., and Michael, A.F. (1990*a*).
Posttransplant anti-glomerular basement membrane nephritis in related males with
Alport syndrome. *Journal of Laboratory and Clinical Medicine*, **116**, 508–15.

Kashtan, C., Kleppel, M.M., Butkowski, R.J., Michael, A.L., and Fish, A.J. (1990*b*).
Alport syndrome, basement membranes and collagen. *Pediatric Nephrology*, **4**,
523–32.

Kashtan, C.E., Michael, A.F., and Kleppel, M.M. (1991). Alport syndrome: association
of deletion in the COL4A5 gene with post transplant anti-GBM nephritis (GN).
Journal of the American Society of Nephrology, **2**, 256.

Kebler, R., Kithier, K., McDonald, FD., and Cadnapaphornchai, P. (1985). Rapidly progressive glomerulonephritis and monoclonal gammopathy. *American Journal of
Medicine*, **78**, 133–8.

Kenouch, S. and Méry, J-Ph. (1992). Sarcoidosis. In *Oxford textbook of clinical nephrology*,
(ed. J.S. Cameron, A.M. Davison, J-P. Grünfeld, D.N.S. Kerr, and E. Ritz)
pp. 576–82. Oxford University Press.

Kingswood, J.C., Banks, R.A, Tribe, C.R., Owen Jones, J., and MacKenzie, J.C. (1984).
Renal biopsy in the elderly: clinicopathological correlations in 143 patients. *Clinical
Nephrology*, **22**, 183–7.

Kitridou, R.C. *et al.* (1986). Renal involvement in mixed connective tissue disease: a longitudinal clinicopathologic study. *Seminars in Arthritis and Rheumatism*, **16**, 135–45.

Klassen, J. *et al.* (1974). Evolution of membranous nephropathy into anti-glomerular-
basement-membrane glomerulonephritis. *New England Journal of Medicine*, **290**,
319–25.

Koethe, J.D., Gerig, J.S., Glickman, J.L., Sturgill, B.C., and Bolton, W.K. (1986).
Progression of membranous nephropathy to acute crescentic rapidly progressive
glomerulonephritis and response to pulse methylprednisolone. *American Journal of
Nephrology*, **6**, 224–8.

Köhler, L.J., Gohara, A.F., Hamilton R.W., and Reeves R.S. (1994). Crescentic fibrillary
glomerulonephritis associated with intermittent rifampicin therapy for pulmonary
tuberculosis. *Clinical Nephrology*, **42**, 263–5.

Korzets, Z. and Bernheim, J. (1987). Rapidly progressive glomerulonephritis (crescentic glomerulonephritis) in the course of type I idiopathic membranoproliferative glomerulonephritis. *American Journal of Kidney Diseases*, **10**, 56–61.

Kurki, P. *et al.* (1984). Transformation of membranous glomerulonephritis into crescentic glomerulonephritis with glomerular basement membrane antibodies: serial determinations of anti-GBM before the transformation. *Nephron*, **38**, 134–7.

Kwan, J., Moore, R.H., Dodd, S.M., and Cunningham, J. (1991). Crescentic transformation in primary membranous glomerulonephritis. *Postgraduate Medical Journal*, **67**, 574–6.

Lai, K.N., Lai, F.M., Leung, A.C., Ho, C.P., and Vallance Owen, J. (1987). Plasma exchange in patients with rapidly progressive idiopathic IgA nephropathy: a report of two cases and review of literature. *American Journal of Kidney Diseases*, **10**, 66–70.

Landwehr, D.M., Cooke, C.L., and Rodriguez, G.E. (1980). Rapidly progressive glomerulonephritis in Behçet's syndrome. *Journal of the American Medical Association*, **244**, 1709–11.

Lapenas, D.J., Drewny, S.J., Luke, R.L., and Leeber, D.A. (1983). Crescentic light chain glomerulopathy. *Archives of Pathology*, **107**, 319–23.

Leaker, B., Fairley, K.F., Dowling, J., and Kincaid-Smith, P. (1987). Lupus nephritis: clinical and pathological correlation. *Quarterly Journal of Medicine*, **62**, 163–79.

Leonard, C.D., Nagle, R.B., Striker, G.E., Cutler, R.E., and Scribner, B.H. (1970). Acute glomerulonephritis with prolonged oliguria: An analysis of 29 cases. *Annals of Internal Medicine*, **73**, 703–11.

Leung, A.C., McLay, A., Dobbie, J.W., and Boulton-Jones, J.M. (1985). Phenylbutazone-induced systemic vasculitis with crescentic glomerulonephritis associated with deficiency of alpha-1-antitrypsin. *Archives of Internal Medicine*, **145**, 685–7.

Lévy, M. (1986). Severe alpha-1-antitrypsin deficiency presenting with cutaneous vasculitis, rapidly progressive glomerulonephritis, and colitis. *American Journal of Medicine*, **81**, 363–64, (letter).

Lévy, M. *et al.* (1985). Berger's disease in children. Natural history and outcome. *Medicine (Baltimore)*, **64**, 157–80.

Lewis, M. *et al.* (1985). Severe deficiency of alpha 1-antitrypsin associated with cutaneous vasculitis, rapidly progressive glomerulonephritis, and colitis. *American Journal of Medicine*, **79**, 489–94.

Lewy, J.E., Salinas-Madrigal, L., Hendron, P.B., Pirani, C.L., and Metcoff, J. (1977). Clinico-pathologic correlations in acute post-streptococcal nephritis. *Medicine (Baltimore)*, **50**, 453–501.

Löhlein, M. (1907). Über die entzündlichen Veränderungen der Glomeruli der menschlichen Nieren und ihre Bedeutung für die Nephritis. *Arbeiten aus dem Pathologischen Institut zu Leipzig*, Vol. 1. Hirzel, Leipzig.

Macarron, P., Garcia Diaz, J.E., Azofra, J.A., and Martin de Francisco, J. (1992). D-pencillamine associated with rapidly progressive glomerulonephritis. *Nephrology Dialysis Transplantation*, **7**, 161–4.

Madiwale, C.V., Mittal, B.V., Dixit, M., and Acharya, V.N. (1994). Acute renal failure due to crescentic glomerulonephritis complicating leprosy. *Nephrology Dialysis Transplantation*, **9**, 178–9.

Magil, A. *et al.* (1988). Prognostic factors in diffuse proliferative lupus nephritis. *Kidney International*, **34**, 511–17.

Majdan, M. *et al.* (1994). Chronic myelogenous leukaemia associated with rapidly progressive glomerulonephritis. *Nephrology Dialysis Transplantation*, **9**, 562–3.

Marcén, R. *et al.* (1991). Recurrence of IgA nephropathy with nephrotic syndrome after kidney transplantation. *Nephron*, **59**, 486–9.

Martini, A., Magrini, U., Scelsi, M., Capelli, V., and Barberis L. (1981). Chronic mesangioproliferative IgA glomerulonephritis complicated by a rapidly progressive course in a 14-year old boy. A case report. *Nephron*, **29**, 164–6.

Mason, P.D. and Lockwood, C.M. (1986). Rapidly progressive nephritis in patients taking hydralazine. *Journal of Clinical Laboratory Immunology*, **20**, 151–3.

Matloff, D.S. and Kaplan, M.M. (1980). D-penicillamine-induced biliary cirrhosis: successful treatment with plasmapheresis and immunosupressives. *Gastroenterology*, **78**, 1046–9.

McCluskey, R.T. and Baldwin, D.S. (1965). The natural history of acute glomerulonephritis. *American Journal of Medicine*, **35**, 213–30.

McCoy, R., Clapp, J., and Seigler, H.F. (1975). Membranoproliferative glomerulonephritis. Progression from the pure form to the crescentic form with recurrence after transplantation. *American Journal of Medicine*, **59**, 288–92.

McCoy, R.C., Johnson, H.K., Stone, W.J., and Wilson, C.B. (1982). Absence of nephritogenic GBM antigen(s) in some patients with hereditary nephritis. *Kidney International*, **21**, 128–37.

McEnery R., McAdams, A.I., and West, C.D. (1985). The effect of prednisone in a high dose alternate day regimen on the natural history of idiopathic membranoproliferative glomerulonephritis. *Medicine (Baltimore)*, **64**, 401–23.

Meyrier, A., Simon, P., Mignon, F., Striker, L., and Ramee, M.P. (1984). Rapidly progressive ('crescentic') glomerulonephritis and monoclonal gammopathies. *Nephron*, **38**, 156–62.

Milliner, D.S., Pierides, A.M., and Holley, K.E. (1982). Renal transplantation in Alport's syndrome. Anti-glomerular basement membrane in the allograft. *Mayo Clinic Proceedings*, **57**, 35–43.

Mitas, J.A., Frank, L.R., Swerdlin, A.R., Johnson, D.L., and Rabetoy, G.M. (1983). Crescentic glomerulonephritis complicating idiopathic membranous glomerulonephropathy. *Southern Medical Journal*, **76**, 664–7.

Mochizuki, T. *et al.* (1994). Identification of mutations in the alpha 3(IV) and alpha 4(IV) collagen genes in autosomal recessive Alport syndrome. *Nature Genetics*, **8**, 77–81.

Modai, D. *et al.* (1985). Biopsy proven evolution of post streptococcal glomerulonephritis to rapidly progressive glomerulonephritis of a post infectious type. *Clinical Nephrology*, **23**, 198–202.

Molina-Perez, M., Gonzales Riemers, E., Santolaria-Fernadez, F., Maceria-Cruz, B., and Ravina-Cabrera M. (1995). Rapidly progressive glomerulonephritis and inflammatory bowel disease. *Diseases of the Colon and Rectum*, **38**, 1006–7.

Montoliu, J., Darnell, A., Torras, A., and Revert, L. (1981). Acute and rapidly progressive forms of glomerulonephritis in the elderly. *Journal of the American Geriatric Society*, **29**, 108–16.

Montseny, J.J., Meyrier, A., Klenikhecht, D., and Callard, P. (1995) The current spectrum of infectious glomerulonephritis: Experience with 76 patients and review of the literature. *Medicine (Baltimore)*, **74**, 63–73.

Moorthy, A.V., Zimmerman, S.W., Burkholder, P.M., and Harrington, A.R. (1976). Association of crescentic glomerulonephritis with membranous glomerulonephropathy: a report of three cases. *Clinical Nephrology*, **6**, 319–25.

Morel-Maroger, L., Kourilsky, O., Mignon, F., and Richet, G. (1974). Antitubular basement membrane antibodies in rapidly progressive poststreptococcal glomerulonephritis: Report of a case. *Clinical Immunology and Immunopathology*, **2**, 185–94.

Morrin, P.A., Hinglais, N., Nabarra, B., and Kreis, H. (1978). Rapidly progressive glomerulonephritis. A clinical and pathologic study. *American Journal of Medicine*, **65**, 446–60.

Murray, A.N., Cassidy, M.J., and Templecamp, C. (1987). Rapidly progressive glomerulonephritis associated with rifampicin therapy for pulmonary tuberculosis. *Nephron*, **46**, 373–6.

Murray, N., Lyons, J., and Chappell, M. (1986). Crescentic glomerulonephritis: A possible complication of streptokinase treatment for myocardial infarction. *British Heart Journal*, **56**, 483–5.

Mustonen, J., Helin, H., Pasternack, A., and Vanttinen, T. (1983). Acute rheumatic fever with extracapillary glomerulonephritis and the nephrotic syndrome. *Annals of Clinical Research*, **15**, 92–4.

Nakamoto, S., Dunea, G., Kolff, W., and McCormack, L. (1965). Treatment of oliguric glomerulonephritis with dialysis and steroids. *Annals of Internal Medicine*, **63**, 359–68.

Naschitz, J.E., Yushurun, D., Scharf, Y., Sajrawi, I., Lazarov, N.B., and Boss, J.H. (1989). Recurrent massive alveolar hemorrhage, crescentic glomerulonephritis, and necrotizing vasculitis in a patient with rheumatoid arthritis. *Archives of Internal Medicine*, **149**, 406–8.

Nässberger, L., Johansson, A-C., Björck S., and Sjöholm, A.G. (1991). Antibodies to neutrophil granulocyte myeloperoxidase and elastase: autoimmune responses in glomerulonephritis due to hydralazine treatment. *Journal of Internal Medicine*, **229**, 261–5.

Neild, G.H. *et al.* (1983). Rapidly progressive glomerulonephritis with extensive glomerular crescent formation. *Quarterly Journal of Medicine*, **52**, 395–416.

Netzer, K. *et al.* (1992). Analysis of COL4A5 gene in patients with Alport syndrome and post-transplant antiglomerular basement membrane disease. *Nephrology Dialysis Transplantation*, **7**, 784 (abstract).

Neugarten, J., Gallo, G.R., and Baldwin, D.S. (1984). Glomerulonephritis in bacterial endocarditis. *American Journal of Kidney Diseases*, **3**, 371–9.

Nguyen, B.P., Reisen, E., and Rodriguez, F.H.J.R. (1988). Idiopathic membranous glomerulopathy complicated by crescentic glomerulonephritis and renal vein thrombosis. *American Journal of Kidney Diseases*, **12**, 326–8.

Niaudet, P. and Lévy, M. (1983). Glomerulonéphrite á croissants diffus. In *Néphrologie Pédiatrique*, (ed. P. Royer, R. Habib, H. Mahieu, and M. Broyer) pp. 381–94. Flammarion, Paris.

Nicholls, K.M., Fairley, K.F., Dowling, J.P., and Kincaid-Smith, P. (1984). The clinical course of mesangial IgA nephropathy. *Quarterly Journal of Medicine*, **53**, 227–50.

Nicholls, K.M. *et al.* (1990). Plasma exchange in progressive IgA nephropathy. *Journal of Clinical Apheresis*, **5**, 128–32.

Nicholson, G.D., Amin, U.F., and Alleyne, G.A. (1975). Membranous glomerulonephropathy with crescents. *Clinical Nephrology*, **4**, 198–201.

Nigam, P. *et al.* (1986). Rapidly progressive (crescenteric) glomerulonephritis in erythema nodosum leprosum: Case report. *Hansenology International*, **11**, 1–6.

Ntoso, K.A., Tomaszewski, J.E., Jimenez, S.A., and Neilson, E.G. (1986). Penicillamine-induced rapidly progressive glomerulonephritis in patients with progressive systemic sclerosis: Successful treatment of two patients and a review of the literature. *American Journal of Kidney Diseases*, **8**, 159–63.

Odum, J., Peh, C.A., Clarkson, A.R. *et al.* (1994). Recurrent mesangial IgA nephritis following renal transplantation. *Nephrology Dialysis Transplantation*, **9**, 309–12.

Ogami, Y. *et al.* (1989). Waldenstrom's macroglobulinemia associated with amyloidosis and crescentic glomerulonephritis. *Nephron*, **51**, 95–8.

Old, C.W., Herrera, G.A., Reimann, B.E., and Latham, R.D. (1984). Acute post-streptococcal glomerulonephritis progressing to rapidly progressive glomerulonephritis. *Southern Medical Journal*, **77**, 1470–2.

Oliver, T.B., Gouldesbrough, D.R., and Swainson, C.P. (1991). Acute crescentic glomerulonephritis associated with antiglomerular basement membrane antibody in Alport's syndrome after second transplantation. *Nephrology Dialysis Transplantation*, **6**, 893–5.

Olsson, P.J., Gaffney, E., Alexander, R.W., Mars, D.R., and Fuller, T.J. (1980). Proliferative glomerulonephritis with crescent formation in Behçet's syndrome. *Archives of Internal Medicine*, **140**, 713–14.

Öner, A., Tinaztepe, K., and Erdogan, Ö. (1995) The effect of triple therapy on the rapidly progressive type of Henoch–Schönlein nephritis. *Pediatric Nephrology* **9**, 6–10.

Panner, B.J. (1980). Rapidly progressive glomerulonephritis and possible amyloidosis. *Archives of Pathology and Laboratory Medicine*, **104**, 603–9.

Parker, M.G., Atkins, M.B., Ucci, A.A., and Levey A.S. (1995). Rapidly progressive glomerulonephritis after immunotherapy for cancer. *Journal of the American Society of Nephrology*, **5**, 1740–4

Peces, R., Riera, J.R., Arboleya, L.R., Lopez-Larrea, C., and Alvarez, J. (1987). Goodpasture's syndrome in a patient receiving penicillamine and carbimazole. *Nephron*, **45**, 316–20.

Petzel, R.A., Brown, D.C., Staley, N.A., McMillen, J.J., Sibley, R.K., and Kjellstrand, C.M. (1979). Crescentic glomerulonephritis and renal failure associated with malignant lymphoma. *American Journal of Clinical Pathology*, **71**, 728–32.

Pirson, Y., Lannoy, N., Smaers, M., Tryggvason, K., and Verellen-Dumoulin, Ch. (1992). Deletion in the COL4A5 gene and outcome of renal transplantation in Alport syndrome. *Nephrology Dialysis Transplantation*, **7**, 785 (abstract).

Pollock, C.A., Ibels, L.S., Levi, J.A., Eckstein, R.P., and Wakeford, P. (1988). Acute renal failure due to focal necrotizing glomerulonephritis in a patient with non-Hodgkin's lymphoma. Resolution with treatment of lymphoma. *Nephron*, **48**, 197–200.

Porter, K.A. *et al.* (1967). Human renal transplants I. Glomerular changes. *Laboratory Investigation*, **16**, 153–81.

Posborg Petersen, V., Kissmeyer-Nielsen, F., and Fjeldborg, O. (1966). Transmission of glomerulonephritis from host to human-kidney allotransplant. *New England Journal of Medicine*, **275**, 1269–73.

Potvliege, P.R., De Roy, G., and Dupuis, F. (1975). Necropsy study on glomerulonephritis in the elderly. *Journal of Clinical Pathology*, **28**, 891–8.

Querin, S. *et al.* (1986). Linear glomerular IgG fixation in renal allografts: incidence and significance in Alport's syndrome. *Clinical Nephrology*, **25**, 134–40.

Rassoul, Z., Al Khader A.A., Al-Sulaiman, M., Dhar, J.M., and Coode, P. (1990). Recurrent allograft antiglomerular basement membrane glomerulonephritis in a patient with Alport's syndrome. *American Journal of Nephrology*, **10**, 73–6.

Reaich, D., Cooper N., and Main J. (1994). Rapid catastrophic onset of Wegener's granulomatosis in a renal transplant. *Nephron*, **67**, 354–57.

Rees, A.J. and Cameron, J.S. (1992). Crescentic glomerulonephritis. In *Oxford textbook of clinical nephrology*, (ed. J.S. Cameron, A.M. Davison, J-P. Grünfeld, D.N.S. Kerr, and E. Ritz) pp. 418–38. Oxford University Press.

Rees, A.J., Lockwood, C.M., and Peters, D.K. (1977). Enhanced allergic tissue damage in Goodpasture's syndrome by intercurrent bacterial infection. *British Medical Journal*, **2**, 723–6.

Richardson, J.A., Rosenau, W., Lee, J.C., and Hopper, J. (1976). Kidney transplantation for rapidly progressive glomerulonephritis. *Lancet*, **ii**, 180–2.

Robles, N.R. *et al.* (1991). IgA nephropathy with rapidly progressive course after kidney transplantation. *Nephron*, **58**, 487–8.

Rosenfeld, J., Levi, J., Robson, M., Pick, A., and Ben-Bassat M. (1970). Fulminating progressive recurrent glomerulonephritis in a renal allograft. *American Journal of Medicine*, **49**, 563–7.

Rosenthal, T., Weiss, P., and Gafni, J. (1978). Renal involvement in Behçets syndrome. *Archives of Internal Medicine*, **138**, 1122–4.

Rovzar, M.A., Logan, J.L., Ogden, D.A., and Graham, A.R. (1986). Immunosuppressive therapy and plasmapheresis in rapidly progressive glomerulonephritis associated with bacterial endocarditis. *American Journal of Kidney Diseases*, **7**, 428–33.

Roy, S., Murphy, W.M., and Arant, B.S. (1981). Post-streptococcal glomerulonephritis in children: Comparison of quintuple therapy versus supportive care. *Pediatrics*, **98**, 403–10.

Sadjadi, S.A., Seelig, M.S., Berger, A.R., and Milstoc, M. (1985). Rapidly progressive glomerulonephritis in a patient with rheumatoid arthritis during treatment with high-dosage D-penicillamine. *American Journal of Nephrology*, **5**, 212–16.

Said, R., Hamzeh, Y., Tarawneh, M., El Khateeb, M., Abdeen, M., and Shaheen, A. (1989). Rapid progressive glomerulonephritis in patients with familial Mediterranean fever. *American Journal of Kidney Diseases*, **14**, 412–16.

Sanz de Castro, S. *et al.* (1988). Recidiva de glomerulonefritis membranoproliferativa tipo II en riñon transplantado con evolución rapidamente progresiva. *Nefrología*, **8**, 70–3.

Schmitt, H. *et al.* (1990). Long term prognosis of membranoproliferative glomerulonephritis type I. Significance of clinical and morphological parameters: an investigation of 220 cases. *Nephron*, **55**, 242–50.

Schmitt, H., Haubitz, M., Mistry, N., Brunkhorst, N., Erbslöh–Möller, and Gross, W.L. (1993). Renal transplantation in Wegener's granulomatosis. *Lancet*, **342**, 860 (letter).

Shah, B., First, M.R., Mendoza, N.C., Clyne, D.H., Alexander, J.W., and Weiss, M.A. (1988). Alport's syndrome: risk of glomerulonephritis induced by anti-glomerular-basement membrane antibody after renal transplantation. *Nephron*, **50**, 34–8.

Sherson, D. and Jorgensen, F. (1989). Rapidly progressive crescenteric glomerulonephritis in a sandblaster with silicosis. *British Journal of Industrial Medicine*, **46**, 675–6.

Singhal, P.C., Chugh, K.S., Kaur, S., and Malik, A.K. (1977). Acute renal failure in leprosy. *International Journal of Leprosy and Other Mycobacterial Diseases*, **45**, 171–4.

Sitprija, V. and Boonpucknavig, V. (1980). Extracapillary glomerulonephritis in Russell's viper bite. *British Medical Journal*, **280**, 1417.

Sonsino, E. *et al.* (1972). Extracapillary proliferative glomerulonephritis: so-called malignant glomerulonephritis. *Advances in Nephrology*, **2**, 121–63

Sopeña, B. *et al.* (1991). Rapidly progressive glomerulonephritis and pulmonary tuberculosis. *Nephron*, **57**, 251–2.

SPNSG (Southwest Pediatric Nephrology Study Group) (1985). A clinopathological study of crescentic glomerulonephritis in 50 children. *Kidney International*, **27**, 450–8.

Srivastava, R.N., Mougdil, A., Bagga, A., Vasudev AS., Bhuyan UN., and Sundraem, K.R. (1992). Crescentic glomerulonephritis in children: a review of 43 cases. *American Journal of Nephrology*, **12**, 155–61.

Steinman, T.J., Jaffe, B., Monaco, A.P., Wolff, S.M., and Fauci, A.S. (1980). Recurrence of Wegener's granulomatosis after kidney transplantation. Successful induction of remission with cyclophosphamide. *American Journal of Medicine*, 68, 458–60.

Streather, C.P. and Scoble, J.E. (1994). Recurrent IgA nephropathy in a renal allograft presenting as crescentic glomerulonephritis. *Nephron*, 66, 113–14.

Sternlieb, I., Bennett, B., and Scheinberg, I.H. (1975). D-penicillamine induced Goodpasture's syndrome in Wilson's disease. *Annals of Internal Medicine*, 82, 673–6.

Stilmant, M.M., Bolton, W.K., Sturgill, B.C., Schmitt, G.W., and Couser, W.G. (1979). Crescentic glomerulonephritis without immune deposits: clinicopathologic features. *Kidney International*, 15, 184–95.

Swainson, C.P. *et al.* (1982). Plasma exchange in the successful treatment of drug induced renal disease. *Nephron*, 30, 244–9.

Tateno, S., Sakai, T., Kobayashi, Y., and Shigematsu, H. (1981). Idiopathic membranous glomerulonephritis with crescents. *Acta Pathologica Japonica*, 31, 211–19.

Taylor, T.K. *et al.* (1979). Membranous nephropathy with epithelial crescents in a patient with pulmonary sarcoidosis. *Archives of Internal Medicine*, 139, 1183–5.

Teruel, J.L., Liaño, F., Mampaso, F., Morteno, J., Querada, C., and Ortuño, J. (1987). Allograft antiglomerular basement membrane glomerulonephritis in a patient with Alport's syndrome. *Nephron*, 46, 43–4.

Tietjen, D.P. and Moore, W.J. (1990). Treatment of rapidly progressive glomerulonephritis due to Behçet's syndrome with intravenous cyclophosphamide. *Nephron*, 55, 69–73.

Treser, G. *et al.* (1969). Antigenic streptococcal component in acute glomerulonephritis. *Science*, 163, 676–9.

Tsunemi, M. *et al.* (1993). A case of crescentic glomerulonephritis associated with polymyositis. *Nephron*, 64, 488–9.

Turner, D.R. *et al.* (1974). Transplantation in mesangiocapillary glomerulonephritis with intramembranous dense 'deposits'. *Kidney International*, 9, 439–48.

Turney, J.H., Adu, D., Michael, J., and McMaster, F. (1986). Recurrent crescentic glomerulonephritis in renal transplant recipient treated with cyclosporin. *Lancet*, i, 1104 (letter).

Van der Heuvel, L.P.W.J. *et al.* (1989). The development of anti-glomerular basement membrane nephritis in two children with Alport's syndrome after renal transplantation: characterization of the antibody target. *Pediatric Nephrology*, 3, 406–13.

Vanhille Ph. *et al.* (1986). Glomérulonéphrite rapidement progressive à dépôts mesangiaux d'IgA au cours d'une sarcoïdose. *Néphrologie*, 5, 207–9.

Velosa, J.A. (1987). Idiopathic crescentic glomerulonephritis or systemic vasculitis? *Mayo Clinic Proceedings*, 62, 145–7.

Vernier, I., Pourrat, J.P., Mignon Conte, M.A., Hemery, M., Dueymes, J.M., and Conte, J.J. (1987). Rapidly progressive glomerulonephritis associated with amyloidosis: Efficacy of plasma exchange. *Journal of Clinical Apheresis*, 3, 226–9.

Wakabayashi, Y., Kobayashi, Y., and Shigematsu, H. (1985). Shunt nephritis: histological dynamics following removal of the shunt. *Nephron*, 40, 111–17.

Walker, P.D., Deeves, E.C., Sahaba, G., Wallin, J.D., and O'Neill, W.M.J.R. (1984). Rapidly progressive glomerulonephritis in a patient with syphilis. Identification of antitreponemal antibody and treponemal antigen in renal tissue. *American Journal of Medicine*, 76, 1106–12.

Weber, M., Kohler, H., Fries, J., Thoenes, W., and Meyer Zum Buschenfelde, K.H. (1985). Rapidly progressive glomerulonephritis in IgA/IgG cryoglobulinemia. *Nephron*, 41, 258–61.

Wegmuller, E., Weidmann, P., Hess, T., and Reubi, F.C. (1985). Rapidly progressive glomerulonephritis accompanying Legionnaire's disease. *Archives of Internal Medicine*, **145**, 1711–13.

Welch, T.R., McAdams, A.J., and Berry, A. (1988). Rapidly progressive IgA nephropathy. *American Journal of Diseases of Childhood*, **142**, 789–93.

Whitworth, J.A., Morel-Maroger, L., Mignon, F., and Richet, G. (1976). The significance of extracapillary proliferation. Clinicopathological review of 60 patients. *Nephron*, **16**, 1–19.

Williams, W.W., Shah, D.J., Morgan, A.G., and Alleyne, G.A.O. (1985). Membranous glomerulopathy with crescents in systemic lupus erythematosus. *American Journal of Nephrology*, **5**, 158–62.

Yeung, C.K., Wong, K.L., Wong, W.S., Ng, M.T., Chan, K.W., and Ng, W.L. (1984). Crescentic lupus glomerulonephritis. *Clinical Nephrology*, **21**, 251–8.

Yoshida, A., Morozumi, K., Takeda, A., and Koyama, K. (1992). A case of rapidly progressive glomerulonephritis associated with bucillamine-treated rheumatoid arthritis. *American Journal of Kidney Diseases*, **20**, 411–13.

Zent, R., van Zyl Smit, R., Duffield, M., and Cassidy M.J.D. (1994). Crescentic nephritis at Groote Schuur hospital, South Africa—not a benign disease. *Clinical Nephrology*, **42**, 22–9.

10

Rapidly progressive glomerulonephritis in children

Michael J. Dillon

Rapidly progressive glomerulonephritis is the clinical correlate of the histologically defined condition of crescentic glomerulonephritis (Heptinstall 1983). It is relatively rare in childhood (Southwest Pediatric Nephrology Study Group, SPNSG 1985; Niaudet and Lévy 1983; Cunningham *et al.* 1980; Anand *et al.* 1975), and is characterized by the presence of extensive crescents in renal biopsy specimens and by a sudden and progressive decline in renal function.

As discussed in previous chapters, crescentic glomerulonephritis can accompany most forms of primary glomerulonephritis in childhood. However, in this age group it is associated also with various systemic diseases, such as systemic lupus erythematosus and several forms of systemic vasculitis (SPNSG 1985; Niaudet and Lévy 1983). The severity of the condition, the multiple aetiologies, and the associated poor prognosis have led to the use of multiple treatment regimens, the efficacy of which has been difficult to assess (Haycock 1988), and there has been lack of clarity in identifying variables with possible therapeutic and prognostic implications.

Definition

Crescentic glomerulonephritis has been defined in a number of ways and this varied nomenclature has created problems in interpreting data and comparing outcome of treatment in patients. It is agreed (Chapter 4) that crescentic glomerulonephritis is defined by the presence of large epithelial crescents within Bowman's space, but their appearance and the number of crescents that is required for the diagnosis is arguable. In childhood, more than 75% (Niaudet and Lévy 1983), 50% or more (SPNSG 1985), and occasionally even 20% of glomeruli affected have been considered to represent crescentic glomerulonephritis (Anand *et al.* 1975). In one series of 39 patients with rapidly progressive glomerulonephritis (RPGN) and extensive crescent formation (Neild *et al.* 1983), 10 patients were under 14 years of age and all had more than 60% of glomeruli affected. In another series of 13 children with RPGN (Cunningham *et al.* 1980), the number of glomeruli affected varied from 10% to 100%. Others emphasize the clinical features of RPGN irrespective of the number of crescents (Robson *et al.* 1981).

In the series reported from Great Ormond Street, London (Jardim *et al.* 1992) crescentic glomerulonephritis was defined as the presence of large epithelial crescents filling Bowman's space in 50% or more of glomeruli present in the biopsy specimen, irrespective of any changes in the underlying glomerular tuft. Crescents were divided into cellular, fibrocellular, or fibrous according to their histological appearance, and further subcategorized according to various criteria, including glomerular tuft changes, immunochemical staining, and clinicopathological correlations. These will be described in more detail later in this chapter.

Incidence

The true incidence of crescentic glomerulonephritis in childhood is unknown. In adults, it comprises 2–5% of all cases of glomerulonephritis (Cole and Salinas-Madrigal 1994) and the calculated annual incidence in Germany is 0.7/100 000 (Andrassy 1991). Of 372 children with glomerular pathology on renal biopsy reported by Miller *et al.* (1984), crescentic lesions were present in 56 patients and in 26 there was a clinical course compatible with RPGN. These data are somewhat similar to those quoted for adults and confirm the relative rarity of the disorder in childhood.

Causes

The diseases causing crescentic glomerulonephritis can be considered in a number of ways. Some classifications subdivide the types of disorder according to three immunofluorescence staining patterns on renal biopsy: (1) anti-glomerular basement membrane (GBM) antibody; (2) no staining or pauci-immune; and (3) immune complex (Bidani and Lewis 1992; Cole and Salinas-Madrigal 1994). Using these criteria the most frequently observed pattern in childhood (in contrast to adults) is immune complex disease, constituting approximately 80% of cases, with pauci-immune and anti-GBM disease making up the remainder in a ratio of 2:1 (Cole and Salinas-Madrigal 1994; Jardim *et al.* 1992; SPNSG 1985).

Other classifications consider rapidly progressive glomerulonephritis/crescentic glomerulonephritis under disease category headings that include: anti-GBM disease, primary systemic vasculitides, systemic disorders such as systemic lupus erythematosus, primary glomerulonephritides, infection-related glomerulonephritides, and various miscellaneous causes (Table 10.1). Considering three large series of childhood patients with crescentic glomerulonephritis reported from the USA, France, and the UK, the pattern of disease was similar, but with some variation between centres (SPNSG 1985; Niaudet and Lévy 1983; Jardim *et al.* 1992).

In 1985, the Southwest Pediatric Nephrology Study Group reported data on 50 children who fulfilled the entry criterion of having 50% or more glomeruli affected by crescents on renal biopsy. Of these, 13 had non-specified immune complex disease, 9 systemic lupus erythematosus, 7 idiopathic (no immune complexes) crescentic glomerulonephritis, 6 poststreptococcal glomerulonephritis, 4 IgA nephropathy, 3 Henoch–Schönlein purpura, 3 vasculitis, 3 possible anti-GBM disease, and 2 dense deposit disease.

Table 10.1 Causes of rapidly progressive glomerulonephritis in childhood

Anti-glomerular basement membrane antibody disease
Goodpasture's syndrome or isolated anti-GBM nephritis.

Primary systemic vasculitis
Henoch–Schönlein purpura, Wegener's granulomatosis, microscopic polyarteritis,
Churg–Strauss syndrome, 'idiopathic'.

Systemic disorders
Systemic lupus erythematosus, Behçet's syndrome, Weber–Christian disease, relapsing
polychondritis, essential mixed cryoglobulinaemia.

Primary glomerulonephritis
Mesangiocapillary glomerulonephritis, IgA nephropathy, membranous nephropathy.

Infection-related glomerulonephritis
Poststreptococcal glomerulonephritis, other post-infectious glomerulonephritides,
bacterial endocarditis, shunt nephritis, hepatitis B nephropathy.

Miscellaneous causes
Drugs (penicillamine, rifampicin, etc.).
Solid tumours and lymphomas.

The paper from Paris by Niaudet and Lévy (1983) reported 41 children with
more than 75% crescents on biopsy. Of these, 11 had Henoch–Schönlein
purpura, 9 membranoproliferative glomerulonephritis, 5 acute glomerulonephritis, 3 anti-GBM disease, 3 IgA nephropathy, 3 polyarteritis, 3 glomerulonephritis
without deposits, 2 immune complex glomerulonephritis, 1 systemic lupus
erythematosus, and 1 shunt nephritis.

The paper from London by Jardim *et al.* (1992) reported 30 children with
crescentic glomerulonephritis, using 50% or more crescents on biopsy as the
inclusion criterion. Of these, 9 had Henoch–Schönlein purpura, 7 mesangiocapillary glomerulonephritis (6 type I and 1 type III), 5 vasculitis (3 microscopic
polyarteritis, 1 polyarteritis nodosa, 1 Wegener's granulomatosis), 4 idiopathic
crescentic nephritis, 2 poststreptococcal glomerulonephritis, 2 anti-GBM
glomerulonephritis, and 1 systemic lupus erythematosus. Table 10.2 compares
the distribution of causes in these three series.

Clinical presentation

The majority of children with crescentic glomerulonephritis present with an
acute nephritic picture, with hypertension, volume overload, renal impairment,
proteinuria, and haematuria. In those in whom the crescentic glomerulonephritis
is secondary to or associated with a systemic disorder, clinical features of this
may also be present and helpful diagnostically. Of the 30 patients reviewed at
Great Ormond Street, London (Jardim *et al.* 1992), oedema was present at onset
in 24 and hypertension in 19. All patients had haematuria and this was macro-

Table 10.2 Causes of crescentic glomerulonephritis in children (%). Comparison of relative occurrences in three large paediatric series

	SWPNSG* (1985) n = 50	Niaudet & Lévy (1983) n = 41	Jardim *et al.* (1992) n = 30
Non-specified immune complex disease	26	4.8	–
Systemic lupus erythematosus	18	2.4	3.3
Idiopathic crescentic glomerulonephritis	14	7.3	13.3
Post-streptococcal glomerulonephritis	12	12.1	6.6
IgA nephropathy	8	7.3	–
Henoch–Schönlein purpura	6	26.8	30
Vasculitis	6	7.3	16.6
Anti-GBM disease	6	7.3	6.6
Mesangiocapillary glomerulonephritis	4	21.9	23.3
Shunt nephritis	–	2.4	–

* SWPNSG, Southwest Pediatric Nephrology Study Group.

scopic in 15. Oliguria requiring peritoneal dialysis for fluid control was present in 15. The glomerular filtration rate (GFR) was less than 30 ml/min per 1.73 m^2 at presentation in 22 patients, and between 30 and 60 ml/min per 1.73 m^2 in the remaining 8. Proteinuria was present in all patients, with nephrotic syndrome present in 14. These data are similar to those recorded in other reports in the literature (SPNSG 1985; Niaudet and Lévy 1983; Cunningham *et al.* 1980), although there is a fairly wide spectrum of presenting features.

Laboratory investigations substantiate the clinical impression of renal impairment and confirm the presence of blood and protein in the urine. Anaemia is frequently present, and may be more marked than anticipated (Cole and Salinas–Madrigal 1994), usually with a normochromic and normocytic blood film. Serological abnormalities vary according to the underlying disease state. Hypocomplementaemia is not uncommon in immune complex disease and systemic lupus erythematosus, whereas in anti-GBM disease there are anti-GBM antibodies in the circulation (Levin *et al.* 1983). Raised antistreptolysin O (ASO) levels with or without raised anti-DNAse B levels are a feature of poststreptococcal glomerulonephritis, but they can be increased coincidentally in other forms of crescentic glomerulonephritis and may, therefore, not be diagnostically helpful. Antinuclear and anti-dsDNA antibodies point to a diagnosis of systemic lupus erythematosus nephritis, and elevated levels of antineutrophil cytoplasmic antibodies (ANCA) may reflect an underlying vasculitic cause (e.g. Wegener's granulomatosis or microscopic polyarteritis, Dillon and Tizard 1991).

In our series (Jardim *et al.* 1992) plasma C3 concentrations were low in 9/30 patients (3 mesangiocapillary glomerulonephritis, 2 idiopathic crescentic nephritis, 2 poststreptococcal glomerulonephritis, 1 systemic lupus erythematosus,

1 anti-GBM nephritis). The ASO titre was raised in 5 patients (2 poststrepto-coccal glomerulonephritis, 1 Wegener's granulomatosis, 1 Henoch–Schönlein purpura, 1 microscopic polyarteritis). Of the 6 patients tested, 3 had raised ANCA (1 Wegener's granulomatosis, 2 microscopic polyarteritis). At that time the ANCA positivity was defined in terms of a crude neutrophil extract ELISA, and it was not possible to distinguish between cytoplasmic and perinuclear stain-ing on indirect immunofluorescence, nor to define which antigen the ANCA were directed towards (proteinase 3 or myeloperoxidase). Subsequently, Wong *et al.* (1993) have shown that in childhood idiopathic crescentic glomerulonephritis tests for ANCA have been positive with a p-ANCA pattern on indirect immunofluorescence, whereas in children with Wegener's granulomatosis a cyto-plasmic staining pattern (c-ANCA) was seen.

Histopathology

The histopathological features seen in renal biopsy material from adults with rapidly progressive glomerulonephritis and crescentic glomerulonephritis have been described in previous chapters. Suffice it to say that there is some contro-versy as to how many glomeruli have to be associated with crescents in order to designate the disease as 'crescentic glomerulonephritis'. Authors vary in their views, and more than 75% (Niaudet and Lévy 1983), 50% or more (SPNSG 1985; Jardim *et al.* 1992), and occasionally even 20% of glomeruli affected have been considered to represent crescentic glomerulonephritis (Anand *et al.* 1975). In addition, there is a need to characterize the nature of the crescents: (1) cellu-lar crescents are those in which there is prominent proliferation of epithelial cells, with some admixture of macrophages and occasionally neutrophils filling the urinary space and compressing the tuft; (2) fibrocellular crescents are those in which strands of membrane-like material and collagen fibres are present among the cells forming the crescent; and (3) fibrous crescents are those in which the cells in the crescent have virtually all disappeared to be replaced by collagen (Jardim *et al.* 1992).

The diagnosis of the underlying renal disease needs to be based on various criteria: (1) the associated changes in the glomerular tuft, such as mesangio-capillary glomerulonephritis; (2) the immunochemical staining, such as the pre-sence of linear IgG staining in anti-GBM glomerulonephritis; and (3) clinicopathological freatures, such as in polyarteritis nodosa, Wegener's granulo-matosis, and microscopic polyarteritis (Jardim *et al.* 1992). However, the identification of the underlying glomerulonephritis is often difficult. Immuno-fluorescence studies prove helpful in, for example, mesangiocapillary glomeru-lonephritis, anti-GBM disease, and IgA nephropathy. Some cases appear to be 'idiopathic', but this remains a diagnosis of exclusion.

On the basis of these criteria, the 30 patients reviewed by Jardim *et al.* (1992) were subdivided into two groups: those with 50–79% crescents and those with 80% or more crescents (Table 10.3). It was clear that the relationship between the nature of the crescents and the subsequent outcome was much more import-

Table 10.3 Clinical, pathological, and management details of 30 children with crescentic glomerulonephritis (from Jardim *et al.* 1992, with permission)

Patient	Age (yrs)	Sex	Diagnosis	Crescents (%)	Fibrous crescents	PD	PE	Steroids	Cyclo	Aza	Anticoag	Follow-up (yrs)	Outcome
Group 1 (50–79% crescents)													
1	15.7	F	SLE	50	–	–	+	+	+	–	–	0.48	(b)
2	3.8	M	HSP	50	+	–	+	+	–	–	+	9.49	ESRF
3	6.6	F	HSP	60	–	–	+	+	–	+	+	1.67	ESRF
4	9.1	M	HSP	60	+	–	+	+	+	+	+	1.76	(c)
5	8.0	F	MCGN III	70	–	–	–	–	–	–	+	3.33	(c)
6	10.4	F	MCGN I	50	–	–	–	+	+	–	–	4.85	(c)
7	10.6	M	MCGN I	50	–	–	+	–	–	–	+	1.80	ESRF
8	12.2	F	MCGN I	55	–	–	+	+	–	+	+	2.48	(c)
9	12.6	F	MCGN I	70	+	+	+	+	+	+	–	0.15	ESRF
10	8.0	M	PSGN	75	–	–	–	MP	–	–	–	2.21	(a)
Group 2 (>80% crescents)													
11	6.6	M	HSP	85	+	–	+	+	+	+	+	5.38	(a)
12	9.3	F	HSP	100	–	–	+	MP	+	–	+	1.14	(b)
13	8.0	M	HSP	80	–	+	+	+	+	–	+	0.97	(b)
14	11.8	M	HSP	80	–	–	+	+	+	+	+	1.64	(a)
15	10.6	F	HSP	80	+	–	+	+	+	–	+	2.25	ESRF
16	8.5	M	HSP	100	+	+	+	+	+	+	+	0.98	ESRF
17	10.7	F	GBM	80	–	+	+	+	+	–	+	0.04	ESRF
18	7.4	F	GBM	100	+	+	+	+	+	+	+	0.97	ESRF
19	9.5	M	PAN	80	–	–	+	+	–	–	+	9.15	(b)
20	11.2	M	Mic Pol	100	–	+	+	+	+	+	+	2.12	(a)
21	10.8	F	Mic Pol	94	+	+	+	+	+	–	+	0.21	ESRF
22	12.3	F	Mic Pol	100	+	+	+	+	+	+	–	0.10	ESRF
23	11.6	F	Wegener's	100	–	–	+	+	+	+	–	1.73	(b)

242

Table 10.3 *(Continued)*

Patient	Age (yrs)	Sex	Diagnosis	Crescents (%)	Fibrous crescents	PD	PE	Steroids	Cyclo	Aza	Anticoag	Follow-up (yrs)	Outcome
24	11.9	M	Idiopathic	100	–	+	+	+	+	+	+	0.73	ESRF
25	6.5	F	Idiopathic	100	–	+	+	+	+	+	+	2.59	(b)
26	7.2	F	Idiopathic	100	+	+	–	+	+	–	+	2.83	ESRF
27	9.8	F	Idiopathic	100	+	+	–	+	–	+	+	0.58	ESRF
28	9.7	M	MCGN I	80	+	+	–	+	+	–	+	0.24	ESRF
29	11.4	f	MCGN I	90	–	+	+	+	+	+	+	2.88	ESRF
30	3.7	M	PSGN	90	–	+	+	+	+	–	+	0.38	ESRF

Abbreviations: PD, peritoneal dialysis; SLE, systemic lupus erythematosus; PE, plasma exchange; HSP, Henoch–Schönlein purpura; MP, methylprednisolone; MCGN, mesangiocapillary glomerulonephritis type I, type III; ESRF, end-stage renal failure; PAN, polyarteritis nodosa; GBM, anti-glomerular basement membrane glomerulonephritis; Mic Pol, microscopic polyarteritis; PSGN, poststreptococcal glomerulonephritis; Cyclo, cyclophosphamide; Aza, azathioprine; Anticoag, anticoagulants; (a), glomerular filtration rate (GFR) >80 ml/min per 1.73 m^2; (b), GFR 30–80 ml/min per 1.73 m^2; (c) GFR <30 ml/min per 1.73 m^2.

ant than the percentage of glomeruli affected by crescents (Jardim *et al.* 1992). Fibrous crescents have a worse prognosis than cellular or fibrocellular crescents. Furthermore, the histological appearances of the crescents can change quite rapidly from cellular to fibrous, especially if therapeutic intervention is delayed and sometimes despite such intervention.

Treatment and outcome

The heterogeneity and poor outcome of childhood crescentic glomerulonephritis have led to multiple treatment regimens. Steroids (oral or high dose intra-venous), cytotoxic agents, anticoagulants, antiplatelet agents, and plasma ex-change, alone or in different combinations, have all been described (SPNSG 1985; Niaudet and Lévy 1983; Haycock 1988; Neild *et al.* 1983; Ferraris *et al.* 1983; Jardim *et al.* 1992).

High-dose intravenous methyl prednisolone, often advocated in adults (Bolton and Sturgill 1989), has been utilized in children with crescentic glomerulonephri-tis (Ferraris *et al.* 1983) coupled with cyclophosphamide; in this series long-term renal recovery occurred in five children after a mean follow-up of 35 months. Methyl prednisolone has also been used alone in 29 children with severe prolifer-ative glomerulonephritis (Robson *et al.* 1981), with a favourable outcome (GFR > 80 ml/min/1.73 m^2) observed in 18 (62%) after a mean follow-up of 35 months.

Results of combined immunosuppressive and anticoagulant therapy have been reported by the SPNSG (1985) with 24 of 47 (52%) patients recovering renal function. The benefit of anticoagulants in this regimen is emphasized by Cunningham *et al.* (1980) who reported renal function recovery in 7 of 13 (54%) patients with crescentic glomerulonephritis. With a similar regimen, Niaudet and Lévy (1983) found renal functional recovery in 19 of 41 (47%) patients.

Treatment regimens used in the study of Jardim *et al.* (1992) included plasma exchange, corticosteroids, anticoagulant and antiplatelet agents, cyclophos-phamide, and azathioprine, in varying combinations (see Table 10.3). Twenty-four patients underwent plasma exchange (mean five sessions each) and of these 13 (54%) progressed to end-stage renal failure (ESRF). Of the 6 children who did not undergo plasma exchange, 3 (50%) also progressed to ESRF. Steroids were used in 27 (2 of whom received intravenous boluses of methyl pred-nisolone), and 22 patients received cyclophosphamide which was changed to aza-thioprine after 8 weeks in 13. Anticoagulant agents were used in 25 patients. Fifteen patients, one from group 1 and 14 from group 2 (Table 10.3) required peritoneal dialysis at onset.

The disease duration between the onset of symptoms and the treatment was less than one month in 19 of 30 patients. Of these 19 patients, 9 had oliguria on presentation and progressed rapidly to ESRF despite treatment, 6 presented with an initial GFR less than 30 ml/min/1.73 m^2 which persisted in 2, and improved to more than 30 ml/min/1.73 m^2 in 4, and in the remaining 4 patients the values of the GFR were above 30 ml/min/1.73 m^2 on presentation and were stable or had increased at the latest follow-up. In 5 of 30 patients the treatment began 1–3 months after disease onset. Of these, 4 had an initial GFR less than 30 ml/min/1.73 m², which improved to values above 80 in 2 patients, remained stable in 1, and deteriorated to ESRF in another. The fifth patient in this group had a reduction in his initial GFR from 37–25 ml/min/1.73 m² at 3 years follow-up. Six children were treated after 3 months of disease evolution and all progressed to ESRF despite an initial GFR above 30 ml/min/1.73 m² in 3.

The benefits of plasma exchange in anti-GBM nephritis have been demonstrated in adult patients (Lockwood *et al.* 1977) and have led to its use in other disorders, such as immune complex-mediated rapidly progressive glomerulonephritis (Lockwood *et al.* 1977). An additional effect of plasma exchange and immunosuppression in adults with RPGN has been described (Thysell *et al.* 1982), but this could not be confirmed by others (Glockner *et al.* 1988). However, one controlled trial suggested that dialysis-dependent patients were more likely to recover renal function if treated with plasma exchange (Pusey *et al.* 1991). Jardim *et al.* (1992) treated 24 children by plasma exchange. Although, statistically, there was no significant difference in the outcome between patients who were and who were not exchanged, 9 of the 10 patients with GFR greater than 30 ml/min/ 1.73 m² at latest follow-up received this treatment. In 7 patients, the presenting GFR was less than 30, and in 2 between 30 and 60 ml/min/1.73 m². Only 1 of the 9 patients had fibrous crescents on presentation. The majority of the 13 patients who progressed to ESRF, despite plasma exchange, had fibrous crescents on presentation, and this may have contributed to the failure of this treatment. Plasma exchange was also used in 7 of 41 patients reported by Niaudet and Lévy (1983). However, only the two patients not requiring dialysis on presentation recovered renal function. The need for dialysis at onset appears to predict a worse outcome. This was shown in the Great Ormond Street series (Jardim *et al.* 1992) and in others (Niaudet and Lévy 1983; Neild *et al.* 1983).

The interval between disease onset and starting treatment has been considered of prognostic value in rapidly progressive glomerulonephritis (Robson *et al.* 1981). In the Great Ormond Street series, the results seem to confirm this. Patients who had treatment initiated 3 months after disease onset developed ESRF. Patients treated 1–3 months from disease onset had variable results (2/5 recovered renal function), but the 12 patients who responded were all treated in the first month of clinical symptoms (Jardim *et al.* 1992).

In the Jardim *et al.* (1992) study, ESRF was associated with mesangiocapillary glomerulonephritis in 4 of 7 patients, and in the remaining 3 follow-up GFR was less than 30 ml/min/1.73 m². The proportion going on to ESRF was less than that reported by Habib *et al.* (1973), in whose study 15 of 16 children progressed to renal failure. Anti-GBM crescentic glomerulonephritis usually rapidly progresses to renal failure, although Lockwood *et al.* (1976) reported functional improvement in adults with plasma exchange instituted early in the disease in non-anuric patients. Even in anuric patients an occasional response, albeit short term, can be achieved by intense plasma exchange as has been demonstrated in the child reported by Levin *et al.* (1983).

It has been accepted that poststreptococcal rapidly progressive glomerulonephritis has a better prognosis, with spontaneous improvement after supportive management (SPNSG 1985; Whitworth *et al.* 1976). No advantage has been found for immunosuppression and anticoagulants over conservative management in children with poststreptococcal crescentic glomerulonephritis (Roy *et al.* 1981). However, progression to renal failure has been reported in children (Niaudet and Lévy 1983; Cunningham *et al.* 1980; Anand *et al.* 1975; Jardim *et al.* 1992).

Conclusion

Rapidly progressive glomerulonephritis associated with crescentic glomerulonephritis on biopsy is relatively rare in children, but does occur. It has multiple aetiologies but, at least in Europe, Henoch–Schönlein purpura and mesangiocapillary glomerulonephritis are the commonest. In spite of therapeutic endeavours, ESRF develops in approximately 50% of patients. Poor prognostic factors include fibrous crescents and the need for dialysis at onset. The number of crescents does not affect outcome. Plasma exchange may have a therapeutic role in children, but results suggest that its benefit may be limited to patients without fibrous crescents at presentation. The association between fibrous crescents and progression to renal failure emphasizes the need for prompt diagnosis and treatment if beneficial results are to be expected.

References

Andrassy, K., Kuster, S., Waldherr, R., and Ritz, E. (1991). Rapidly progressive glomerulonephritis: analysis of prevalence and clinical course. *Nephron*, **59**, 206–12.

Anand, S.K., Trygstad, C.W., and Sharma, H.M., and Northway, J.D. (1975). Extracapillary proliferative glomerulonephritis in children. *Pediatrics*, **56**, 434–42.

Bidani, A.K. and Lewis, E.J. (1992). Idiopathic rapidly progressive glomerulonephritis and Goodpasture's syndrome. In *Pediatric kidney disease* (2nd edn), (ed. C.M. Edelmann) pp. 1223–45. Little, Brown, Boston.

Bolton, W.K. and Sturgill, B.C. (1989). Methylprednisolone therapy for acute crescentic rapidly progressive glomerulonephritis. *American Journal of Nephrology*, **9**, 368–75.

Cole, B.R. and Salinas-Madrigal, L. (1994). Acute proliferative glomerulonephritis and crescentic glomerulonephritis. In *Pediatric nephrology* (3rd edn), (ed. M.A. Holliday, T.M. Barratt, and E.D. Avner), pp. 697–718. Williams & Wilkins, Baltimore.

Cunningham, R.J., Gilfoil, M., Cavallo, T., Brouhard, B., Travis, L., Berger, M. *et al.* (1980). Rapidly progressive glomerulonephritis in children: a report of thirteen cases and a review of the literature. *Pediatric Research*, **14**, 128–32.

Dillon, M.J. and Tizard, E.J. (1991). Antineutrophil cytoplasmic antibodies and anti-endothelial cell antibodies. *Pediatric Nephrology*, **5**, 256–9.

Ferraris, J.R., Gallo, G.E., Ramirez, J., Iotti, R., and Gianantonio, C. (1983). 'Pulse' methylprednisolone therapy in the treatment of acute crescentic glomerulonephritis. *Nephron*, **34**, 207–8.

Glockner, W.H., Sieberth, H.G., Wichmann, H.E., Backes, E., Bambauer, R., Boesken, W.H. *et al.* (1988). Plasma exchange and immunosuppression in rapidly progressive glomerulonephritis: a controlled, multi-centre study. *Clinical Nephrology*, **29**, 1–8.

Habib, R., Kleinknecht, C., Gubler, M.C., and Levy, M. (1973). Idiopathic membranoproliferative glomerulonephritis in children. Report of 105 cases. *Clinical Nephrology*, 1, 194–14.

Haycock, G.B. (1988). The treatment of glomerulonephritis in children. *Pediatric Nephrology*, 2, 247–55.

Heptinstall, R.H. (1983). Crescentic glomerulonephritis. In *Pathology of the kidney* (3rd edn), (ed. R.H. Heptinstall) pp. 443–7. Little, Brown, Boston.

Jardim, H.M.P.F., Leake, J., Risdon, R.A., Barratt, T.M., and Dillon, M.J. (1992). Crescentic glomerulonephritis in children. *Pediatric Nephrology*, 6, 231–5.

Levin, M., Rigden, S.P.A., Pincott, J.R., Lockwood, C.M., Barratt, T.M., and Dillon, M.J. (1983). Goodpasture's syndrome: treatment with plasmapheresis, immunosuppression, and anti-coagulation. *Archives of Diseases in Childhood*, 58, 697–702.

Lockwood, C.M., Rees, A.J., Pearson, T.A., Evans, D.J., Peters, D.K., and Wilson, C.B. (1976). Immunosuppression and plasma exchange in the treatment of Goodpasture's syndrome. *Lancet*, I, 711–15.

Lockwood, C.M., Rees, A.J., Pinching, A.J., Pussell, B., Sweny, P., Uff, J. *et al.* (1977). Plasma exchange and immunosuppression in the treatment of fulminating immune-complex mediated crescentic nephritis. *Lancet*, i, 63–7.

Miller, M.N., Baumal, R., Poucell, S., and Steele, B.T. (1984). Incidence and prognostic importance of glomerular crescents in renal disease of childhood. *American Journal of Nephrology*, 4, 244.

Neild, G.H., Cameron, J.S., Ogg, C.S., Turner, D.R., Williams, D.G., Brown, C.B. *et al.* (1983). Rapidly progressive glomerulonephritis with extensive glomerular crescent formation. *Quarterly Journal of Medicine*, 52, 395–416.

Niaudet, P. and Lévy, M. (1983). Glomérulonéphrites à croissants diffus. In *Néphrologie pédiatrique* (3rd edn), (ed. P. Royer, R. Habib, H. Mathieu, and M. Broyer) pp. 381–94. Flammarion, Paris.

Pusey, C.D., Rees, A.J., Evans, D.J., Peters, O.K., and Lockwood, C.M. (1991). Plasma exchange in focal necrotizing glomeselomphritis without anti-GBM antibodies. *Kidney International*, 40, 757–63.

Robson, A.M., Rose, G.M., Cole, B.R., and Ingelfinger, J.R. (1981). The treatment of severe glomerulopathies in children with intravenous methylprednisolone pulses. *Proceedings of the 8th International Congress on Nephrology, Athens*, pp. 305–11. Karger, Basel.

Roy III, S., Murphy, W.M., and Arant, B.S. (1981). Poststreptococcal crescentic glomerulonephritis in children: comparison of quintuple therapy versus supportive care. *Journal of Pediatrics*, 98, 403–10.

SPNSG (Southwest Pediatric Nephrology Study Group) (1985). A clinicopathological study of crescentic glomerulonephritis in 50 children. *Kidney International*, 27, 450–8.

Thysell, H., Bygren, P., Bengtsson, U., Lindholm, T., Norlin, M., Jonsson, M. *et al.* (1982). Immunosuppression and the additive effect of plasma exchange in treatment of rapidly progressive glomerulonephritis. *Acta Medica Scandinavica*, 212, 107–14.

Whitworth, J.A., Morel-Maroger, L., Mignon, F., and Richet, G. (1976). The significance of extracapillary proliferation: Clinico-pathological review of 60 patients. *Nephron*, 16, 1–19.

Wong, S-N., Shah, V., Dillon, M.J. (1993). The spectrum of anti-neutrophil cytoplasmic antibodies (ANCA) in childhood systemic vasculitis. *Clinical and Experimental Immunology*, 93(suppl. 1), 30 (abstract).

11

Novel treatment strategies in rapidly progressive glomerulonephritis

Peter W. Mathieson and C. Martin Lockwood

There is no other area in nephrology in which such radical transformation in prognosis has occurred during the last 20 years as it has for patients with rapidly progressive glomerulonephritis (RPGN). In 1973, the outlook for kidney survival was dismal (Cameron 1978). Now nephrologists expect most patients with RPGN to achieve sustained recovery of renal function, even if they present dependent on dialysis. What has led to these increased expectations? Undoubtedly, a major factor has been the recognition that autoimmune mechanisms play an important role in the development of almost all forms of RPGN, leading to the realization that treatment with immunosuppressive drugs can be swiftly effective. Contributory also must be the improvement in management of patients with renal failure, particularly in dialysis technology, as well as better monitoring capabilities, which incorporate measurements of circulating surrogate markers of autoimmune injury so that treatment may be adjusted appropriately. Therefore, is there a requirement to develop other therapies and if so, what are the prospects of success? This chapter examines the reasons for the need and describes the progress towards the development of strategies which may achieve more specific forms of immunotherapy for RPGN than available hitherto, first, in experimental models and, second, albeit more preliminarily, in the clinical setting.

More specific immunotherapy for RPGN: a case for need

RPGN can develop in the context of a number of different diseases. Those considered here are those in which components of the glomerulus, be they the endothelial cells or the underlying glomerular capillary basement membrane (GBM), bear the brunt of an autoimmune attack by autoantibodies which may be vasculotoxic or nephrotoxic, respectively. In the case of the endothelial cell, autoantibody-mediated injury may be promoted by the presence of neutrophil polymorphonuclear leucocytes (Ewert *et al.* 1992). These cells bear antigens identical to those that can be induced on the endothelial cell surface by cytokines, such as tumour necrosis factor (Mayet *et al.* 1993). Autoantibodies to neutrophil cytoplasm antigens (ANCA) are closely associated with the development of systemic vasculitides, such as Wegener's granulomatosis and microscopic polyangiitis, in which the autoantibodies have a predominant specificity for the antigens proteinase-3 and myeloperoxidase, respectively, and in which renal vasculitis is usually a prominent feature (Gross *et al.* 1993). Similar autoantibodies, usually with specificity for myeloperoxidase are found in patients with idiopathic RPGN, which is now considered to be a 'forme fruste' of microscopic polyangiitis, or renal-limited vasculitis (Falk and Jenette 1988).

Diagnosis and monitoring of systemic vasculitis

The specificity and sensitivity of c-ANCA in unselected patients have been questioned by Rao *et al.* (1995). However, these authors placed considerable reliance on the semantics of different vasculitis syndromes, with strict criteria for a diagnosis of Wegener's granulomatosis, and did not give information on other diagnoses. It is possible that the value of c-ANCA for a specific diagnosis of WG has been over-emphasized, and tissue histology should remain the 'gold standard'. However, if systemic vasculitis is considered a disease spectrum embracing several different entities, ANCA remains a useful diagnostic tool. There seems little doubt of the value of ANCA in monitoring of patients with known systemic vasculitis; most disease relapses are associated with ANCA positivity (De'Oliviera *et al.* 1995; Jayne *et al.* 1995). Soluble adhesion molecules do not seem to be reliable indicators of disease activity (John *et al.* 1994; Mrowka and Sieberth 1995). Other more recently reported markers, such as neopterin (Nassonov *et al.* 1995), await validation in larger studies. Circulating proteins such as these may simply be surrogate markers of the inflammatory process; it remains unlikely that therapy aimed at any of these single proteins or groups of proteins will provide effective disease-modifying therapy.

Although activation of polymorphs by ANCA, with consequent release of toxic oxygen radicals at inappropriate sites, such as juxtaposed to the glomerular endothelial cell surface, was believed to be the main route by which glomerular injury could be initiated, growing evidence suggests that direct injury of the endothelial cell itself, as described above, may also be important. In the case of the glomerular basement membrane, access of circulating autoantibodies to the GBM is provided by fenestrae, which are gaps between the endothelial cells, found in the renal microvasculature (Turner *et al.* 1993). ANCA-positive vasculitis and anti-GBM nephritis account for the majority of patients presenting with RPGN. The rarer forms of RPGN, which may accompany crescentic change in primary forms of glomerulonephritis, such as membranous or IgA nephritis, or which occur in the context of systemic lupus erythematosus, will not be considered further.

Although the finding of circulating vasculotoxic or nephrotoxic autoantibodies has greatly facilitated the diagnosis of RPGN, their presence has assumed an even greater importance since they carry clinical implications, both with regard to treatment and to prognosis. Patients with ANCA-positive renal vasculitis respond well to conventional immunosuppressive drug therapy with cytotoxic drugs and steroids, and escalation of treatment to include, for example, intensive plasma exchange is rarely required, unless the patient is dialysis-dependent, when it may be beneficial (Pusey *et al.* 1991*a*). Such treatment regimens usually bring about substantial recovery in patients with renal vasculitis, despite the severity of nephritis at presentation, whether it is judged biochemically by plasma creatinine level or histologically by extent of glomerular necrosis and crescent formation. This is not the case for anti-GBM nephritis, when a similar therapeutic approach rarely leads to recovery of independent renal function in the dialysis-dependent patient, and where additional plasma exchange is felt by many nephrologists to be essential to the successful treatment of patients, even though they present with nephritis of lesser severity (Turner *et al.* 1993).

As far as prognosis is concerned, with adequate treatment approximately 90% of patients with systemic vasculitis will go into remission, albeit in 80% this may take up to 12 months. However, almost half the patients will relapse, sometimes several years after presentation (Jayne *et al.* 1995). Thus, treatment may be required in the long term for a substantial proportion of patients, with all that this entails in terms of cumulative drug toxicity (see below). In contrast, anti-GBM nephritis is a self-limiting disease. Untreated, circulating anti-GBM antibody is usually detectable for about 18 months, but this can be reduced to approximately 2 months in patients treated with cytotoxic drugs, steroids, and intensive plasma exchange. Once antibodies have been eliminated, disease stabilizes in most patients and recurrence of anti-GBM antibody is extremely unusual (Turner *et al.* 1993).

Thus the design of specific immunotherapy for RPGN needs to take into account the fact that relatively long-term treatment, or treatment on multiple occasions, may be necessary for patients with systemic vasculitis, whereas short-term treatment, once only, may suffice for patients with anti-GBM nephritis.

Conventional therapy for RPGN

The drugs conventionally used for RPGN are broadly similar for both anti-GBM nephritis and renal vasculitis. High-dose steroids, together with cytotoxic agents, such as cyclophosphamide, form the mainstay of treatment. For anti-GBM nephritis, which is a short-term disease capable of a fulminating course, the aim is to remove circulating anti-GBM antibody by intensive daily plasma exchange, and so tide the patient over, while immunosuppressive drugs act to suppress further anti-GBM antibody formation. Empirically it has been found that for an adult patient the most effective therapy consists of a two-week course of daily whole volume plasma exchange, together with cyclophosphamide at 3mg/kg/day and prednisolone at 60 mg/day. Cyclophosphamide is reduced to 2 mg/kg/day in elderly patients (>55 years) or temporarily discontinued if leucopenia or severe infection occurs. Steroids are tapered so that at two months patients are receiving a daily dose of prednisolone 10 mg. On this regimen, circulating anti-GBM antibody is usually no longer detectable after two months. Once anti-GBM antibodies are eliminated drug therapy can safely be withdrawn (Turner *et al.* 1993). None of the components of this therapeutic regimen have been formally evaluated by adequate controlled trials, no doubt because of the rarity of the condition and the difficulties surrounding the comparison of severely ill patients. A small trial to assess the contribution of plasma exchange did suggest a trend whereby plasma exchange hastened the disappearance of circulating anti-GBM antibodies.

For renal and systemic vasculitis, cytotoxic drugs and steroids are usually combined at the same dose as for anti-GBM nephritis initially, in an induction regimen, to gain effective control of the disease at presentation. This is followed after a short period, usually two to three months later, by a lower dose, maintenance regimen in which other immunosuppressive agents, such as azathioprine, may substitute for cyclophosphamide. At the same time, the steroid treatment may be converted to an alternate day regimen. A prospective randomised controlled trial, in which patients were stratified at entry for levels of renal function, confirmed the benefit of additional plasma exchange for patients with severe (dialysis-dependent) renal vasculitis (Pusey *et al.* 1991*a*). Satisfactory evaluation of the contribution of individual drugs is still awaited and several studies are underway.

Problems with conventional therapy

This is particularly a problem for patients with systemic vasculitis due to the frequent need to use immunosuppressive drugs long term. In a study of a large group of patients with Wegener's granulomatosis ($n = 158$) treated with cyclophosphamide and steroids, the morbidity due to treatment toxicity alone is shown in Table 11.1 (Hoffmann *et al.*) This table of complications excludes those in which the disease and treatment may have combined to contribute to the morbidity, for example, the development of an intercurrent chest infection as a consequence of lung cavity formation due to disease, and the association of this with immunosuppression due to cyclophosphamide.

Table 11.1   Direct complications of conventional immunosuppression (after Hoffman *et al.* 1992)

Wegener's granulomatosis ($n = 158$)			
Cyclophosphamide (%)		Prednisolone (%)	
Female infertility	57	Cushingoid features	100
Cyclophosphamide cystitis	43	Cataracts	21
Hair loss	17	Fractures	11
Bladder cancer	3	(aseptic necrosis: 3%)	
Myelodysplasia	2	Diabetes mellitus	8
Development of malignancy[*]	↑ × 2.4	(requiring insulin: 3%)	
Development of bladder cancer[*]	↑ × 33		

[*] Related to an age- and sex-matched population.

Ideally, a new strategy would implement regulation at any of (or all) three stages of the autoimmune response: (1) at the induction phase, by interference with T cell orchestration of B cell function; (2) at the propagation phase, by selective removal of effectors of the autoimmune injury; (3) at the mediation phase, by restriction of target tissue injury, for example, by down-regulation of specific receptors for potentially injurious cells, antibodies, or cytokines. We will review how far this has been possible in experimental and human crescentic nephritis.

Lessons from experimental models

Novel therapies for RPGN are likely to evolve fairly slowly because of the relative success of conventional therapy and the difficulties in performing controlled trials in these uncommon and rapidly evolving conditions. For many immunologically mediated human diseases, the study of experimental models has provided valuable information on pathogenetic mechanisms and led to the development of novel therapeutic strategies. As well as enabling identification of suitable targets for therapy, animal studies provide a means of testing the efficacy and safety of novel forms of treatment. RPGN is no exception, but the available animal models have many differences from human RPGN, and caution must therefore be exercised in extrapolating from the experimental models to the analogous human diseases.

Experimental models of anti-GBM disease

Most animal models of anti-GBM disease involve infusion of pre-formed anti-GBM antibodies, or deliberate immunization with GBM to induce such antibodies. These models therefore provide little or no information about the factors operating early in the induction of a spontaneous anti-GBM autoantibody response. However, the models have been very helpful in the analysis of effector mechanisms operating once such a response has developed.

'Nephrotoxic', nephritis is the term used to describe the renal disease that results when heterologous anti-GBM antibodies are infused into animals; there is linear deposition of the infused immunoglobulin along the GBM and development of a proliferative nephritis with crescents, especially if the animals are pre-immunized against immunoglobulin from the donor species (so-called 'accelerated' nephrotoxic nephritis). Nephrotoxic nephritis has been used extensively to study the mechanisms where anti-GBM antibodies induce tissue injury, but at present the observations made have not been used to guide novel forms of therapy. For example, neutrophils (Naish *et al.* 1975) and complement (Unanue and Dixon 1967) have been shown to play a role in the mediation of tissue injury in nephrotoxic nephritis. Corticosteroids have effects on neutrophil function, but to date no more specific therapy directed against neutrophils has been tested in RPGN. Possibilities include monoclonal antibodies designed to deplete neutrophils—although the tremendous capacity of the bone marrow to increase production of neutrophils, and the rapid turnover of these cells, will always limit the effectiveness of such an approach. Agents directed against key molecules in neutrophil function provide another strategy, for example, the surface proteins that mediate neutrophil adhesion to endothelium, or cytokines important in neutrophil activation such as interleukin-8 (IL-8) (Mulligan *et al.* 1993; Adams *et al.* 1994; Broaddus *et al.* 1994).

A powerful method of inducing selective neutropenia is illustrated by experiments in which dogs were immunized with recombinant granulocyte-macrophage colony-stimulating factor (GM-CSF). The resulting antibody response led to neutralization of endogenous GM-CSF and profound long-lasting suppression of neutrophil numbers (Hammond *et al.* 1991). The possible duration of this effect, and the likely consequences for susceptibility to infection, remain completely unknown, but this example does illustrate the potential power of this type of approach. Macrophages also play an important role in nephrotoxic nephritis, and similar strategies could be directed at this cell type. Administration of a prostaglandin E1 analogue to rats with accelerated nephrotoxic nephritis reduced macrophage accumulation in glomeruli without affecting circulating or deposited anti-GBM antibodies (Cattell *et al.* 1990). Regarding complement, potent inhibitors of complement activation are now becoming available (Fearon 1991) and show promise in experimental models of both immunological (Pruitt *et al.* 1991) and non-immunological tissue injury (Weisman *et al.* 1990). As yet, there are no examples of application of complement-inhibition to RPGN, but this is an area which could be explored in the near future.

The role of the coagulation cascade has been extensively studied in accelerated nephrotoxic nephritis, in which deposition of fibrin is a prominent feature. Defibrination with ancrod protects renal function in this model (Thomson *et al.* 1976) and heparin has a lesser effect (Thomson *et al.* 1975a). Fibrinolytic therapy with streptokinase is effective if started early (Tipping and Holdsworth 1986); newer agents such as recombinant tissue plasminogen activator may also have useful effects (Zoja *et al.* 1990; Mathieson *et al.* 1991a). Therapy directed against the coagulation system has some advocates in human glomerulonephritis (Kincaid-Smith 1984), but has not been widely adopted. Recent studies have demonstrated a role for platelets in nephrotoxic nephritis and depletion of platelets (Wu *et al.* 1993), or administration of a platelet-activating factor (PAF) receptor antagonist (Kakuta 1993), may influence favourably experimental renal injury. There is some evidence that peptide growth factors such as platelet-derived growth factor (PDGF) and the insulin-like growth factors are important in renal disease (Frampton *et al.* 1988; Segal 1989), but few selective antagonists of these agents are available. There is one report of the use of a PDGF antagonist in nephrotoxic nephritis in rabbits, without significant benefit (Shinkai and Cameron 1987), but this is an area where further research may be fruitful. The renal cortical enzyme cathepsin L, a cysteine proteinase, has recently been implicated in causation of tissue injury in experimental anti-GBM disease, since a specific inhibitor of this enzyme reduced proteinuria (Baricos *et al.* 1991). This type of highly specific therapy is attractive, but it is noteworthy that the agent did not influence renal excretory function or histology (Baricos *et al.* 1991), so the potency of this approach remains in doubt.

Nephrotoxic nephritis has provided valuable information on the relationship of anti-GBM antibody to tissue injury, with both the amount of antibody bound (Unanue and Dixon 1967; Huland 1973), and the rate of antibody binding (Van Zyl Smit *et al.* 1983) being important. The amount of injury resulting from binding of a defined amount of antibody can be increased by acute phase stimuli such as bacterial lipopolysaccharide or the pro-inflammatory cytokines tumour necrosis factor and IL-1 (Tomosugi *et al.* 1989). This phenomenon probably explains the clinical observation that intercurrent infection increases tissue injury in this disease (Rees *et al.* 1977). An interesting illustration of the possible pathogenetic role of infection is provided by the report that animals immunized against streptococcal antigens developed pulmonary haemorrhage in association with antibodies which bound to both GBM and ABM (Fitzsimons and Large 1991). Antimicrobial drugs alone may have useful therapeutic effects in systemic vasculitis (Deremee 1989) but have not been tested in anti-GBM disease. Anti-GBM antibodies cross-react with the pulmonary alveolar basement membrane (ABM); there is experimental evidence that lung inflammation and/or pulmonary haemorrhage results only when alveolar capillary permeability is increased, so that the antibodies can gain access to the ABM *in vivo* (Jennings *et al.* 1981; Downie *et al.* 1982). This may explain the clinical observation that pulmonary haemorrhage is more common in cigarette smokers (Donaghy and Rees 1983). In a murine model of anti-GBM disease, binding to the ABM and resultant pneumonitis and pulmonary haemorrhage were enhanced by the cytokines IL-2 and interferon-α (Quelez *et al.* 1990). An analogous role for cytokines in the human disease is plausible, suggesting that therapy aimed at key cytokines could be useful.

Standard therapy for anti-GBM disease is centered around attempts to remove the pathogenic antibody and suppress its further synthesis, and the data from animal models certainly support this strategy. More selective ways in which this could be achieved remain desirable; immunoadsorption with protein-A provides a slightly more selective method than plasma exchange (Bygren *et al.* 1985; Esnault *et al.* 1993*a*), but the ideal would be to remove only the pathogenic antibody. Now that the molecular nature of the autoantigen recognized by anti-GBM antibodies is known in considerable detail (Turner *et al.* 1992; Hudson *et al.* 1993), it should be possible to produce large quantities of pure autoantigen using recombinant DNA technology. In theory, such a preparation could be used to construct antigen columns for the adsorption of specific antibody by affinity chromatography, although the technical and economic problems with such an approach remain formidable. A system has been developed which allows testing of immunoadsorption strategies in conscious unrestrained rats (Pusey *et al.* 1991*b*), and this may allow the use of animal models to test the efficacy of novel methods of antibody removal.

Nephrotoxic nephritis has also been used to study the progressive glomerular and interstitial sclerosis that occurs after acute inflammation has subsided. Studies using nephritic kidneys transplanted into syngeneic individuals have shown that progressive glomerular scarring is not dependent on persistence of circulating anti-GBM antibodies, but continues independently (El Nahas *et al.*

1985). Thus, it may be amenable to non-immunological intervention, as in other forms of renal disease (Fine 1988).

Another animal model of anti-GBM disease involves the immunization of susceptible rats with homologous GBM (Pusey *et al.* 1991*c*), which leads to deposition of anti-GBM antibodies in the kidney and resultant proteinuria. This model has been used to examine the effects of cyclosporin, which mainly acts on T lymphocytes, with encouraging results (Reynolds *et al.* 1991). There are anecdotal reports of the effectiveness of this agent in human anti-GBM disease when conventional therapy has failed (Querin *et al.* 1992). Treatment with a monoclonal antibody to CD4+ T cells has also been shown to be effective in this model (Reynolds and Pusey 1994). Another relatively specific anti-T cell agent, FK506, is effective in accelerated nephrotoxic nephritis (Hara *et al.* 1990). Depletion of CD8+ cells prevented proteinuria and crescent formation in this model (Kawasaki *et al.* 1992). These observations support a role for T cells in the pathogenesis of anti-GBM disease and suggest that therapy aimed at this cellular compartment may be worthy of detailed testing.

Experimental models of systemic vasculitis

Necrotizing vasculitis occurs in a number of experimental situations (Mathieson *et al.* 1993*a*) but none of these closely resemble vasculitis in humans. Certain experimental viral infections may be complicated by vasculitis, for example in mice with tumours induced by polyoma virus (Dawe *et al.* 1987), in mice with murine leukaemia virus infections (Miyazama *et al.* 1987), and in Aleutian disease of mink (Henson and Gorham 1973). It has recently been suggested that some human vasculitic diseases may be associated with parvovirus infections and that the therapeutic efficacy of pooled immunoglobulin can be accounted for by antiviral activity (Finkel *et al.* 1994). As already mentioned, antimicrobial drugs alone may have useful therapeutic effects in systemic vasculitis (Deremee 1989), but specific antiviral agents have not yet been tested.

Necrotizing vasculitis occurs, especially in the gut, in Brown–Norway rats treated with the polyclonal B cell activator mercuric chloride (Mathieson *et al.* 1992). These animals develop a number of autoantibodies including antibodies to myeloperoxidase (MPO) (Esnault *et al.* 1992), and the tissue injury is ameliorated by treatment with antimicrobial drugs (Mathieson *et al.* 1992, 1993*b*). Despite these similarities with systemic vasculitis, this model has weaknesses: especially the presence of multiple autoantibodies, the atypical organ distribution of tissue injury, and the lack of nephritis. Nevertheless, the model has been used to test the efficacy of novel treatment approaches such as antioxidant drugs (Qasim *et al.* 1993*a*), and therapies aimed at neutrophils (Qasim *et al.* 1993*b*) and T cells or subsets thereof (Mathieson *et al.* 1991*b*, 1993*a,b*; Qasim *et al.* 1993*c*). Each of these approaches shows some promise, but the extent to which these observations can be extrapolated to human systemic vasculitis remains uncertain.

Most experimental models of crescentic glomerulonephritis feature prominent immune deposits, but there are two recent reports of experimental models where the nephritis does appear to be 'pauci-immune'. One (Kinjoh *et al.* 1993) is in recombinant inbred mice which were derived from a lupus-prone strain, with selection for further breeding based on the frequency of crescent formation. The resulting mice rapidly develop a florid crescentic nephritis with scanty immune deposits. Intriguingly, these mice also develop extra-renal vasculitis, suggesting that the genetic factors predisposing to the crescentic nephritis are the same as, or closely linked to, those responsible for susceptibility to vasculitis in other organs. The other model (Brouwer *et al.* 1993), involves immunization of rats with MPO, followed by direct perfusion of the kidney with various injurious agents, including hydrogen peroxide plus MPO or other neutrophil constituents. The resulting nephritis may not be truly pauci-immune, in that there *is* initial deposition of IgG and C3 (Brouwer *et al.* 1993; Yang *et al.* 1993).

Shoenfeld and colleagues recently reported an intriguing model in which mice are immunized with IgG from vasculitis patients with ANCA. These mice develop antibodies with reactivity against mouse neutrophils, and these antibodies are capable of inducing a respiratory burst in neutrophils *in vitro*. Furthermore, the mice develop perivascular mononuclear cell infiltrates in the lungs (Blank *et al.* 1995; Tomer *et al.* 1995) The authors invoke an idiotype/anti-idiotype explanation for this phenomenon and regard their results as supportive of a pathogenetic role for ANCA. However, the animals do not have overt vasculitis and no causative link between the immunization with ANCA and the development of perivascular inflammation can be proved. There are, as yet, no reports of the effects of immunotherapy in this experimental model.

The utility of these experimental models for the further study of pathogenetic mechanisms and for testing of novel forms of therapy will be examined in the next few years. At present, however, no entirely satisfactory animal model of systemic vasculitis is available.

Experimental models of other forms of nephritis

Study of animal models of lupus, in which there is typically a proliferative glomerulonephritis, have suggested many useful therapeutic targets for the analogous human disease. These include treatments directed at inflammatory mediators, such as products of arachidonic acid metabolism, which are involved in inflammation in human (Patrono *et al.* 1985), and animal (Kelley *et al.* 1986) nephritis. Diets rich in eicosapentaenoic acid ameliorate experimental lupus in mice (Kelley *et al.* 1985). Cytokines, such as IL-1 and tumour necrosis factor (TNF), are integral components of inflammatory reactions and their production by mononuclear cells may also be amenable to dietary manipulation (Endres *et al.* 1989). This may explain the beneficial effect on experimental lupus nephritis of diets supplemented with polyunsaturated fatty acids (Prickett *et al.* 1987). Another therapeutic strategy which has been shown to be useful is an anti-CD4 antibody, which can reverse advanced lupus nephritis in one murine model (Wofsey and Seaman 1987). Benefit from defibrination with ancrod has been reported in murine lupus nephritis (Cole *et al.* 1990), and this agent has been used in some preliminary human studies (Pollak *et al.* 1982; Segasothy *et al.* 1986; Kim *et al.* 1988). However, ancrod is unlikely to find a major role in clinical practice since it is highly immunogenic. However, the potential usefulness of defibrination should not be forgotten; if more acceptable agents could be developed, such therapy might provide a useful adjunct to immunosuppressive drugs in a number of forms of nephritis.

Administration of anti-thymocyte antibodies to rats induces a mesangial proliferative glomerulonephritis Renal injury in this model can be markedly ameliorated by an antibody to transforming growth factor-beta 1 (TGFβ1) (Border *et al.* 1990), but whether this approach could be effective in other forms of nephritis is unknown. A PAF receptor antagonist is also protective in this model (Stahl *et al.* 1991).

A proliferative immune complex nephritis arises in animals immunized with bovine serum albumin (BSA); effective therapies in this model include ancrod (Thomson *et al.* 1975b) and cyclosporin (Fujita *et al.* 1991). Another experimental model of immune complex nephritis results when dogs are immunized with concanavalin A; useful histological improvement and reduction in proteinuria has been reported with a thromboxane synthetase inhibitor (Longhofer *et al.* 1991).

Future therapeutic strategies

Monoclonal antibodies (mAbs) offer the possibility of a highly specific form of therapy for a wide variety of human diseases. Xenogeneic mAbs, raised in rodents, are liable to induce allergic reactions; furthermore, neutralizing antibodies produced by the recipient may lead to loss of efficacy in prolonged or repeated courses of treatment. Genetic engineering techniques are now available that enable the 'humanization' of rodent mAbs, so that the structural parts of the antibody molecule can be rendered less antigenic (Reichmann *et al.* 1988). Suitable targets for mAb therapy include lymphocyte subsets, for example CD4+ T cells (Mathieson *et al.* 1990), or specific cytokines (Strom and Kelley 1989; Moreland *et al.* 1993). The ultimate specificity in anti-T cell therapy would be to target only autoreactive T cell clones. This ideal appears to have been achieved in one experimental model of autoimmune disease, experimental allergic encephalomyelitis (Acha-Orbea *et al.* 1988; Vandenbark *et al.* 1989), but as yet there is insufficient knowledge of autoreactive T cells in man for this approach to be contemplated in any form of human renal disease.

There have been several recent publications continuing the debate on the role of T cells in systemic vasculitis. As outlined earlier, therapy aimed at T cells has considerable potential, but direct demonstration of autoreactive T cells *in vitro* has proved difficult. Three recent studies have reported proliferation of patients' T cells in response to PR3 or to MPO (Brouwer *et al.* 1994; Ballieux *et al.* 1995; Griffith *et al.* 1996). However, in each case there was considerable overlap between patients and controls, and the relevance of the findings to the pathogenesis of systemic vasculitis has been questioned (Mathieson and Oliviera 1995).

Two recent studies have reported restricted usage of T cell receptor variable genes in patients with systemic vasculitis (Giscombe *et al.* 1995; Simpson *et al.* 1995); if this can be confirmed, selective therapy aimed at these T cells (using mAbs or peptides) may be worth testing.

Proteinase-3 (PR3) is one of the major antigenic targets for ANCA. Two recent observations concern the interaction of PR3 with its main inhibitor, α-1-antitrypsin (α1AT), and the relationship that this may have to the pathogenesis of systemic vasculitis. The first is that anti-PR3 antibodies inhibit the formation of the PR3–α1AT complex, possibly potentiating the enzymic activity of PR3; furthermore the inhibitory capacity of anti-PR3 antibodies seems to correlate more closely with disease activity than does the actual autoantibody titre (Dolman *et al.* 1993). The second is that genetic polymorphisms of α1AT that result in relative deficiencies of this protease inhibitor may be associated with a predisposition to the development of anti-PR3 autoantibodies (Esnault *et al.* 1993*b*). The suggestion that the proteolytic activity of ANCA autoantigens may play some role in tissue injury in systemic vasculitis provides a novel disease mechanism and suggests another target for therapy.

The predisposition to systemic vasculitis, which is associated with certain α-1-antitrypsin phenotypes, has been confirmed in further studies (Lhotta *et al.* 1994; Savige *et al.* 1995). However, in one of these studies (Savige *et al.* 1995), there was a poor correlation between phenotype and the serum level of α1AT. Also, both studies examined large numbers of individuals with severe α1AT deficiency and found no cases of systemic vasculitis or ANCA positivity, so the strength of any aetiological link between α1AT activity and systemic vasulitis must remain in doubt. The importance of this association for pathogenesis of systemic vascul-itis, and in particular the therapeutic potential of treatment aimed at α1AT, remains uncertain.

In view of the intensity of inflammation that occurs in systemic vasculitis and the presumed immunological disturbance which underlines the condition, it is not surprising that elevated levels of various cytokines, adhesion molecules, and other inflammatory markers have been reported (Lai and Lockwood 1993; Wang *et al.* 1993). If such observations are to shed light on pathogenesis and/or suggest suitable targets for therapy, some specificity for the disease process is a prerequisite. In this connection, the report of high levels of IL-8 (a key cytokine in neutrophil and endothelial cell activation) in systemic vasculitis and the corre-lation between IL-8 levels and disease activity (Arimura *et al.* 1993) are poten-tially exciting. Monoclonal antibodies to IL-8 show promise in experimental models of neutrophil-mediated inflammation (Mulligan *et al.* 1993; Broaddus *et al.* 1994), and may be worthy of investigation in systemic vasculitis.

Granulocyte colony-stimulating factor (G-CSF) is a cytokine that stimulates the development of cells of the granulocyte lineage from bone marrow progeni-tors. Recombinant G-CSF is now widely used in clinical practice, and there have been reports of vasculitis developing as an adverse effect of this form of therapy[8] (Farhey and Herman 1995). Furthermore, G-CSF has been implicated in the pathogenesis of Sweet's syndrome, a cutaneous disease in which there is perivascular inflammation but no actual vasculitis, and in which ANCA have been reported (Reuss-Borst *et al.* 1994). Therapy aimed at endogenous G-CSF would obviously be expected to induce granulocytopenia (Hammond *et al.* 1991); this could provide a potent form of therapy targeted towards the neutrophil, but the consequences for defence against bacterial infection would require careful assessment.

Another humoral factor which has been studied recently is haptoglobin, a plasma α2-glycoprotein. Cid *et al.* (1993) reported that haptoglobin stimulates angiogenesis (the formation of new blood vessels) *in vivo* and *in vitro*, that sera from patients with systemic vasculitis contain elevated levels of haptoglobin, and that the level of this protein correlates with disease activity and with the capacity of the serum to induce angiogenesis. However, since haptoglobin is known to be an acute phase reactant (Kushner 1982; Hansen *et al.* 1987), and since the report by Cid and colleagues did not include any disease controls, the significance of their findings for systemic vasculitis remains unproven. Nevertheless, angiogenesis is a widespread phenomenon and may be an important mode of tissue repair in response to inflammation (Folkman and Klagsbrun 1987); therapeutic measures designed to harness the body's normal repair mechanisms would have considerable potential.

Activation of endothelial cells has been demonstrated in skin biopsies from patients with systemic vasculitis (Bradley *et al.* 1994). One key mediator of endothelial activation is the transcription factor NF-kappa B (Ferran *et al.* 1995); this factor may be amenable to specific blockade since it acts via reactive oxygen intermediates. *In vitro*, the antioxidant pyrrolidine dithiocarbamate markedly inhibits endothelial activation (Ferran *et al.* 1995). Targeted delivery of this agent or similar compounds to sites of disease activity could provide a novel form of therapy. Neutrophil cytotoxicity towards umbilical vein endothelial cells mediated by lipoxin A4 *in vitro* involves neutrophil adherence via CD18, endogenous production of platelet-activating factor (PAF), and pertussis-sensitive intracellular G proteins (Bratt *et al.* 1995). Cytotoxicity can be abrogated using selective inhibitors of each of these (Bratt *et al.* 1995), and, in theory, these forms of therapy could be used *in vivo*, although, again, selective delivery to sites of disease may be difficult.

A further approach to more selective intervention in autoimmune disease would be to manipulate endogenous immunoregulatory systems. Indirect evidence of the importance of immunoregulatory mechanisms in man is provided by anti-GBM disease, where in contrast to most autoimmune diseases relapse is very rare (Savage *et al.* 1986), suggesting the re-establishment of immunoregulatory control. If such endogenous immunoregulatory mechanisms could be harnessed, a powerful and specific form of therapy would result. In anti-tubular basement membrane (TBM) nephritis in mice it is possible to activate antigen-specific suppressor cells by injecting the animals with syngeneic lymphocytes which have been conjugated with the TBM antigen used to induce the disease (Neilson *et al.* 1985). These suppressor cells are able to attenuate renal injury even when induced up to six weeks after the onset of the autoimmune process. A similar approach is, in principle, feasible in man, but would depend on the availability of sufficient amounts of the relevant autoantigen.

Specific immunotherapy for human RPGN

The advent of 'humanized' monoclonal antibodies with specificity for lymphocytes, particularly encompassing T lymphocytes, provided a therapeutic opportunity to target those cells selectively and so perhaps interfere with the propagation of the autoimmune response. The four patients who received this treatment initially were patients with a long history of intractable multi-system vasculitis and in whom there was biopsy evidence that lymphocytic involvement appeared to be important in disease pathogenesis (Lockwood *et al.* 1993). Although all four were refractory to steroid and cytotoxic drug regimens, as used for patients with RPGN, their prompt response to monoclonal antibody therapy indicated the potential this approach might have for interrupting T cell-dependent B cell function in autoimmune nephritis. We therefore considered the use of this form of immunotherapy as supplementary treatment for patients with RPGN in which the autoimmune response proved difficult to control by conventional means.

Monoclonal antibodies

The anti-T cell monoclonal antibodies used were humanised anti-CD52 (CAMPATH-1H) and an anti-CD4; CD52 is a glycoprotein complex carried on most lymphocytes but not natural killer (NK) cells. The anti-CD52 is lytic, and the anti-CD4 is a blocking antibody; both are isotype IgG1. Similar antibodies to these have been shown to act synergistically in animal models of tolerance induction and the two together, but not individually, can arrest the progression of experimental autoimmune arthritis, whereas either alone can prevent its induction (Hom *et al.* 1988). This combination therapy seemed to be the optimal strategy for human disease which is usually well established by the time the patient is referred for treatment. The monoclonals were given intravenously on a daily basis using doses up to 40 mg/day for up to 10 days. The effect of treatment was monitored by lymphocyte counts (those for CD4 being most useful), standard tests of organ function, and levels of autoantibody.

Patients

Initially, two patients with RPGN who were resistant to conventional therapy, were given additional 'humanized' monoclonal antibody therapy. Both patients had Wegener's granulomatosis with anti-PR3 antibodies; one of these also had anti-GBM antibodies.

Patient 1

This 56-year-old man presented with proteinuria in May 1992. ANCA serology was positive for circulating anti-PR3 autoantibodies and renal biopsy showed a focal necrotizing glomerulonephritis, both compatible with the diagnosis of Wegener's granulomatosis (WG). He was started on conventional therapy with cyclophosphamide 150 mg once daily and prednisolone 60 mg once daily. However, because the plasma creatinine, which was 307 μmol/l at presentation, continued to rise despite two weeks of immunosuppressive drug treatment, and a short course of plasma exchange revealed that autoantibody synthesis was still active, he was referred for further management. An autologous isotope-labelled polymorph scan showed nasal and lung involvement consistent with WG, isotope EDTA glomerular filtration rate (GFR) was 5ml/min, and renal biopsy showed acute necrotizing glomerulonephritis with crescent formation.

CAMPATH-1H was given at 4 mg/day for 10 days. However, a further course of plasma exchange revealed that antibody synthesis still continued and so CAMPATH-1H, as additional immunosuppression, was given at 40 mg/day for 6 days, after which antibody levels fell, remaining near the normal range until discharge from hospital (see Fig. 11.1). A repeat white cell scan was normal. Renal biopsy after treatment showed merely scarred glomeruli compressed by old fibrous crescents, without any active glomerulonephritis. Isotope GFR showed a value of 12 ml/minute; the patient thereafter required haemodialysis twice weekly and is well on follow-up. Maintenance prednisolone continued at 10 mg/day. In this patient, measurements of ANCA were used as surrogates of disease activity and helped determine the treatment strategy. Although the auto-

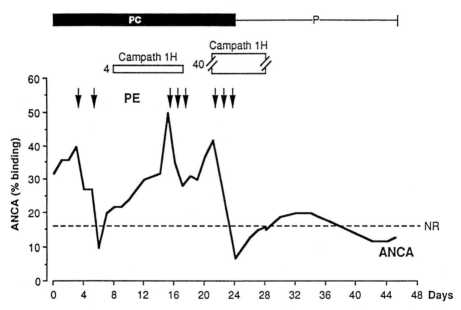

Mab therapy : ANCA +ve RPGN

Fig. 11.1 *Patient 1.* Effect of monoclonal antibody therapy on ANCA production. The patient had already received induction therapy with prednisolone (P) and cyclophosphamide (C) for two weeks before referral (day 0). As shown by arrows, plasma exchange (PE) was followed by active ANCA synthesis despite CAMPATH-1H 4 mg daily; after the dose was increased to 40 mg/day there was successful control of ANCA production.

immune response was eventually controlled, irreversible destruction of glomerular archi-tecture probably precluded substantial recovery of renal function.

Patient 2

This 66-year-old man presented in August 1992 with a six-month history of night sweats, cough with expectoration of white sputum, and a two-week history of diarrhoea with weight loss. On admission he was found to have a creatinine of 1547 μmol/l, and a renal biopsy showed evidence of a recent florid, uniformly crescentic glomerulonephritis with an accompanying vasculitis. Immunofluorescence showed linear IgG deposited along the GBM. Serologically, he was found to have both circulating ANCA (anti-PR3) and anti-GBM antibodies. Autologous isotope-labelled polymorph scan showed diffuse uptake in both lungs, together with increased uptake in the region of the right maxillary sinus, appearances which were consistent with diagnosis of WG. He was commenced on pred-nisolone and cyclophosphamide in conventional dosage and although this led to reduction in ANCA levels, anti-GBM antibody synthesis was still active, even after two weeks of immunosuppression. He was then referred for monoclonal antibody treatment in the hope that, because of the recent onset of the nephritis and the coincidental vasculitis, control of both of these might avoid permanent loss of renal function.

Attempts to control anti-GBM antibody synthesis were made with CAMPATH-1H at 40 mg/day for 5 days, followed by anti-CD4 20 mg/day for 5 days. After the monoclonal antibody treatment, a further short course of plasma exchange showed that anti-GBM antibody synthesis had ceased (see Fig. 11.2); thereafter, levels of anti-GBM antibody fell

Mab therapy : Anti GBM disease

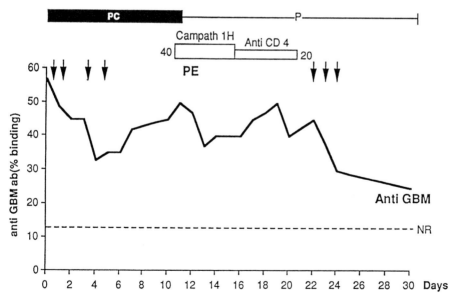

Fig. 11.2 *Patient 2.* Effect of CAMPATH-1H and anti-CD4 on anti-GBM antibody production. Anti-GBM antibody synthesis ceased after combination CAMPATH-1H and anti-CD4 treatment.

to background and have not been detected during follow-up. The cyclophosphamide therapy was discontinued after only 18 days (an event necessitated by the development of leucopenia and thrombocytopenia). Steroids were withdrawn gradually and discontinued after three months. There was no recovery of renal function and the patient remains on renal dialysis therapy. The rapid termination of anti-GBM antibody production, however, suggested that earlier intervention in the course of anti-GBM nephritis might produce better renal recovery.

Comments and conclusion

Monoclonal antibody therapy was used in these pilot studies as a supplement to conventional immunosuppression to try to control the autoimmune responses occurring in these two patients with RPGN. What impact was made by this approach is difficult to interpret, since it could be argued that the effects on autoantibody production were merely those consequent on an overly delayed response to the cyclophosphamide and steroids. Nevertheless, the close temporal association to the administration of the monoclonal therapy, together with the evident dose dependence in Patient 1, argues that autoantibody synthesis was finally terminated by the additional treatment. In both patients, autoantibodies served as surrogate markers for the disease and were useful guides to management. Whether control of their production represents complete arrest of the disease process cannot be determined at this stage. Better techniques for assessing treatment effects other than by repeated biopsy are urgently required.

Thus far, this is but preliminary experience of the possible value of 'humanized' monoclonal anti-T cell antibody therapy for RPGN. However, the treatment was simple to administer, well tolerated, and was not complicated by opportunistic infection. The success of monoclonal antibody therapy in 6 other patients with Wegener's granulomatosis refractory to conventional treatment has recently been reported by Lockwood *et al.* (1996). Further persuasive evidence for such a therapeutic approach is now required from studies in patients in which monoclonal antibody therapy can be used alone and/or in patients in whom the state of the disease activity can be monitored more directly. This may then make this form of specific immunotherapy both feasible and attractive for RPGN.

References

Acha-Orbea, H., Mitchell, D.J., Timmerman, L. *et al.* (1988). Limited heterogeneity of T cell receptors from lymphocytes mediating autoimmune encephalomyelitis allows specific immune intervention. *Cell*, **54**, 263–73.

Adams, D.H. and Shaw S. (1994). Leucocyte-endothelial interactions and regulation of leucocyte migration. *Lancet*, **343**, 831–6.

Arimura, Y., Minoshima, S., Nagasawa, T. *et al.* (1993). Serum IL-8, soluble ICAM-1, glomerular expression of cellular adhesion molecules and myeloperoxidase (MPO) release from the neutrophils in MPO-ANCA associated crescentic glomerulonephritis (CRGN). *Clinical and Experimental Immunology*, **93** (suppl 1), 27, (abstract).

Ballieux, B.E.P.B., van den Burg, S.H., Hagen, E.C., Van der Woude, F.J., Melief, C.J.M., and Daha, M.R. (1995). Cell-mediated autoimmunity in patients with Wegener's granulomatosis. *Clinical and Experimental Immunology*, **100**, 186–93.

Baricos, W.H., Cortez, S.L., Le, Q.C. *et al.* (1991). Evidence suggesting a role for cathepsin G in an experimental model of glomerulonephritis. *Archives in Biochemistry and Biophysics*, **288**, 468–72.

Blank, M., Tomer, Y., Stein, M. *et al.* (1995). Immunization with anti-neutrophil cytoplasmic antibody (ANCA) induces the production of mouse ANCA and perivascular lymphocyte infiltration. *Clinical and Experimental Immunology*, **102**, 120–30.

Border, W.A., Okuda, S., Languino, L.R. *et al.* (1990). Suppression of experimental glomerulonephritis by antiserum against transforming growth factor beta 1. *Nature*, **346**, 371–4.

Bradley, J.R., Lockwood, C.M., and Thiru, S. (1994). Endothelial cell activation in patients with systemic vasculitis. *Quarterly Journal of Medicine*, **87**, 741–5.

Bratt, J., Lerner, R., Ringertz, B., and Palmblad, J. (1995). Mechanisms for lipoxin A4-induced neutrophil-dependent cytotoxicity for human endothelial cells. *Journal of Laboratory and Clinical Medicine*, **126**, 36–43.

Broaddus, V.C., Boylan, A.M., Hoeffel, J.M. *et al.* (1994). Neutralization of IL-8 inhibits neutrophil influx in a rabbit model of endotoxin-induced pleurisy. *Journal of Immunology*, **152**, 2960–67.

Brouwer, E., Huitema, M.G., Klok, P.A. *et al.* (1993). Antimyeloperoxidase-associated proliferative glomerulonephritis: an animal model. *Journal of Experimental Medicine*, **177**, 905–14.

Brouwer, E., Stegeman, C.A., Huitema, M.G., Limburg, P.C., and Kallenberg, C.G.M. (1994). T cell reactivity to proteinase 3 and myeloperoxidase in patients with Wegener's granulomatosis (WG). *Clinical and Experimental Immunology*, **98**, 448–53.

Bygren, P., Freiburghaus, C., Lindholm T. *et al.* (1985). Goodpasture's syndrome treated with staphylococcal protein A immunoadsorption. *Lancet*, **ii**, 1295–6.

Cameron, J.S. (1978). The natural history of glomerulonephritis. In *Progress in glomerulonephritis*, (ed: P. Kincaid Smith, A.J.F. d'Apice, and R.C. Atkins) pp. 1–27. Wiley, New York.

Cattell, V., Smith, J., and Cook, H.T. (1990). Prostaglandin E1 suppresses macrophage infiltration and ameliorates injury in an experimental model of macrophage-dependent glomerulonephritis. *Clinical and Experimental Immunology*, **79**, 260–5.

Cid, M.C., Grant, D.S., Hoffman, G.S. *et al.* (1993). Identification of haptoglobin as an angiogenic factor in sera from patients with systemic vasculitis. *Journal of Clinical Investigation*, **91**, 977–85.

Cole, E.H., Glynn, M.F.X., Laskin, C.A. *et al.* (1990). Ancrod improves survival in murine systemic lupus erythematosus. *Kidney International*, **37**, 29–35.

Dawe, C.J., Freund, R., Barncastle, J.P. *et al.* (1987). Necrotizing arterial lesions in mice bearing tumors induced by polyoma virus. *Journal of Experimental Pathology*, **3**, 177–201.

De'Oliviera, J., Gaskin, G., Dash, A., Rees, A.J., and Pusey, C.D. (1995). Relationship between disease activity and anti-neutrophil cytoplasmic antibody concentration in long-term management of systemic vasculitis. *American Journal of Kidney Diseases*, **25**, 380–9.

Deremee, R.A. (1989). The treatment of Wegener's granulomatosis with trimethoprim/sulfamethoxazole: illusion or vision? *Arthritis and Rheumatism*, **31**, 1068–72.

Dolman, K.M., Stegeman, C.A., van de Wiel, B.A. *et al.* (1993). Relevance of c-ANCA mediated inhibition of proteinase-3-alpha-1-antitrypsin complexation to disease activity in Wegener's granulomatosis. *Clinical and Experimental Immunology*, **93**, (suppl. 1), 18, (abstract).

Donaghy, M. and Rees, A.J. (1983). Cigarette smoking and lung haemorrhage in glomerulonephritis caused by autoantibodies to glomerular basement membrane. *Lancet*, ii, 1390–3.

Downie, G.M., Roholt, O.A., Jennings, L. *et al.* (1982). Experimental anti-alveolar basement membrane antibody-mediated pneumonitis: II. Role of endothelial damage and repair, induction of autologous phase, and kinetics of antibody deposition in Lewis rats. *Journal of Immunology*, **129**, 2647–52.

El Nahas, A.M., Lechler, R., Zoob, S.N., *et al.* (1985). Progression to renal failure after nephrotoxic nephritis in rats studied by renal transplantation. *Clinical Science*, **68**, 15–21.

Endres, S., Ghorbani, R., Kelley, V.E. *et al.* (1989). The effect of dietary supplementation with n-3 polyunsaturated fatty acids on the synthesis of interleukin-1 and tumor necrosis factor by mononuclear cells. *New England Journal of Medicine*, **320**, 265–71.

Esnault, V.L.M., Mathieson, P.W., Thiru, S. *et al.* (1992). Autoantibodies to myeloperoxidase in Brown Norway rats treated with mercuric chloride. *Laboratory Investigation*, **67**, 114–20.

Esnault, V.L., Testa, A., Jayne D.R. *et al.* (1993a). Influence of immunoadsorption on the removal of immunoglobulin G autoantibodies in crescentic glomerulonephritis. *Nephron*, **65**, 180–4.

Esnault, V.L.M., Testa, A., Audrain, M., *et al.* (1993b). Alpha-1-antitrypsin genetic polymorphism in ANCA-positive systemic vasculitis. *Kidney International*, **43**, 1329–32.

Ewert, B.H., Jennette, J.C., and Falk, R.J. (1992). Antimyeloperoxidase antibodies stimulate neutrophils to damage human endothelial cells. *Kidney International*, **41**, 375–83.

Falk, R.J. and Jennette, J.C. (1988). Antineutrophil cytoplasmic antibodies with specificity for myeloperoxidase in patients with systemic vasculitis and idiopathic necrotising and crescentic glomerulonephritis. *New England Journal of Medicine*, **318**, 1651–7.

Farhey, Y.D. and Herman, J.H. (1995). Vasculitis complicating granulocyte colony stimulating factor treatment of leukopenia and infection in Felty's syndrome. *Journal of Rheumatology*, **22**, 1179–82.

Fearon, D.T. (1991). Anti-inflammatory and immunosuppressive effects of recombinant soluble complement receptors. *Clinical and Experimental Immunology*, **86** (suppl. 1), 43–6.

Ferran, C., Millan, M.T., Csizmadia, V. *et al.* (1995). Inhibition of NF-kappa B by pyrrolidine dithiocarbamate blocks endothelial cell activation. *Biochemical and Biophysical Research Communications*, **214**, 212–23.

Finkel, T.H., Torok, T.J., Ferguson, P.J. *et al.* (1994). Chronic parvovirus B19 infection and systemic necrotising vasculitis: opportunistic infection or aetiological agent? *Lancet*, **343**, 1255–8.

Fine, L.G. (1988). Preventing the progression of human renal disease: Have rational therapeutic principles emerged? *Kidney International*, **33**, 116–28.

Fitzsimons, E.J. and Lange, C.F. (1991). Hybridomas to specific streptococcal antigen induce tissue pathology *in vivo*: autoimmune mechanisms for post-streptococcal sequelae. *Autoimmunity*, **10**, 115–24.

Folkman, J. and Klagsbrun, M. (1987). Angiogenic factors. *Science*, **235**, 442–7.

Frampton, G., Hildreth, G., Hartley, B. *et al.* (1988). Could platelet-derived growth factor have a role in the pathogenesis of lupus nephritis? *Lancet*, **ii**, 343.

Fujita, M., Iida, H., Asaka, M. *et al.* (1991). Effects of the immunosuppressive agent, ciclosporin, on experimental immune complex glomerulonephritis in rats. *Nephron*, **57**, 201–5.

Giscombe, R., Grunewald, J., Nityanand, S., and Lefvert, A.K. (1995). T cell receptor (TCR) V gene usage in patients with systemic necrotizing vasculitis. *Clinical and Experimental Immunology*, **101**, 213–19.

Griffith, M.E., Coulthart, A., and Pusey, C.D. (1996). T cell responses to myeloperoxidase (MPO) and proteinase 3 (PR3) in patients with systemic vasculitis. *Clinical and Experimental Immunology*, **103**, 253–8.

Gross, W.L., Schmitt, W.H., and Csernok, E. (1993). ANCA and associated diseases: immunodiagnostic and therapeutic aspects. *Clinical and Experimental Immunology*, **91**, 1–12.

Hammond, W.P., Csiba, E., Canin, A. *et al.* (1991). Chronic neutropenia. A new canine model induced by human granulocyte colony stimulating factor. *Journal of Clinical Investigation*, **87**, 704–10.

Hansen, J.E.S., Iversen, J., Lihme, A. *et al.* (1987). Acute phase reaction, heterogeneity and microheterogeneity of serum proteins as non-specific tumor markers in lung cancer. *Cancer*, **60**, 1630–5.

Hara, S., Fukatsu, A., Suzuki, N. *et al.* (1990). The effects of a new immunosuppressive agent, FK506, on the glomerular injury in rats with accelerated nephrotoxic serum glomerulonephritis. *Clinical Immunology and Immunopathology*, **57**, 351–62.

Henson, J.B. and Gorham, J.R. (1973). Animal model of human disease. Persistent viral infections, immunologically mediated glomerulonephritis and arteritis, dysgammopathies. Animal model: Aleutian disease of mink. *American Journal of Pathology*, **71**, 345–8.

Hoffmann, G.S., Kerr, G.S., Leavitt, R.Y. *et al.* (1992). Wegener's granulomatosis: analysis of 158 patients. *Annals of Internal Medicine*, **116**, 488–98.

Hom, J.T., Butler, L.D., Riedl, P.E., and Bendele, A.M. (1988). The progression of the inflammation in established collagen induced arthritis can be altered by treatment with immunological or pharmacological agents which inhibit T cell activities. *European Journal of Immunology*, **18**, 881–8.

Hudson, B.G., Kalluri, R., Gunwar, S. *et al.* (1993). Molecular characteristics of the Goodpasture autoantigen. *Kidney International*, **43**, 135–9.

Huland, H. (1973). Kasuistischer Beitrag zur Ätiologie des Goodpasture-syndroms. *Med. Klin.*, **68**, 437.

Jayne, D.R., Gaskin, G., Pusey, C.D., and Lockwood, C.M. (1995). ANCA and predicting relapse in systemic vasculitis. *Quarterly Journal of Medicine*, **88**, 127–33.

Jennings, L., Roholt, O.A., Pressman, D. *et al.* (1981). Experimental anti-alveolar basement membrane antibody-mediated pneumonitis. I. The role of increased permeability of the alveolar capillary wall induced by oxygen. *Journal of Immunology*, **127**, 129–34.

John, S., Neumayer, H.H., and Weber, M. (1994). Serum circulating ICAM-1 levels are not useful to indicate active vasculitis or early renal allograft rejection. *Clinical Nephrology*, **42**, 369–75.

Kakuta, S. (1993). Effects of reactive oxygen species scavenger and platelet activating factor antagonist on accelerated nephrotoxic nephritis. *Nippon Jinzo Gakkai Shi*, **35**, 115–24.

Kawasaki, K., Yaoita, E., Yamamoto, T. *et al.* (1992). Depletion of CD8 positive cells in nephrotoxic serum nephritis of WKY rats. *Kidney International*, **41**, 1517–26.

Kelley, V.E., Ferreti, A., Izui, S. *et al.* (1985). A fish oil diet rich in eicosapentaenoic acid reduces cyclooxygenase metabolites, and suppresses lupus in MRL-lpr mice. *Journal of Immunology*, **134**, 1914–19.

Kelley, V.E., Sneve, S., and Musinski, S. (1986). Increased renal thromboxane production in murine lupus nephritis. *Journal of Clinical Investigation*, **77**, 252–9.

Kim, S., Wadhwa, N.K., Kant, K.S. *et al.* (1988). Fibrinolysis in glomerulonephritis treated with Ancrod: renal functional, immunologic and histopathologic effects. *Quarterly Journal of Medicine*, **69**, 879–95.

Kincaid-Smith, P. (1984). Anticoagulants are of value in the treatment of renal disease. *American Journal of Kidney Diseases*, **3**, 299–307.

Kinjoh, K., Kyogoku, M., and Good, R.A. (1993). Genetic selection for crescent formation yields mouse strain with rapidly progressive glomerulonephritis and small vessel vasculitis. *Proceedings of the National Academy of Science USA*, **90**, 3413–17.

Kushner, I. (1982). The phenomenon of the acute phase response. *Annals of the New York Academy of Science*, **389**, 39–48.

Lai, K.N. and Lockwood, C.M. (1993). Serum soluble interleukin 2 receptor levels in anti-neutrophil cytoplasmic autoantibodies-positive systemic vasculitis. *Postgraduate Medical Journal*, **69**, 708–11.

Lhotta, K., Vogel, W., Meisl, T. *et al.* (1994). Alpha-1-antitrypsin phenotypes in patients with anti-neutrophil cytoplasmic antibody-positive vasculitis. *Clinical Science*, **87**, 693–5.

Lockwood, C.M., Thiru, S., Isaacs, J.D., Hale, G., and Waldmann, H. (1993). Humanised monoclonal antibody therapy for intractable systemic vasculitis. *Lancet*, **341**, 1620–2.

Lockwood, C.M., Thiru, S., Stewart, S., Hale. G., Isaacs, J., Wraight, P., *et al.* (1996). Treatment of refractory Wegener's granulomatosis with humanized monoclonal antibodies. *Kidney International*, **89**, 903–12.

Longhofer, S.L., Frisbie, D.D., Johnson, H.C. *et al.* (1991). Effects of thromboxane synthetase inhibition on immune complex glomerulonephritis. *American Journal of Veterinary Research*, **52**, 480–7.

Mayet, W.J., Csernok, E., Szymkowialk, C. *et al.* (1993). Human endothelial cells express proteinase 3, the target antigen of anticytoplasmic antibodies in Wegener's granulomatosis. *Blood*, **82**, 1221–9.

Mathieson, P.W., Cobbold, S.P., Hale, G. *et al.* (1990). Monoclonal antibody therapy in systemic vasculitis. *New England Journal of Medicine*, **323**, 250–54.

Mathieson, P.W., Thiru, S., Peters, D.K. *et al.* (1991*a*). Effects of Ancrod and rTPA on fibrin accumulation, glomerular inflammation and renal function in nephrotoxic nephritis. *International Journal of Experimental Pathology*, **72**, 679–93.

Mathieson, P.W., Stapleton, K.J., Oliveira, D.B.G. *et al.* (1991*b*). Immunoregulation of mercuric chloride-induced autoimmunity in Brown Norway rats: a role for CD8 + T cells revealed by *in vivo* depletion studies. *European Journal of Immunology*, **21**, 2105–9.

Mathieson, P.W., Thiru, S., and Oliveira, D.B.G. (1992). Mercuric chloride-treated Brown Norway rats develop widespread tissue injury including necrotizing vasculitis. *Laboratory Investigation*, **67**, 121–9.

Mathieson, P.W., Qasim, F.J., Esnault, V.L.M. *et al.* (1993*a*). Animal models of systemic vasculitis. *Journal of Autoimmunity*, **6**, 251–64.

Mathieson, P.W., Thiru, S., and Oliveria, D.B.G. (1993*b*). Regulatory role of OX22 + T cells in mercury-induced autoimmunity in the Brown Norway rat. *Journal of Experimental Medicine*, **177**, 1309–16.

Mathieson, P.W. and Oliveira, D.B.G. (1995). The role of cellular immunity in systemic vasculitis. *Clinical and Experimental Immunology*, **100**, 183–5.

Miyazama, M., Nose, M., Kawashima, M., *et al.* (1987). Pathogenesis of arteritis of SL/Ni mice. Possible lytic effect of anti-gp 70 antibodies on vascular smooth muscle cells. *Journal of Experimental Medicine*, **166**, 890–908.

Moreland, L.W., Heck, L.W., Jr., Sullivan, W. *et al.* (1993). New approaches to the therapy of autoimmune diseases: rheumatoid arthritis as a paradigm. *American Journal of Medicine*, **305**, 40–51.

Mrowka, C. and Sieberth, H.G. (1995). Detection of circulating adhesion molecules ICAM-1, VCAM-1 and E-selectin in Wegener's granulomatosis, systemic lupus erythematosus amd chronic renal failure. *Clinical Nephrology*, **43**, 288–96.

Mulligan, M.S., Jones, M.L., Bolanowski, M.A. *et al.* (1993). Inhibition of lung inflammatory reactions in rats by an anti-human IL-8 antibody. *Journal of Immunology*, **150**, 5585–95.

Naish, P.F., Thomson, N.M., Simpson, I.J. *et al.* (1975). Role of polymorphonuclear leucocytes in the autologous phase of nephrotoxic nephritis. *Clinical and Experimental Immunology*, **22**, 102–11.

Nassonov, E., Samsonov, M., Beketova, T., Semenkova, L., Wachter, H., and Fuchs, D. (1995). Serum neopterin concentrations in Wegener's granulomatosis correlate with vasculitis activity. *Clinical and Experimental Rheumatology*, **13**, 353–6.

Neilson, E.G., McCafferty, E., Mann R. *et al.* (1985). Tubular antigen-derivatized cells induce a disease-protective, antigen-specific, and idiotype-specific suppressor T cell network restricted by I-J and Igh-V in mice with experimental interstitial nephritis. *Journal of Experimental Medicine*, **162**, 215–30.

Patrono, C., Ciabattoni, G., and Remuzzi, G. (1985). Functional significance of renal prostacyclin and thromboxane A2 production in patients with systemic lupus erythematosus. *Journal of Clinical Investigation*, **76**, 1011–18.

Pollak, V.E., Glueck, H.I., Weiss, M.A. *et al.* (1982). Defibrination with ancrod in glomerulonephritis. Effect on clinical and histologic findings and on blood coagulation. *American Journal of Nephrology*, **2**, 195–207.

Prickett, J.D., Robinson, D.R., and Steinberg, A.D. (1981). Dietary enrichment with the polyunsaturated fatty acid eicosapentaenoic acid prevents proteinuria and prolongs survival in NZBxNZW F1 mice. *Journal of Clinical Investigation*, **68**, 556–9.

Pruitt, S.K., Baldwin, W.M., Marsh, H.C., Jr. *et al.* (1991*b*). The effect of soluble complement receptor type 1 on hyperacute xenograft rejection. *Transplantation*, **52**, 868–73.

Pusey, C.D., Rees, A.J., Evans, D.J., Peters, D.K., and Lockwood, C.M. (1991*a*). Plasma exchange in focal necrotising glomerulonephritis without anti-GBM antibodies. *Kidney International*, **40**, 757–63.

Pusey, C.D., Aslam, M., Cohen, J. *et al.* (1991*b*). Experimental models of plasma perfusion. *Journal of Clinical Apheresis*, **6**, 99–102.

Pusey, C.D., Holland, M.J., Cashman, S.H. *et al.* (1991*c*). Experimental autoimmune glomerulonephritis induced by homologous and isologous glomerular basement membrane in Brown Norway rats. *Nephrology Dialysis Transplantation*, **6**, 457–65.

Qasim, F.J., Thiru, S., Mathieson, P.W. *et al.* (1993*a*). The effect of antioxidant therapy on experimental vasculitis. *Clinical and Experimental Immunology*, **93** (Suppl. 1), 28 (abstract).

Qasim, F.J., Thiru, S., Sgotto, B. *et al.* (1993*b*). The effect of antibodies against neutrophils on experimental vasculitis. *Clinical and Experimental Immunology*, **93** (Suppl. 1), 22 (abstract).

Qasim, F.J., Thiru, S., Mathieson, P.W. *et al.* (1993*c*). Effects of cyclosporin A on experimental vasculitis. *Clinical and Experimental Immunology*, **93** (Suppl. 1), 28 (abstract).

Queluz, T.H., Pawlowski, I., Brunda, M.J. *et al.* (1990). Pathogenesis of an experimental model of Goodpasture's hemorrhagic pneumonitis. *Journal of Clinical Investigation*, **85**, 1507–15.

Querin, S., Schurch, W., and Beaulieu, R. (1992). Cyclosporin in Goodpasture's syndrome. *Nephron*, **60**, 355–9.

Rao, J.K., Allen, N.B., Feussner, J.R. and Weinberger, M. (1995). A prospective study of antineutrophil cytoplasmic antibody (c-ANCA) and clinical criteria in diagnosing Wegener's granulomatosis. *Lancet*, **346**, 926–31.

Rees, A.J., Lockwood, C.M., and Peters, D.K. (1977). Enhanced allergic tissue injury in Goodpasture's syndrome by intercurrent bacterial infection. *British Medical Journal*, ii, 723–36.

Reuss-Borst, M.A., Muller, C.A., and Waller, H.D. (1994). The possible role of G-CSF in the pathogenesis of Sweet's syndrome. *Leukaemia Lymphoma*, **15**, 261–4.

Reynolds, J., Cashman, S.J., Evans, D.J. *et al.* (1991). Cyclosporin A in the prevention and treatment of experimental autoimmune glomerulonephritis in the brown Norway rat. *Clinical and Experimental Immunology*, **85**, 28–32.

Reynolds, J., and Pusey, C.D. (1994). In vivo treatment with a monoclonal antibody to T helper cells in experimental autoimmune glomenelonephritis in the BN rat. *Clinical and Experimental Immunology*, **95**, 122–7.

Riechmann, L., Clark, M., Waldmann, H. *et al.* (1988). Reshaping human antibodies for therapy. *Nature*, **332**, 323–7.

Savage, C.O.S., Pusey, C.D., Bowman, C. *et al.* (1986). Antiglomerular basement membrane antibody mediated disease in the British Isles 1980–4. *British Medical Journal*, **292**, 301–4.

Savige, J.A., Chang, L., Cook, L., Burdon, J., Daskalakis, M., and Doery, J. (1995). Alpha-1-antitrypsin deficiency and anti-proteinase 3 antibodies in anti-neutrophil cytoplasmic antibody (ANCA)-associated systemic vasculitis. *Clinical and Experimental Immunology*, **100**, 194–7.

Segal, R. and Fine, L.G. (1989). Polypeptide growth factors and the kidney. *Kidney International*, **36**, (suppl. 1), 2–10.

Segasothy, M., Kong, C.T., Morad, Z. *et al.* (1986). Rapidly progressive glomerulonephritis: treatment with combined immunosuppression and anticoagulation with arvin. *Singapore Medical Journal*, **27**, 422–7.

Shinkai, Y. and Cameron, J.S. (1987). Trial of platelet-derived growth factor antagonist, trapidil, in accelerated nephrotoxic nephritis in the rabbit. *British Journal of Experimental Pathology*, **68**, 847–52.

Simpson, I.J., Skinner, M.A., Geursen, A. *et al.* (1995). Peripheral blood T lymphocytes in systemic vasculitis: increased T cell receptor V beta 2 gene usage in microscopic polyarteritis. *Clinical and Experimental Immunology*, **101**, 220–6.

Stahl, R.A., Thaiss, F., Oberle, G. *et al.* (1991). The platelet activating factor antagonist WEB 2170 improves glomerular hemodynamics and morphology in a proliferative model of mesangial cell injury. *Journal of the American Society of Nephrology*, **2**, 37–44.

Strom, T.B. and Kelley, V.E. (1989). Towards more selective therapies to block undesired immune responses. *Kidney International*, **35**, 1026–33.

Thomson, N.M., Simpson, I.J., and Peters, D.K. (1975a). A quantitative evaluation of anticoagulants in experimental nephrotoxic nephritis. *Clinical and Experimental Immunology*, **19**, 301–8.

Thomson, N.M., Simpson, I.J., Evans, D.J. *et al.* (1975b). Defibrination with ancrod in experimental chronic immune complex nephritis. *Clinical and Experimental Immunology*, **20**, 527–35.

Thomson, N.M., Moran, J., Simpson, I.J. *et al.* (1976). Defibrination with ancrod in nephrotoxic nephritis in rabbits. *Kidney International*, **10**, 343–7.

Tipping, P.G. and Holdsworth, S.R. (1986). Fibrinolytic therapy with streptokinase for established experimental glomerulonephritis. *Nephron*, **43**, 258–64.

Tomer, Y., Gilburd, B., Black, M. *et al.* (1995). Characterization of biologically active antineutrophil cytoplasmic antibodies induced in mice. Pathogenetic role in experimental vasculitis. *Arthritis and Rheumatism*, **38**, 1375–81.

Tomosugi, N.I., Cashman, S.J., Hay, H. *et al.* (1989). Modulation of antibody-mediated glomerular injury in vivo by bacterial lipopolysaccharide, tumour necrosis factor, and IL-1. *Journal of Immunology*, **142**, 3083–90.

Turner, N., Mason, P.J., Brown, R. *et al.* (1992). Molecular cloning of the human Goodpasture antigen demonstrates it to be the alpha 3 chain of type IV collagen. *Journal of Clinical Investigation*, **89**, 592–601.

Turner, N., Lockwood, C.M., and Rees, A.J. (1993). Antiglomerular basement membrane antibody mediated nephritis. In *Diseases of the kidney*, (ed. R.W. Schrier and C.W. Gottschalk) pp. 929–69. Little, Brown, Boston.

Unanue, E.R. and Dixon, F.J. (1967). Experimental glomerulonephritis: Immunological events and pathogenetic mechanisms. *Advances in Immunology*, **6**, 1–90.

Vandenbark, A.A., Hashim, G., and Offner, H. (1989). Immunization with a synthetic T-cell receptor V-region peptide protects against experimental autoimmune encephalomyelitis. *Nature*, **341**, 541–4.

Van Zyl Smit, R., Rees, A.J., and Peters, D.K. (1983). Factors affecting severity of injury during nephrotoxic nephritis in rabbits. *Clinical and Experimental Immunology*, **54**, 366–72.

Wang, C.R., Liu, M.F., Tsai, R.T. *et al.* (1993). Circulating intercellular adhesion molecules-1 and autoantibodies including anti-endothelial cell, anti-cardiolipin, and anti-neutrophil cytoplasm antibodies in patients with vasculitis. *Clinical Rheumatology*, **12**, 375–80.

Weisman, H.F., Bartow, T., Leppo M.K. *et al.* (1990). Soluble human complement receptor type 1: *in vivo* inhibitor of complement suppressing post-ischemic myocardial inflammation and necrosis. *Science*, **249**, 146–51.

Wofsey, D. and Seaman, W.E. (1987). Reversal of advanced murine lupus in NZB/NZW F1 mice by treatment with monoclonal antibody to L3T4. *Journal of Immunology*, **138**, 3247–53.

Wu X., Pippin, J., and Lefkowith, J.B. (1993). Platelets and neutrophils are critical to the enhanced glomerular arachidonate metabolism in acute nephrotoxic nephritis in rats. *Journal of Clinical Investigation*, **91**, 766–73.

Yang, J.J., Tuttle, R., Jennette, C.J. *et al.* (1993). Glomerulonephritis in rats immunized with myeloperoxidase (MPO). *Clinical and Experimental Immunology*, **93**, (Suppl. 1), 22, (abstract).

Zoja, C., Corna, D., Macconi, D. *et al.* (1990). Tissue plasminogen activator therapy of rabbit nephrotoxic nephritis. *Laboratory Investigation*, **62**, 34–40.

INDEX